theclinics.com

Agnes E. Rupley, DVM, Dipl. ABVP–Avian
CONSULTING EDITOR

VETERINARY CLINICS OF NORTH AMERICA

Exotic Animal Practice

Common Procedures

GUEST EDITOR
Chris Griffin, DVM, Dipl. ABVP–Avian

May 2006 • Volume 9 • Number 2

SAUNDERS

An Imprint of Elsevier, Inc.
PHILADELPHIA   LONDON   TORONTO   MONTREAL   SYDNEY   TOKYO

W.B. SAUNDERS COMPANY
A Division of Elsevier Inc.

Elsevier, Inc., 1600 John F. Kennedy Blvd., Suite 1800, Philadelphia, PA 19103-2899

http://www.vetexotic.theclinics.com

VETERINARY CLINICS OF NORTH AMERICA: Volume 9, Number 2
EXOTIC ANIMAL PRACTICE ISSN 1094-9194
MAY 2006 ISBN 1-4160-3580-X
Editor: John Vassallo

Copyright © 2006 by Elsevier Inc. All rights reserved. No part of this publication may be reproduced or transmitted in any form or by any means, electronic or mechanical, including photocopy, recording, or any information retrieval system, without written permission from the publisher.

Single photocopies of single articles may be made for personal use as allowed by national copyright laws. Permission of the publisher and payment of a fee is required for all other photocopying, including multiple or systematic copying, copying for advertising or promotional purposes, resale, and all forms of document delivery. Special rates are available for educational institutions that wish to make photocopies for nonprofit educational classroom use. Permissions may be sought directly from Elsevier's Rights Department in Philadelphia, PA, USA: phone: (+1) 215 239 3804, fax: (+1) 215 239 3805, e-mail: healthpermissions@elsevier.com. Requests may also be completed on-line via the Elsevier homepage (http://www.elsevier.com/locate/permissions). In the USA, users may clear permissions and make payments through the Copyright Clearance Center, Inc, 222 Rosewood Drive, Danvers, MA 01923, USA; phone: (978) 750-8400; fax: (978) 750-4744, and in the UK through the Copyright Licensing Agency Rapid Clearance Service (CLARCS), 90 Tottenham Court Road, London W1P 0LP, UK; phone: (+44) 171 436 5931; fax: (+44) 171 436 3986. Others countries may have a local reprographic rights agency for payments.

Reprints. For copies of 100 or more of articles in this publication, please contact the commercial Reprints Department, Elsevier Inc., 360 Park Avenue South, New York, New York 10010-1710. Tel: (212) 633-3813 Fax: (212) 633-1935, e-mail: reprints@elsevier.com

The ideas and opinions expressed in *Veterinary Clinics of North America: Exotic Animal Practice* do not necessarily reflect those of the Publisher. The Publisher does not assume any responsibility for any injury and/or damage to persons or property arising out of or related to any use of the material contained in this periodical. The reader is advised to check the appropriate medical literature and the product information currently provided by the manufacturer of each drug to be administered to verify the dosage, the method and duration of administration, or contraindications. It is the responsibility of the treating physician or other health care professional, relying on independent experience and knowledge of the patient, to determine drug dosages and the best treatment for the patient. Mention of any product in this issue should not be construed as endorsement by the contributors, editors, or the Publisher of the product or manufacturers' claims.

Veterinary Clinics of North America: Exotic Animal Practice (ISSN 1094-9194) is published in January, May, and September by Elsevier, Inc.; Business and Editorial offices: 1600 John F. Kennedy Blvd., Suite 1800, Philadelphia, PA 19103-2899. Customer Service Office: 6277 Sea Harbor Drive, Orlando, FL 32887-4800. Subscription prices are $135.00 per year for US individuals, $230.00 per year for US institutions, $70.00 per year for US students and residents, $160.00 per year for Canadian individuals, $265.00 per year for Canadian institutions, $170.00 per year for international individuals, $265.00 per year for international institutions and $85.00 per year for Canadian and foreign students/residents. To receive student/resident rate, orders must be accompanied by name of affiliated institution, date of term, and the *signature* of program/residency coordinator on institution letterhead. Orders will be billed at individual rate until proof of status is received. Foreign air speed delivery is included in all *Clinics* subscription prices. All prices are subject to change without notice.

POSTMASTER: Send address changes to *Veterinary Clinics of North America: Exotic Animal Practice*; Elsevier Periodicals Customer Service, 6277 Sea Harbor Drive, Orlando, FL 32887-4800. **Customer Service: 1-800-654-2452 (US). From outside of the US, call 1-407-345-1000.**

Veterinary Clinics of North America: Exotic Animal Practice is covered in *Index Medicus*.

Printed in the United States of America.

COMMON PROCEDURES

CONSULTING EDITOR

AGNES E. RUPLEY, DVM, Diplomate, American Board of Veterinary Practitioners–Avian; and Director and Chief Veterinarian, All Pets Medical & Laser Surgical Center, College Station, Texas

GUEST EDITOR

CHRIS GRIFFIN, DVM, Diplomate, American Board of Veterinary Practitioners–Avian, Griffin Avian and Exotic Veterinary Hospital, Kannapolis, North Carolina

CONTRIBUTORS

THOMAS H. BOYER, DVM, Pet Hospital of Penasquitos, San Diego, California

MATTHEW E. BRAUN, MS, PhD, DVM, Department of Clinical Sciences, College of Veterinary Medicine, Auburn University, Auburn, Alabama

JOHN CHITTY, BvetMed, CertZooMed, Cbiol, MIBiol, MRCVS, Strathmore Veterinary Clinic, Andover, Hants, United Kingdom

BYRON J. S. DE LA NAVARRE, DVM, Chief of Exotic Animal Service, Animal House of Chicago, Complete Veterinary Care, Inc, Chicago, Illinois

RICARDO EMANUEL CASTANHEIRA DE MATOS, LMV, Avian Medicine and Surgery Resident, Section of Wildlife and Exotic Medicine, Department of Clinical Sciences, College of Veterinary Medicine, Cornell University, Ithaca, New York

JENNIFER GRAHAM, DVM, Diplomate, American Board of Veterinary Practitioners–Avian; Affiliate Assistant Professor, Department of Comparative Medicine, University of Washington, Seattle; VCA Veterinary Specialty Center of Seattle, Lynnwood, Washington

CHRIS GRIFFIN, DVM, Diplomate, American Board of Veterinary Practitioners–Avian, Griffin Avian and Exotic Veterinary Hospital, Kannapolis, North Carolina

J. JILL HEATLEY, DVM, MS, Diplomate, American Board of Veterinary Practitioners–Avian; Department of Clinical Sciences, College of Veterinary Medicine, Auburn University, Auburn, Alabama

CATHY A. JOHNSON-DELANEY, DVM, Diplomate, American Board of Veterinary Practitioners–Avian; Eastside Avian and Exotic Animal Medical Center, Kirkland, Washington

VICTORIA JOSEPH, DVM, Diplomate, American Board of Veterinary Practitioners–Avian, Bird and Pet Clinic of Roseville, Roseville, California

ERIC KLAPHAKE, DVM, Diplomate, American Board of Veterinary Practitioners–Avian; Associate Veterinarian, Avian Health Clinic, Reynoldsburg, Ohio

ANGELA M. LENNOX, DVM, Diplomate, American Board of Veterinary Practitioners–Avian; Avian and Exotic Animal Clinic of Indianapolis, Indianapolis, Indiana

JAMES K. MORRISEY, DVM, Diplomate, American Board of Veterinary Practitioners–Avian; Lecturer, Section of Wildlife and Exotic Medicine, Department of Clinical Sciences, College of Veterinary Medicine, Cornell University, Ithaca, New York

DEBBIE A. MYERS, DVM, Louisiana State University, Baton Rouge, Louisiana

LAUREN V. POWERS, DVM, Diplomate, American Board of Veterinary Practitioners–Avian; Carolina Veterinary Specialists, Huntersville, North Carolina

DRURY R. REAVILL, DVM, Diplomate, American Board of Veterinary Practitioners–Avian; Diplomate, American College of Veterinary Pathologists; Zoo/Exotic Pathology Service, West Sacramento, California

COMMON PROCEDURES

CONTENTS

Preface xi
Chris Griffin

Clinical Techniques of Invertebrates 205
Matthew E. Braun, J. Jill Heatley, and John Chitty

This article highlights techniques and equipment needed to successfully restrain, diagnose, and treat gastropods (including snails and slugs) and arthropods (including spiders, scorpions, honeybees, cockroaches, silkworms, phasmids, centipedes, and millipedes). A review of current clinical techniques for invertebrates kept as pets and those kept for agricultural use is provided. The specific techniques of restraint, assessment of hydration, fluid therapy, diagnostic sampling, imaging, exoskeleton repair, ectoparasite control and removal, euthanasia, and postmortem examination are reviewed for use in the invertebrate patient. The authors intend this article to stimulate further research and reporting on appropriate and humane techniques for use in these species and to increase the ability of the veterinary practitioner to successfully attend to these animals.

Common Diagnostic and Clinical Techniques for Fish 223
Drury R. Reavill

Fish medicine has common diagnostic and clinical procedures that are essential for disease diagnosis and patient management. With a few modifications for handling of the fish patient, these resemble procedures performed in most veterinary hospitals and clinics in our other companion species. The predictive value of these diagnostic methods is improving with the ever-increasing number of publications in fish medicine. Training in aquatic clinical procedures is offered at most large continuing education conferences and as specialty courses. These basic procedures are the important first steps toward improving the health of our aquatic companion animals.

Common Procedures in Reptiles and Amphibians 237
Byron J. S. de la Navarre

> Reptiles and amphibians continue to be popular as pets in the United States and throughout the world. It therefore behooves veterinarians interested in caring for these exotic species to continually gather knowledge concerning both their proper husbandry and the conditions that require medical and/or surgical intervention. This article covers husbandry, physical examination, and clinical and diagnostic techniques in an effort to present guidelines for the evaluation of the reptile or amphibian patient. Gathering clinical data will aid veterinarians in arriving at the proper diagnosis, increasing the chances of success with treatment protocols, and educating the clients in proper nutrition and husbandry for their pets.

Common Procedures with Venomous Reptiles 269
Thomas H. Boyer

> Venomous reptiles should be handled in a safe and consistent manner, even after death. Owners and staff should be warned not to handle the venomous reptile, and one should have emergency protocols in place before the properly bagged and encased reptile is presented. It is important to know what one is treating as well as one's limitations. After being carefully removed from the bag, the venomous reptile may be transferred to a handling container, tubed, or squeezed with the appropriate equipment. The author usually induces injectable or gas anesthesia at this point. Veterinarians who are inexperienced with venomous reptiles should learn how to handle them through a reputable seminar or class before electing to see them in their practice.

Common Procedures in Psittacines 287
Lauren V. Powers

> General techniques performed on psittacine birds are described in this article, including restraint, handling, and grooming. Procedures to collect diagnostic samples and to administer therapeutic agents are detailed, including fluid therapy and nutritional support.

Common Procedures in Other Avian Species 303
Angela M. Lennox

> Although psittacine species represent the majority of avian patients seen in most exotic animal practices, nonpsittacine species such as passerines and galliformes may be presented as pets, as members of zoo collections, or as injured or ill wildlife. Many features of handling, restraint, sample collection, medicine, and surgery are similar in psittacine and nonpsittacine species. In many cases, the equipment required will be similar as well, with a few modifications.

Raptor Medicine: An Approach to Wild, Falconry, and Educational Birds of Prey 321
Victoria Joseph

> A veterinarian receiving birds of prey (raptors) will often be presented with wild, educational, or falconry raptors. Raptors trained for the sport of falconry and educational raptors are handled in a precise manner, often differently from the wild raptors. It is imperative for veterinarians treating raptors to be familiar with the equipment and terminology used by the individuals caring for these birds. The hospital staff must also be educated to handle the raptors properly, both wild and tame, because differences do exist between the approaches. Raptor medicine requires a thorough diagnostic work-up and aggressive therapeutic plan to help ensure a fast and complete recovery.

Common Procedures in the Pet Ferret 347
Ricardo Emanuel Castanheira de Matos and
James K. Morrisey

> The domestic ferret is an increasingly popular pet in North America and Europe and may easily be incorporated into the structure and workings of most small animal hospitals. Not only does treatment of ferrets provide case diversity and intellectual challenges to the veterinarian but it may increase revenue, because most ferret owners have several ferrets. The diagnostic and supportive care procedures used commonly in ferrets are similar to those used in dogs and cats. This article presents the common diagnostic and supportive care procedures used in ferrets, with special emphasis on some of the unique aspects that make these procedures easier to learn and perform.

Common Procedures in Rabbits 367
Jennifer Graham

> Rabbits are popular companion animals that present to veterinary clinics for routine and emergency care. Clinics equipped for treating dogs and cats may be easily adapted to accommodate rabbits. This article reviews common procedures performed by the clinician specific to rabbits. Topics include handling and restraint, triage and patient assessment, sample collection, and supportive care techniques. Miscellaneous procedures, including anesthetic delivery, nasolacrimal duct flushing, and ear cleaning, are also discussed.

Common Rodent Procedures 389
Eric Klaphake

> Rodents are commonly owned exotic animal pets that may be seen by veterinary practitioners. Although most owners presenting their animals do care about their pets, they may not be aware of the diagnostic possibilities and challenges that can be offered by rodents

to the veterinarian. Understanding clinical anatomy, proper handling technique, realistic management of emergency presentations, correct and feasible diagnostic sampling, anesthesia, and humane euthanasia procedures is important to enhancing the doctor-client-patient relationship, especially when financial constraints may be imposed by the owner.

Common Procedures in Hedgehogs, Prairie Dogs, Exotic Rodents, and Companion Marsupials 415
Cathy A. Johnson-Delaney

Nondomesticated species are commonly being kept as companion animals. These include the African pygmy hedgehog (*Atelerix albiventris*), the North American black-tailed prairie dog (*Cynomys ludovicianus*), and exotic rodents such as the degu (*Octodon degus*) and duprasi or fat-tailed gerbil (*Pachyuromys duprasi*). Common companion marsupials include the sugar glider (*Petaurus breviceps*), Bennett's or Tammar (Dama) wallabies (*Macropus rufogriseus rufogriseus and Macropus eugenii*, respectively), the Brazilian or South American gray short-tailed opossum (*Monodelphis domestica*), and the North American Virginia opossum (*Didelphis virginiana*). Although many of these animals are now bred domestically and are fairly docile when human-raised, they are essentially wild animals and hence have strong instincts to hide illness and pain.

Common Procedures and Concerns with Wildlife 437
Debbie A. Myers

Wildlife patients have special needs compared with pet patients in regard to handling and restraint, the importance of the stress response, physical examination, and neonatal concerns. Because many wildlife patients present with wounds and fractures, a good understanding of the pathophysiology of these processes is also important. The primary goal of all wildlife rehabilitation procedures is the ultimate release of the animal back into its natural environment.

Index 461

GOAL STATEMENT

The goal of the *Veterinary Clinics of North America: Exotic Animal Practice* is to keep practicing veterinarians up to date with current clinical practice in exotic animal medicine by providing timely articles reviewing the state of the art in exotic animal care.

ACCREDITATION

The *Veterinary Clinics of North America: Exotic Animal Practice* offers continuing education credits, awarded by Cummings School of Veterinary Medicine at Tufts University, Office of Continuing Education.

Cummings School of Veterinary Medicine at Tufts University is a designated provider of continuing veterinary medical education. Veterinarians participating in this learning activity may earn up to 6 credits per issue up to a maximum of 18 credits per year. Credits awarded may not apply toward license renewal in all states. It is the responsibility of each participant to verify the requirements of their state licensing board.

Credit can be earned by reading the text material, taking the examination online at ***http://www.theclinics.com/home/cme***, and completing the program evaluation. Following your completion of the test and program evaluation, and review of any and all incorrect answers, you may print your certificate.

TO ENROLL

To enroll in the *Veterinary Clinics of North America: Exotic Animal Practice* Continuing Veterinary Medical Education Program, call customer service at 1-800-654-2452 or sign up online at ***http://www.theclinics.com/home/cme***. The CVME program is now available at a special introductory rate of $49.95 for a year's subscription.

FORTHCOMING ISSUES

September 2006
Case Reports: The Front Line in Exotic Medicine
Robert J.T. Doneley, BVSc, FACVSc
(Avian Health), *Guest Editor*

January 2007
Cytology
Michael M. Garner, DVM, Dipl. ACVP
Guest Editor

May 2007
Critical Care
Marla Lichtenberger, DVM
Guest Editor

RECENT ISSUES

January 2006
Renal Disease
M. Scott Echols, DVM, Dipl. ABVP–Avian
Guest Editor

September 2005
The Exotic Pet Practice
Angela M. Lennox, DVM, Dipl. ABVP–Avian
Guest Editor

May 2005
Gastroenterology
Tracey K. Ritzman, DVM, Dipl. ABVP–Avian
Guest Editor

The Clinics are now available online!

Access your subscription at
www.theclinics.com

Preface

Common Procedures

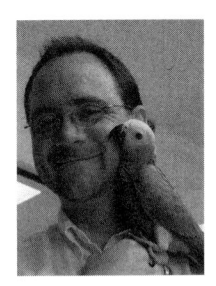

Chris Griffin, DVM, DABVP–Avian
Guest Editor

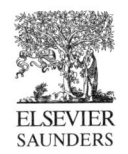

Dr. Agnes Rupley approached me a few years ago and suggested that I consider being the guest editor of an issue of *Veterinary Clinics of North America: Exotic Animal Practice*. I was, and still am, flattered that she believed I had the ability and contacts needed to put together an issue on any topic covering our exotic animal patients. I had my doubts as to either qualification, especially when I considered available topics. Feeling that each of the possible topics might have been beyond my comfort zone and experience, I tried to find something I was comfortable with... and voila! An issue on a topic with which I have some experience came to mind: Common Procedures.

I considered this topic and thought, "This will be an excellent opportunity to put a lot of great, practical tips together in one place, something that will benefit every facet of exotic pet care in veterinary hospitals." My vision was a publication that was based in practical (and well-conceived) techniques, accessible not only to veterinarians but also to technicians, veterinary nurses, and other support staff who routinely take part in patient care, diagnostic sample collection, and therapeutic delivery. It was a grand vision.

Then we got down to the business of actually getting all of this done. I asked many well-respected colleagues in our profession to share their wealth of knowledge and expertise within various fields. I begged others to do the same. I even promised ice cream to a few of the potential authors, trying my best to ensure the best possible panel of contributors I could find. (I am up for a trip to Baskin Robbins or Ben and Jerry's in Baltimore!) My selections were based on two things: (1) the potential authors had to be excellent veterinarians and wonderful people (they all are); (2) they had to be well-versed in these procedures. The resulting mix of private practitioners, university-based clinicians, and research-oriented investigators has brought us this wonderful issue.

The major problem with this issue was trying to decide how many procedures should be considered "common" for each species. After determining that a complete, exhaustive accounting of all these procedures would result in a tome of more than 4500 pages, the authors and I tried to streamline our effort into a more reasonable length. It is not our intent to state that these procedures are the only common ones that may be performed during the course of exotic pet practice—only that they are among the most common.

This issue may be the least scientific (yet medical) issue of this series that Elsevier has ever published. In a way, I hope that is the case. The information provided herein is meant to educate and guide everyone in a practice that interacts with exotic pets (from spiders, fish, pet parrots, tortoises, wallabies, and canaries to raptors, wildlife, and venomous reptiles). Reading this issue will not make anyone an expert on the treatment or handling of these animals; the hope is that reading the following pages will equip even the novice veterinary staff (doctors included) to be better prepared to perform these "common procedures" on exotic patients. It is my hope that even the most experienced exotic pet veterinarians will take away something positive from every article and that the less experienced exotic pet veterinarians will use this issue as one of the core guides for safe handling and treatments techniques.

Special thanks to all of the excellent authors. Without you, there would be nothing after this wandering preface. Your work, insight, and experience make this issue everything I wanted it to be... and more. I am honored to be associated with this work, and I hope that everyone who reads even a part of this issue can sense the passion, intelligence, and focus that permeate each topic. Thanks to my parents (they are my daily inspiration) and April Strickland and the rest of the wonderful staff at my practice, who have supported me and lived through this adventure while making sure I was still practicing (and doing many of the common procedures found in this issue). Thanks also to you, Scooby Doo, our little Grey Girl (January 14, 2005–February 27, 2006, pictured). It is because of angels like you that we all strive to do our part a little better every day. As more procedures become more common in our exotic patients, I hope to see a "Common Procedures: Part Deux" in the near future!

Chris Griffin, DVM, DABVP–Avian
Griffin Avian and Exotic Veterinary Hospital
2100 Lane Street
Kannapolis, NC 28083, USA

E-mail address: info@griffinexotics.com

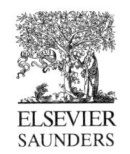

Clinical Techniques of Invertebrates

Matthew E. Braun, MS, PhD, DVM[a],*, J. Jill Heatley, DVM, MS, DABVP–Avian[a], John Chitty, BvetMed, CertZooMed, Cbiol, MIBiol, MRCVS[b]

[a]*Department of Clinical Sciences, 612 Hoerlein Hall, College of Veterinary Medicine, Auburn University, Auburn, AL 36849, USA*
[b]*Strathmore Veterinary Clinic, London Road, Andover, Hants SP10 2PH, United Kingdom*

As technology and knowledge grow in veterinary medicine, so too does the number of species to which the veterinarian has a responsibility to attend. Invertebrates have been ignored to some extent by veterinary medicine, although they constitute almost 90% of the animal kingdom [1,2]. Dissemination of appropriate techniques for treating these creatures is necessary based on the increased interest in ownership of invertebrate exotic pets and the resultant demand for veterinary care. These animals offer advantages in our increasingly mobile society, whose members also live in smaller quarters. Invertebrates have relatively short lifespans, can be interactive, and require minimal but specific care. Invertebrates have the advantages of small size and portable habitats, while still being interesting and novel when compared with more conventional mammalian and avian pets. Producers of invertebrate products should also have adequate care available to their invertebrate "herds," just as services are provided for other production animals, such as cattle, swine, or poultry. Efficient production of goods such as honey and silk depends on healthy, cohesive colonies and healthy individuals. The veterinarian has an obligation to know current clinical techniques for this economically important class of animals.

Challenges to treating invertebrates arise from the characteristics of these species that differ from those of familiar mammalian and avian species. The most notable difference is that invertebrates, like reptiles and amphibians, are ectotherms that depend on environmental temperatures to regulate thermal homeostasis. Many members of the group possess exoskeletons or shells, which necessitate particular therapeutic skills. Contact with some

* Corresponding author.
E-mail address: braunme@auburn.edu (M.E. Braun).

species of invertebrates poses the risk of envenomation, stings, and irritation. The small size of these creatures also makes visualization and manipulation challenging. Fortunately, all these challenges may be overcome by employing the appropriate technique.

This article highlights techniques and equipment needed to successfully restrain, diagnose, and treat gastropods (including snails and slugs) and arthropods (including spiders, scorpions, honeybees, cockroaches, silkworms, phasmids [stick and leaf insects], centipedes, and millipedes). A review of current clinical techniques for invertebrates kept as pets and those kept for agricultural use is provided. The specific techniques of restraint, assessment of hydration, fluid therapy, diagnostic sampling, imaging, exoskeleton repair, ectoparasite control and removal, euthanasia, and postmortem examination are reviewed for use in the invertebrate patient. The authors intend this article to stimulate further research and reporting on appropriate and humane techniques for use in these species and to increase the ability of the veterinary practitioner successfully to attend to these animals.

Handling, restraint, and anesthesia

All good clinical techniques begin with adequate restraint, whether chemical or manual, and similar techniques may be used for most invertebrate species. Techniques for manual restraint must provide safety to the patient and the clinician as well as adequate patient immobilization. Knowledge of defensive or aggressive postures of these species can be helpful to avoid being harmed by these patients. For example, the aggressive tarantula may first flick hair and then lift its front legs to expose its fangs to warn the handler before biting [3]. Exercising good technique in restraint allows for safe and effective examination and therapy.

Direct handling of invertebrates should be done not far above a soft surface [1,2,4]. Careless handling resulting in a fall of the patient can damage the invertebrate's exoskeleton, causing loss of hemolymph and even death. When handling many invertebrates, one must also consider one's safety and the risk for bites and stings. Several pieces of equipment assist with arthropod restraint and reduce the risk of bites and stings. Urticarial hairs (setae) on tarantulas and some caterpillars may be avoided by wearing latex gloves and eye protection or by using padded forceps [5,6]. Latex, lightweight leather, or cloth gloves should be worn when handling millipedes, centipedes, and other species that exude noxious, irritant, or venomous secretions. Latex gloves used with tarantulas should be rinsed free of powder before handling to protect the spider's book lung, which is a paired organ located in the cranioventral opisthosoma that consists of numerous layers of thin tissue in an air-filled atrium, enabling diffusion of oxygen into the hemolymph [5].

Transparent containers allow close examination with only minor manipulation. Clear plastic tubes, such as those used for venomous snakes, and clear plastic boxes are excellent for handling and obtaining external visualization of many species (Fig. 1). For more invasive restraint, arthropods may be immobilized by using cellophane, transparent plastic, or plexiglass to pin the patient gently in one position (Fig. 2). This method offers good visualization for examinations and good restraint for drug administration and other treatments. Snails, millipedes, and slugs are easily handled by grasping at the midbody or allowing the animal to rest on the gloved hand. One should not grasp large spiders but rather entice them to crawl onto the hand by prodding the abdomen [7]. In general, handling of the invertebrates by the extremities is not recommended given the frailty of the limbs, but scorpions may be picked up with padded forceps by the base of the tail (Fig. 3). Another method for handling tarantulas consists of a gauze sling looped beneath the pedicel or waist of the spider between the cephalothorax and abdomen while the forefinger applies gentle downward pressure on the cephalothorax to immobilize the spider [3]. Tarantulas will stop moving their legs as they are suspended slightly above the table for this method, which is useful for drawing hemolymph, administering fluid and medications, and examining the ventrum.

Hypothermia is another option for immobilization of terrestrial invertebrates. A patient may be placed in a refrigerator for approximately 30 minutes to take advantage of the invertebrate's inability to regulate its body temperature. The patient may then be allowed to warm slowly without ill effects. This method should not be used for surgical procedures or techniques that cause pain [4]. Analgesia is not provided by this technique, and its effect on the immune system of invertebrates is, to the authors' knowledge, unknown.

Chemical restraint agents commonly used include inhalant and injectable anesthetics [1,2,4]. Gas anesthesia may be the most technically simple and effective method of restraint for terrestrial invertebrates. Enclose the patient

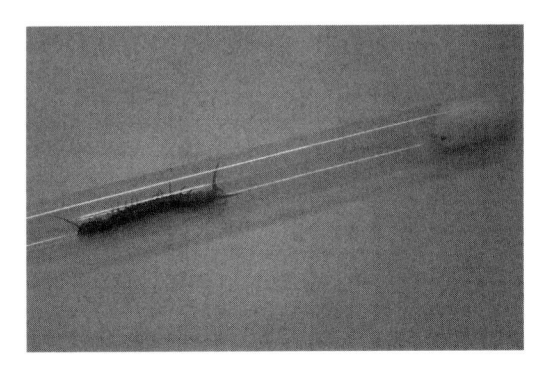

Fig. 1. Clear plastic tube used to facilitate visual examination of a centipede (*Scolopenda* spp).

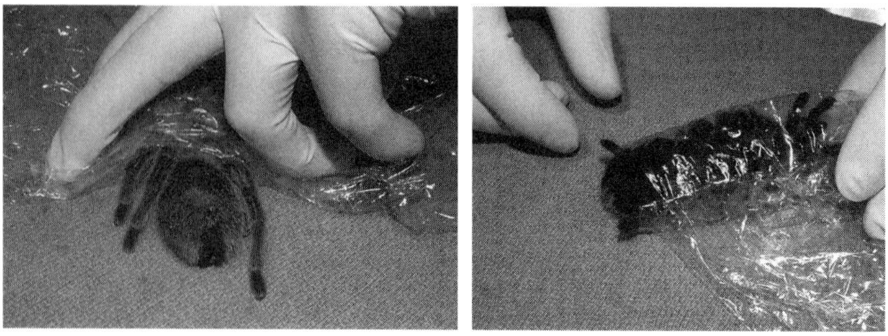

Fig. 2. Plastic food wrap may be used for restraint of tarantulas.

in a gas delivery chamber and deliver the agent by a direct method or, preferably, with a vaporizer (Fig. 4). In the tarantula, recommended anesthetic protocols include carbon dioxide at 10% to 20% for 3 to 5 minutes, halothane at 4% for 5 to 10 minutes, methoxyflurane at 4% for 10 to 30 minutes, and isoflurane at 3% to 4% for 10 to 15 minutes [3]. For direct delivery, a cotton ball or sponge may be soaked in anesthetic agent and placed in the chamber. To ensure that the patient cannot come into contact with the anesthetic agent, a specially built induction chamber is required for the direct method [4].

Several drugs are available for the immobilization of aquatic patients. Common immobilization agents used are tricaine methanesulfonate (MS-222) (Finquel, Foster and Smith, Rhinelander, Wisconsin), benzocaine, clove oil (eugenol), and ethanol. MS-222 is commonly added to water in a concentration of 100 mg/1 L of water. Buffering MS-222 with the addition of sodium bicarbonate is recommended for use in invertebrates with sensitive skin, such as snails and slugs. Benzocaine is probably the best choice of available anesthetics, but it must be made as a stock solution in ethanol

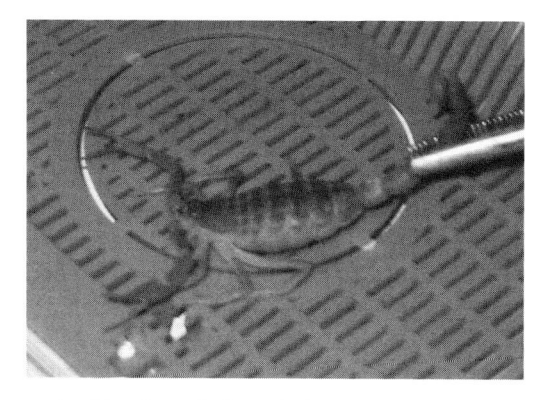

Fig. 3. Scorpion restraint. The pincers indicate the hazards of handling this animal. The stinger is gently restrained with forceps, ideally ones that have been padded.

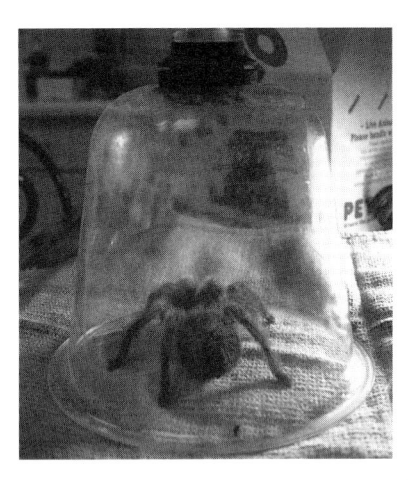

Fig. 4. Chilean rose haired tarantula (*Grammostola rosea*) being induced in a standard large dog anesthesia mask with isoflurane gas.

and stored away from light. The commonly used inhalant anesthetics, such as isoflurane, may be used in aquatic invertebrates by bubbling them through water. Immerse the entire patient (or just the foot of gastropods) in the anesthetic solution until it is immobile, then remove it. To keep the patient moist and sedate, a misting of anesthetic solution may be applied periodically; by varying this solution's concentration, one can control anesthetic depth [4]. Although the aforementioned agents will provide the sedation needed properly to handle the patient, the analgesic effects have not yet been determined for invertebrates [4,8].

Cardiovascular system monitoring of some terrestrial and aquatic invertebrates is possible using an 8-MHz Doppler probe [9]. Determination of depth of anesthesia in invertebrates may be challenging. In terrestrial invertebrates, the righting reflex, immobility, and response or lack thereof to gentle prodding or other aversive stimuli are generally used to determine the depth of anesthesia. In leeches, attachment to the surface, swimming motion, muscle tone, sucker function, and response to stimulation were assessed for determination of anesthetic depth [4]. Reversal of anesthesia in aquatic species is simple and rapid when they are returned to normal water. Oxygen supplementation of both terrestrial and aquatic species is recommended for anesthetic recovery or in the event of anesthetic complication.

Assessment of hydration and fluid therapy

Hydration status is as important to invertebrate well-being as it is to conventional domestic animals. Dehydrated arthropods may be sluggish or anorexic or have a shriveled opisthosoma or abdomen. Mollusks will also exhibit sluggishness and anorexia and have shriveled, desiccated soft tissues. Debilitated arthropods can rehydrate themselves but may not be able to obtain water on their own. Tarantulas, for instance, are dependent on hemolymph pressure for movement. Flexor muscles pulling on the cuticle of the exoskeleton induce flexion of the limbs, but hemolymph pressure is necessary for limb extension. Adequate hemolymph pressure in the appendages cannot be achieved when the animal is suffering from volume depletion due to dehydration [10]. Therefore, when locomotion is compromised, the animal cannot reach a water source to rehydrate. The clinician can rehydrate the patient by simply introducing water to its mouthparts. A spoon, shallow bowl, or syringe may be used to administer fluids to a tarantula's pharynx. However, care must be taken not to allow the patient, in its compromised state, to become submerged, or it may be unable to remove itself from the water and drown [1,10,11]. Mollusks can be rehydrated by submerging the patient in water [12].

In severe cases of dehydration, intracoelomic or intracardiac injection may be employed for fluid administration. Fluid choices include lactated Ringer's solution, normal saline, or, in the case of tarantulas, a Spider's Ringer's solution consisting of sodium chloride 11.104 g/L, potassium chloride 0.149 g/L, calcium chloride dehydrate 0.588 g/L, magnesium chloride hexahydrate 0.813 g/L, and sodium phosphate heptahydrate 0.268 g/L [10].[1] Fluid is administered through a 27-gauge needle with an insulin syringe. The amount varies based on the species. In tarantulas, a 10% hydration deficit is approximately 2% to 4% of the spider's body weight. In a 30-g tarantula that is 10% dehydrated, administration of 0.9 mL of fluids is appropriate to replace the deficit. The three anatomic options for fluid administration are into the heart, into the coelom of the opisthosoma, and into the ventral joint membranes. Pericardial or cardiac injection is accomplished with introduction of the needle on the dorsal midline of the opisthosoma at an angle of 45° to 60° from vertical (Fig. 5). The advantage to the pericardial method is that a large volume may be infused quickly and that exact placement is not crucial because extracardiac administration is not harmful. Spiders have an open venous system, which allows absorption in the event of extracardiac leak. Because of the risk for cardiac laceration with the needle, this method is reserved for immobilized or anesthetized animals [10]. The intracoelomic injection is administered along the transverse plane in the lateral opisthosoma (see Fig. 5). Either opisthosomal injection site must be repaired with cyanoacrylate, as described for exoskeleton repair. For injection into the ventral joint membrane of the limbs, the patient need not be anesthetized. Insert a needle shallowly into the ventral joint membrane of any leg (Fig. 6). The rate of administration is much slower using this method because of the small space available in the limb. If damage

---

[1] This comes sold as a research product.

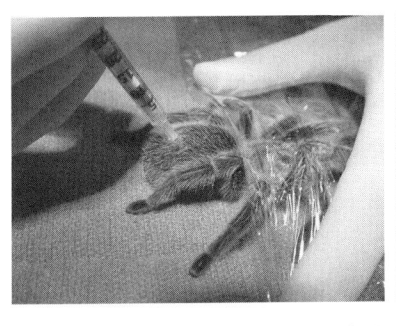

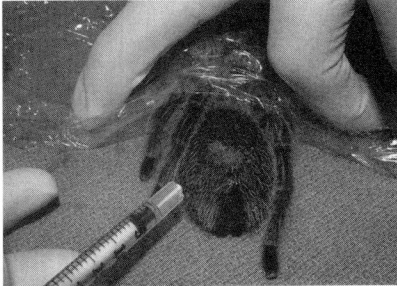

Fig. 5. Pericardial (*left*) and intracoelomic (*right*) injection of fluids in the Chilean rose haired tarantula (*Grammostola rosea.*)

occurs, the limb may be autotomized and the stump sealed with cyanoacrylate [10]. Methods for intracoelomic and ventral joint injection in spiders may be applied to other arthropods. Additionally, methods outlined earlier for fluid therapy may be used for drug administration. Use of intravenous formulations of drugs and dosages modified from those in other poikilotherms has been advocated for invertebrate therapeutics [3].

Diagnostic sampling

Proper sampling technique must be observed to obtain diagnostic results. Invertebrate patient size demands sampling be performed with the fewest possible attempts. Although a comprehensive review of invertebrate sampling is available, a summary is provided here [13].

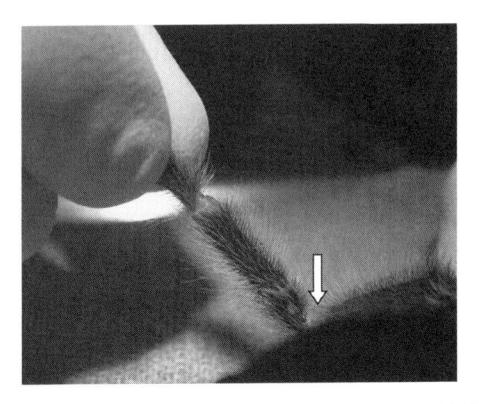

Fig. 6. When the tarantula is placed in dorsal recumbency, the ventral joint membrane may be used for injection. Arrow denotes the injection site.

Hemolymph collection

To assess physiologic parameters, hemolymph samples may be obtained. The small sample amount, not to exceed 10% of patient body weight, can make sampling difficult. In mollusks, hemolymph may be obtained from the heart or cephalopod sinus by means of a capillary tube or 25-gauge needle and syringe. To access the heart, a hole may be made in the shell using a dental drill. Alternatively, hemolymph can be sampled from the cephalopedal sinus in anesthetized patients. In bivalve mollusks, once the adductor muscle is transected and the left valve is removed, the heart can be found by its beating [13]. Alternatively, one may file a notch in each valve to create an opening and then insert the needle into the adductor sinus through the adductor muscle [13]. Another method for bleeding snails may be done without shell perforation. Locate the pneumostome (respiratory opening) as a landmark by watching for the appearance of bubbles (Fig. 7). In snails weighing less than 50 g, the needle insertion point is approximately 5 mm below the pneumostome, and in snails weighing between 50 g and 200 g the point is approximately 20 mm below the pneumostome. Hemolymph may be aspirated using a 25-gauge needle and syringe [14].

Hemolymph can be collected from arthropods by direct withdrawal from the heart, coelom, or legs. Methods for hemolymph collection are similar to those described for fluid administration, with aspiration of these sites substituted for injection.

Integumental diagnostics

The observation of integumental lesions may require samples to be taken for isolation of bacterial, fungal, or viral agents. With appropriate

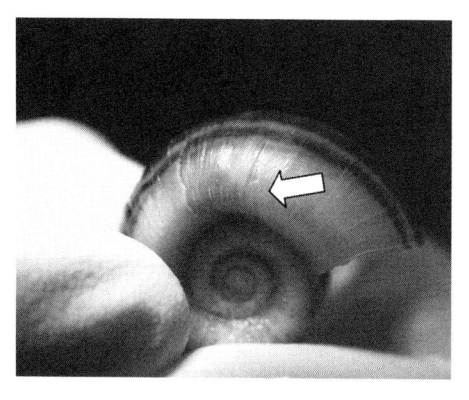

Fig. 7. Pneumostome in the snail may be found by looking for the expulsion of air bubbles. Arrow denotes the light shadow of the air bubbles visualized through the right side of the shell.

handling and restraint, techniques used in mammals for diagnosis of skin disease may be used to take samples from arthropods. Clinical signs of infectious skin diseases of mollusks and arthropods have been reviewed [11]. Disease from an infectious agent in an invertebrate colony generally indicates overpopulation or hygiene problems [1,12,13]. Skin scrapings, swabs, and touch preparations from ulcerated lesions may be used for culture and cytology for diagnosis and identification of bacterial, fungal, and viral infections. Similar diagnostics along with excision of deeper lesions may be used for histopathology [11,15]. Commensal and symbiotic organisms that may live on these animals can make result interpretation challenging. Culturing techniques need to take into account the ectothermic nature of the host. Standard incubation temperatures of 37°C may not be the optimum range for some invertebrate pathogens [13]. After sampling, lesions should be irrigated with saline to minimize dehydration and facilitate healing [11].

Fecal examination

Fecal samples are useful for examination of gut flora [13]. Fresh samples can simply be collected from the habitat of an individual or taken from a sample of a colony population. Colonies of invertebrates often have to be regarded as a whole organism. In these cases, culling samples of sick and healthy individuals can allow for diagnosis with minimal loss [16,17]. When the small size of the patient will not allow for taking adequate sample amounts, whole body extracts may also be used diagnostically to determine the causes of dysecdysis and European foulbrood, a disease of honeybees [12,13,16]. Samples may also be diluted to obtain adequate sample volumes [12,13]. Although we still need to increase our knowledge of normal invertebrate physiology and expand our clinical pathology capabilities, interpretation of several diagnostic samples is now available to the veterinarian. Quality samples are essential for definitive diagnosis and guidance of treatment.

Imaging

Radiography is a useful tool in invertebrate medicine. Invertebrates with a solid exoskeleton are more appropriate subjects for diagnostic radiography than are soft-bodied species. Snails and millipedes contain large airspaces that show up well on radiographs (Fig. 8). Feeding a preferred dietary item, such as fruit or other invertebrates, containing barium allows for contrast radiography and better visualization of the alimentary tracts of invertebrates (Fig. 9; see Fig. 8).

Endoscopy can also provide needed information about our invertebrate patients. Laparoscopy may be appropriate in some large-bodied species.

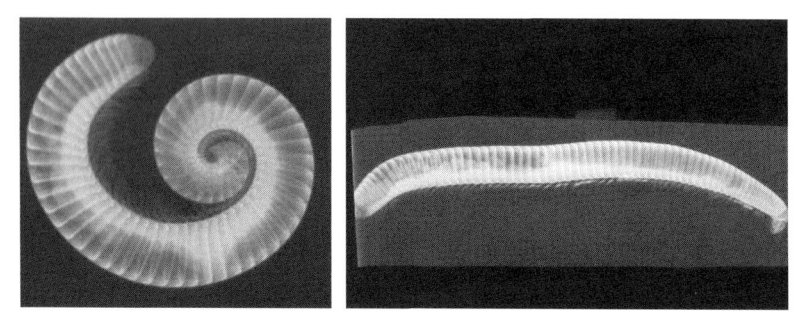

Fig. 8. Ventrodorsal and lateral radiographic views of a giant millipede. In the lateral view, barium enhances the gastrointestinal tract in the ventral aspect of the body, and large dorsal airspace is also apparent. This specimen has been anesthetized with isoflurane.

However, there are dangers associated with entering the central chambers filled with hemolymph.

Endoscopy of external orifices is safe and extremely useful, owing in large part to the excellent magnification obtained by this procedure. In particular, much may be visualized by performing endoscopy of the snail pneumostome. This imaging technique also facilitates sample taking.

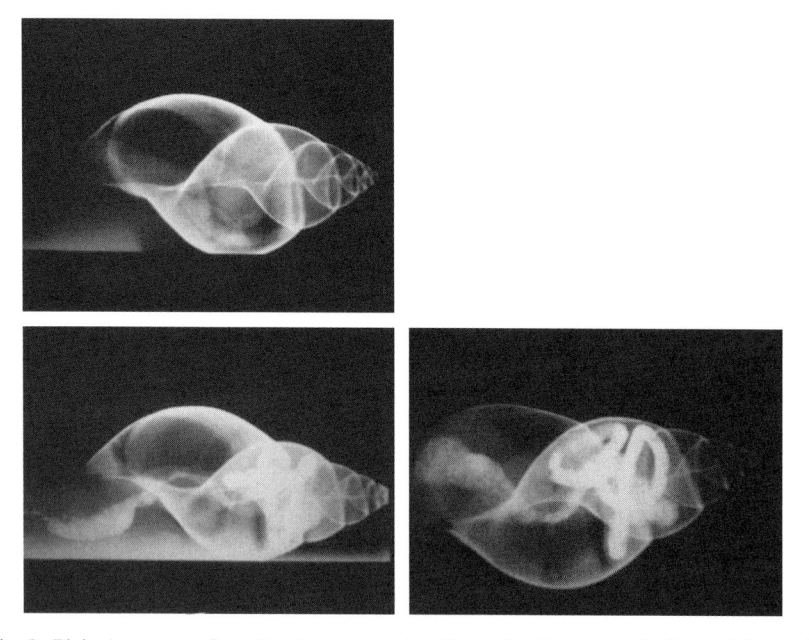

Fig. 9. Plain (*upper panel*) and barium contrast radiography (*lower panel*) views of the snail, *Achatina fulica*, are useful to visualize the gastrointestinal tract.

Integumental disorders and exoskeleton repair

The authors consider the anatomy of the exoskeleton here because invertebrates suffer many similar integumental diseases based on the presence of their exoskeletons. In the arthropod, the exoskeleton consists of an epicuticle, a procuticle (the thickest layer), and an epidermal cell layer. The procuticle is the chitinous layer providing protection and support, whereas the epicuticle is the nonchitinous layer responsible for waterproofing, hormone production, and antimicrobial properties. In mollusks, the protective shell is secreted as a layered structure by the epidermis. The prostratum is composed of sclerotized protein, with underlying layers being composed of calcium carbonate crystals. Crustaceans also incorporate a calcified cuticle into their exoskeletons [12]. These exoskeletal systems are the primary protection for these species, but exoskeleton compromise by trauma, infection, or dysecdysis can be life threatening.

Prevention of integumental disease relies primarily on the ability of owners to maintain proper environmental conditions for their animals. Maintaining both temperature and humidity within the optimal limits for a given species may prevent many skin ailments. Maintaining appropriate hygiene in the habitat by removing old food, feces, and bedding will reduce the likelihood of parasitic infestation and infectious disease. Periodic cleaning of the entire habitat with disinfectants is especially important for the control of myiasis. Avoiding overpopulation and providing adequate open space for molting are essential for maintaining healthy captive invertebrates. Treatment of integumental disease can be an emergency.

Exoskeleton or shell trauma

The assessment of an invertebrate integumental injury is important to the patient's appropriate and successful treatment. When a traumatic insult occurs to an arthropod's integument from a fall, predation, or surgical intervention, several issues must be addressed to correct the problem. The break in the protective outer layer may cause hemolymph loss and dehydration and create an avenue for infection. On injury to the exoskeleton, an increased heart rate increases hemolymph pressure and hence the possibility of hemolymph loss [12]. Loss of hemolymph can be immediately fatal, making quick action to repair the defect essential. As with other patients, immediate hemolymph stasis may be achieved by direct pressure. Other methods to stop loss of hemolymph are the use of sugar icing, talcum powder, paraffin wax, beeswax, plasticine, or tape to seal the hole in the exoskeleton temporarily [11].

The most effective method of exoskeleton repair involves use of a cyanoacrylate adhesive, such as tissue adhesive (Vetbond, 3M Animal Care Products, St. Paul, Minnesota), Instant Krazy Glue (Elmer's Products, Inc., Columbus, Ohio), or Super Glue (Pacer Technologies, Rancho Cucamonga, California), to seal wounds or reduce shell fractures [18]. Invertebrate patients with exoskeleton repairs should be monitored through the next molt to confirm that dysecdysis has not occurred at the repair site. Exoskeleton repair with suture material (Vicryl, Ethicon, Somerville, New Jersey) resulted in death of tarantula patients [18]. Placement of sutures in the opisthosomal (caudal body segment) was difficult, as was good tissue purchase, and this method of closure did not prevent serious hemolymph loss. Tarantulas died as a result of hemolymph loss immediately postoperatively and also died after ecdysis when the sutures tore through the opisthosoma. Suturing may be effective with injuries of the prosoma because of the greater tissue density of that body segment; however, dysecdysis may also be likely [18].

Complete or partial limb loss of an arthropod generally does not require treatment. Although this is a compromise of the exoskeleton, no great loss of hemolymph generally occurs, and patient survival without ill effects is likely. Many arthropods, especially the young, can regenerate lost limbs as they grow and molt [1].

The risk for hemolymph loss in a mollusk with a damaged shell is dependent on the location of the fracture. However, the risks for dehydration and infection are great, so shell damage in a mollusk is an emergency. Soft tissue injuries to mollusks can often be fatal because of the large amount of hemolymph that is rapidly lost. If immediate treatment is not possible, the patient may be placed in a bowl of normal saline or clean water [1]. Any patient exhibiting an exoskeleton or shell injury should be rehydrated and given prophylactic antibiotic therapy. To repair a compromised shell, reduce the fractures and apply an adhesive product, such as cyanoacrylate glue, to maintain the fragments in apposition. The shell is then reinforced with scaffolding material (Figs. 10 and 11) that will absorb the adhesive and provide support and stability while the fractures heal [19]. Although this method is similar to the repair of a turtle shell, the weight of the repair and the character of the scaffolding should be appropriate to the size of the patient. Mollusks with shell injury will benefit from dietary calcium supplementation [19]. Persistent shell abnormalities can occur when the mantle of a mollusk is damaged [1].

Dysecdysis

The ability to molt properly is essential to the growth, development, and healing of many species of invertebrates, particularly insects, spiders, centipedes, millipedes, and scorpions. Dysecdysis in captive invertebrates occurs in several forms stemming from multiple causes. The most common causes of dysecdysis are hormonal abnormalities caused by low levels of humidity, overcrowding (ie, lack of space suitable for molting), nutritional problems, and infection. Dysecdysis can manifest as incomplete or abnormal molting, inappropriately frequent molting, or molt arrest [12]. Frequent molting may be caused by eyestalk injuries in certain crustaceans and is used intentionally to increase body size in shrimp and lobster farming [20]. The hormone

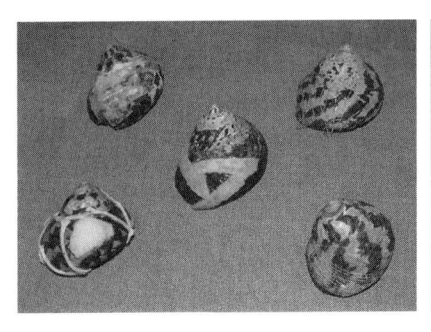

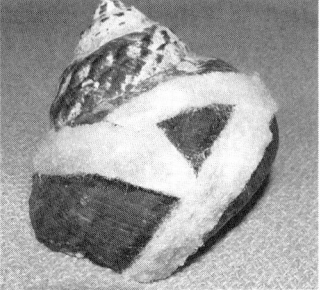

Fig. 10. Methods of snail shell repair (*left panel*). These snail shells were broken and then repaired with cyanoacrylate glue and tissue paper (*upper right*), thread (*upper left*), felt (*center*), household cotton twine (*lower left*), and roll gauze (*lower right*). On the authors' hands the felt technique (*right panel*) appeared to have the best holding power while being lightweight.

ecdysone, responsible for molt induction, can be affected by stressors such as repeated handling [21]. For colonial invertebrates with dysecdysis, culling a sample of animals to determine the levels of endogenous ecdysone from total body extracts may be diagnostic [21].

Patients with retained portions of integument require treatment and a review (and correction) of current husbandry practices as necessary. Enclosure humidity should be increased to greater than 85%, and a thermal gradient should be provided to include the top end of the animal's preferred optimum temperature zone [1,11]. Apply glycerine to retained epidermis to loosen and remove it by teasing the pieces away with forceps or a cotton-tipped applicator. Removal is similar to that of the retained spectacle of the snake; overzealous traction may damage the underlying exoskeleton.

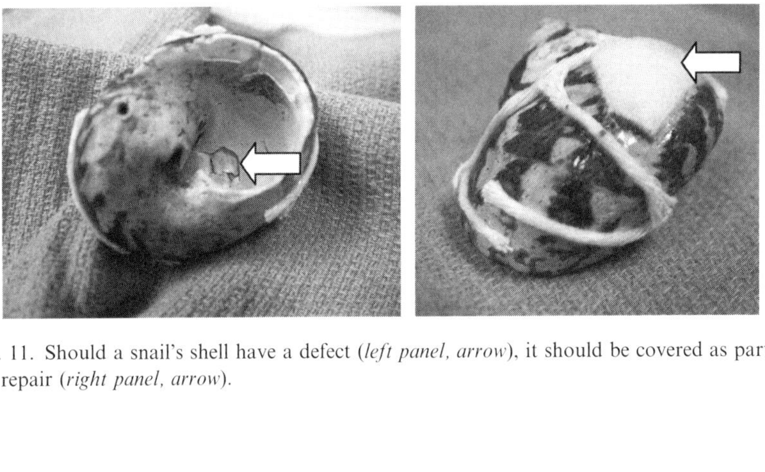

Fig. 11. Should a snail's shell have a defect (*left panel, arrow*), it should be covered as part of the repair (*right panel, arrow*).

Ectoparasite control and removal

Parasitic infestation may cause integumental disorders or dysecdysis. Several species of mite can infest arthropods, but mites should be identified as pathogens before removal. In many species, such as hissing cockroaches and millipedes, the mites and host form a symbiotic relationship as the mites feed on organic matter gathered in the joints or between the body plates (Fig. 12). Killing these mites leaves the host vulnerable to bacterial or fungal infections.

Ectoparasitic mites of spiders and other arthropods are thought to come from food sources such as crickets and meal worms. Hence, cleaning debris of past meals from the habitat in a timely manner is recommended. Treatment of parasitic conditions in arthropods is challenging because of the close taxonomic relationship between the parasite and the host [6]. Drugs effective against the mite infestation can also kill the arthropod patient. Unlike arthropods, snails with ectoparasite infestation may be safely treated with pyrethroids [11].

Manual removal of parasites has the greatest efficacy in arthropods. Most patients must be anesthetized for mite removal [6]. For arthropods such as cockroaches, phasmids, mantids, and scorpions, shaking the arthropod gently in a bag of flour may dislodge the mites [22]. Swabbing with a soft paintbrush or cotton ball may also dislodge the mites from arthropods [6]. Mite removal from spiders may require manual removal with ophthalmic forceps and magnification. A cotton-tipped applicator coated with vaseline may also be used to entrap the mites and lift them from the exoskeleton. Anesthesia of the patient may facilitate mite removal by also anesthetizing the mites. Flumethrin strips are effective against infestation when placed in the vivarium. Other suggested methods of mite removal in tarantulas may have severe consequences and are not endorsed by the authors. Application of a drop of mineral oil on the spider, to capture the mites as they roam, is not efficacious and may compromise the spider's

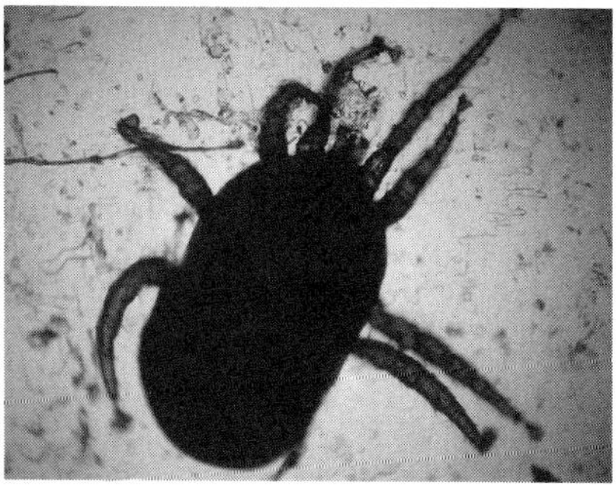

Fig. 12. A commensal millipede mite; the mites are nonpathogenic, and mite removal may harm the host indirectly.

book lung. Bathing a tarantula in a dilute soap solution for mite removal may also potentially compromise the book lung. The use of predatory mites, *Hyoapsis,* can be an alternative treatment of mite infestation, but these mites are not universally available owing to certain national environmental policies [6].

Although it is not an integumental disorder, infestation of apiaries with the *Varroa jacodsoni* mite causes economic loss to honey manufacturers [12,16]. Diagnosis of this disease, varrosis, can be difficult because the mite undergoes most developmental stages in the sealed cells of the hive. As the mite population nears 1000, signs of the infestation can be seen. The mites feed on the pupal hemolymph in the sealed cell, causing stunting, deformities, or death. The presence of adult mites on adult bees is diagnostic for the infestation (Fig. 13). However, this is only seen late in infestation, when it may be too late to save the hive. Many beekeepers will place flumethrin strips inside the hive and count the number of mites gathered on the strip (Fig. 14). The number of mites accumulated indicates the need for treatment. As fewer bees reach adulthood as a result of infection, the social cohesion of the hive breaks down and the colony collapses. The hive disbands, and the members of the hive disperse to other hives. Dispersing members carry the mite with them and spread the disease [16]. Treatment with pyrethroids, flumethrin, and tau-fluvalinate will prevent colony collapse and infestation of other hives [12,16]. Practitioners should familiarize themselves with the appropriate drug withdrawal times for the honey produced.

Euthanasia and postmortem examination

Euthanasia is a procedure that must be performed humanely. Whether canine or arachnid, swine or snail, it is the veterinarian's obligation to provide quick and painless euthanasia to ailing, cull, food, and research

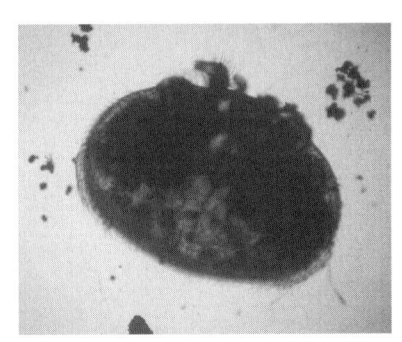

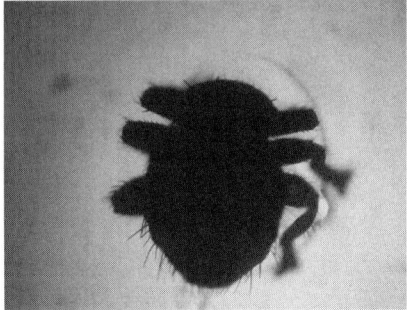

Fig. 13. Adult *Varroa* spp mite of the honeybee (*left*) and a bee louse (*right*). Nonpathogenic bee lice can often be found in the debris beneath the hive.

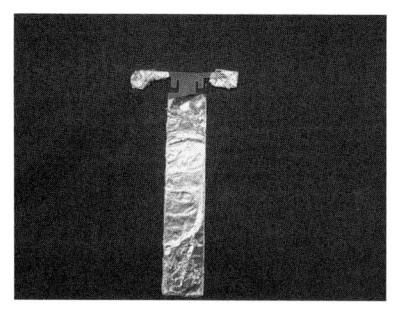

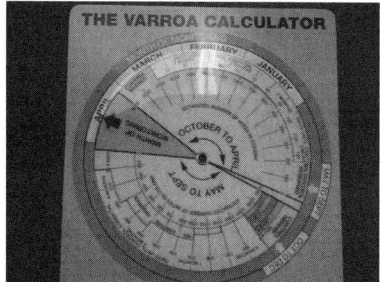

Fig. 14. Bayvarol (Bayer, Leverkusen, Germany) strip (*left*) for Varroaiasis diagnosis and control and calculator (*right*) for assessing mite numbers and the necessity of treatment.

animals. Guidelines have been set for acceptable methods of euthanasia for mammalian species, and the same is true for some invertebrates. A list of acceptable euthanasia options has been published for snails [17]. Among these options are freezing, immersion in boiling water, and overdosing with the chemical anesthetics outlined in the restraint section. Euthanasia with an anesthetic overdose is the best method for enabling postmortem examination. Crushing is an acceptable alternative for euthanasia of snails, but this option does not preserve the carcass for necropsy. Pain control should be considered when performing euthanasia of invertebrates. Do not freeze the unanesthetized invertebrate patient [17].[2] These methods can be applied and should be sufficient to achieve humane euthanasia in all invertebrates. Further advice is available in the British and Irish Association of Zoo and Aquaria's guide to invertebrate euthanasia [23].

Summary

In the growing population of captive invertebrates, many species can meet many needs. Whether invertebrates are pets, research animals, or production animals, these creatures need adequate and informed veterinary care. Although more is known about these interesting species than formerly, a great deal of research has yet to be done. The techniques outlined here will aid in the diagnosis and treatment of many common ailments of invertebrate patients. It is to be hoped that distribution of this knowledge will improve care for captive invertebrates and create a body of skilled individuals who may be called on to care for the rare or endangered invertebrate species. Our goal should be to set a standard for invertebrate veterinary medicine that is as high as that set for our more conventional mammalian and avian patients.

---

[2] Freezing of anesthetized patients is legal and endorsed, but freezing should not be used as a method without prior anesthesia.

Acknowledgments

The authors wish to acknowledge Petco, Opelika, Alabama for the donation of snail shells in Figs. 10 and 11 for practice and demonstration of fracture repair techniques in these animals.

References

[1] Cooper JE. Emergency care of invertebrates. Vet Clin North Am Exot Anim Pract 1998;1(1): 251–64.
[2] Cooper JE. Invertebrate care. Vet Clin North Am Exot Anim Pract 2004;7(2):473–86.
[3] Johnson-Delaney C. Invertebrates. In: Delaney CJ, editor. Exotic companion medicine handbook. Lake Worth (FL): Zoological Education Network; 1998. p. 1–13.
[4] Cooper JE. Invertebrate anesthesia. Vet Clin North Am Exot Anim Pract 2001;4(1):57–67.
[5] Blaikie AJ, Ellis J, Sanders R, et al. Eye disease associated with handling pet tarantulas: three case reports. Br Med J 1997;314(7093):1524–5.
[6] Varga MJ. Mites in a cobalt blue "tarantula" (*Haplopelma lividum*). Veterinary Invertebrate Society Newsletter 2004;2(20):2–6.
[7] Cooper JE. A veterinary approach to spiders. J Small Anim Pract 1987;28:229–39.
[8] Judge SE. General anaesthetic action in the field of invertebrate central nervous system. Gen Pharmacol 1980;11(4):337–41.
[9] Rees Davies R, Chitty J, Saunders R. Cardiovascular monitoring of an Achatina snail with a Doppler ultrasound probe. Presented at the Autumn Meeting of the British Veterinary Zoological Society. London, 2002.
[10] Pizzi R. Treating dehydration in tarantulas (*Theraphosidae*). Veterinary Invertebrate Society Newsletter 2005;2(21):2–7.
[11] Cooper JE. Skin disease in invertebrates. In: Locke PH, Harvey RG, Mason IS, editors. Manual of small animal dermatology. Cheltenham, England: BSAVA; 1993.
[12] Williams DL. Integumental disease in invertebrates. Vet Clin North Am Exot Anim Pract 2001;4(2):309–20.
[13] Williams DL. Sample taking in invertebrate veterinary medicine. Vet Clin North Am Exot Anim Pract 1999;2(3):777–801.
[14] Cooper JE. Bleeding of pulmonate snails. Lab Anim 1994;28(3):277–8.
[15] Cooper JE. Oncology of invertebrates. Vet Clin North Am Exot Anim Pract 2004;7(3): 697–703.
[16] Williams DL. A veterinary approach to the European honey bee (*Apis mellifera*). Vet J 2000; 160(1):61–73.
[17] Cooper JE, Knowler C. Snails and snail farming: an introduction for the veterinary profession. Vet Rec 1991;129(25–6):541–9.
[18] Pizzi R, Ezendam T. Spiders and sutures: or how to make wounds a whole lot worse. Veterinary Invertebrate Society Newsletter 2005;2(21):18–20.
[19] Connolly C. Repair of the shell of a Giant African Landsnail (*Achatina fulicia*), using Leucopor tape and Nexabond tissue adhesive. Veterinary Invertebrate Society Newsletter 2004; 2(20):8–11.
[20] Williams DL. Biology and pathology of the invertebrate eye. Vet Clin North Am Exot Anim Pract 2002;5(2):407–15.
[21] Bonaric JC, Reggi MD. Changes in ecdysone levels in the spider *Pisaura mirabilis* nymphs (Araneae, Pisaridae). Bulletin de la Société Zoologique de France 1977;107:449–52.
[22] Darmo L, Ludwig F. Madagascan giant hissing roaches. Carolina Tips 1995;58(2):5–6.
[23] British and Irish Association of Zoos and Aquariums. Guide to invertebrate euthanasia. London: British and Irish Association of Zoos and Aquaria.

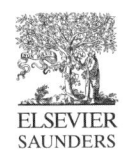

Common Diagnostic and Clinical Techniques for Fish

Drury R. Reavill, DVM, DABVP–Avian, DACVP

Zoo/Exotic Pathology Service, 2825 KOVR Drive, West Sacramento, CA 95605, USA

Fish medicine has common diagnostic and clinical procedures that are essential for disease diagnosis and patient management. With a few modifications for handling of the fish patient, these resemble procedures performed in most veterinary hospitals and clinics in our other companion species. The predictive value of these diagnostic methods is improving with the ever-increasing number of publications in fish medicine. Training in aquatic clinical procedures is offered at most large continuing education conferences and as specialty courses. These basic procedures are the important first steps toward improving the health of our aquatic companion animals.

Triage and patient assessment

Safe handling

The most difficult part of fish evaluation and collection of diagnostic samples can be getting the patient and the veterinarian together. It is possible to move most aquarium fish in water-filled plastic bags or other water-safe containers. The client should be instructed to place the fish in one bag or other suitable container with an adequate amount of water and to collect a second water sample, for testing water quality. Placing both these bags in a Styrofoam or similar insulated container will help maintain the water temperature. Within the clinic, it is recommended to maintain tanks that may be set up quickly for freshwater or salt-water fish. The minimum equipment needed is a pump, air stone, water conditioning chemicals, and heater (see Box 1 for a more comprehensive list).

An assessment of clinical signs may be made during the initial phone consultation, as the owner is being instructed on how to bring in the fish. Some

---

E-mail address: dreavill@zooexotic.com

> **Box 1. Suggested equipment**
>
> - Air pump with tubing and an airstone
> - MS-222 stock solution
> - Two buckets or other similar containers
> - Plastic bags
> - Thermometer
> - Aquarium heater
> - Large syringe or turkey baster
> - Clean, dechlorinated water
> - Commercial dechlorinating agent
> - Fine net(s)
> - Surgical latex gloves with talc removed
> - Oxygen tank
> - High-detail intensifying screens and detail film, without a grid
> - Ultrasound with 7- and 5-MHz transducer

grave clinical signs that suggest the fish may not survive transportation include curling, where the fish is bending head to tail; drifting, which is an aimless, unpropelled motion; and head standing, where the fish is head down in a vertical position. Even given a poor prognosis, evaluation of the fish may be helpful in determining the risk to the remaining animals within the aquarium system.

The veterinarian is encouraged to consider safe handling of the fish with regard to the owner, the patient, and anyone assisting in restraint, diagnostics, or treatments. Some fish, such as the scorpion fish, are venomous. The venom is in the spines on the dorsal, anal, and pelvic fins. This toxin can be painful and cause severe swelling. Even after death, this toxin retains potency for as long as 48 hours. If stung, the affected area should be immediately washed in hot water (105°F) for 30 to 90 minutes, because the venom is heat labile and will be inactivated [1]. Other fish that are difficult to handle include many of the fresh-water catfish and marine fish that support various spines (surgeonfish) or those that have sharp teeth, such as triggerfish and eels. These fish not only can inflict significant damage but also can become entangled in nets, resulting in trauma.

Handling of these animals with gloved hands, preferably rinsed examination gloves, is recommended. This measure will help protect the fish handler from zoonotic fish diseases, such as *Nocardia* spp and *Mycobacterium marinum* [2,3]. Both of these bacteria, entering cuts on the hand, can cause a chronic granulomatous lesion that is difficult to control. Salt water itself is abrasive and can irritate the skin and eyes. Although gloves will reduce the exposure, it is also suggested that the handler wash after handling the fish. The safety of the fish is another concern: gloves may reduce the degree of trauma to the scales and fins, as well as lessening removal of the important protective mucous barrier on the surface of the fish [4].

For physical restraint, the fish may be placed in thick towels or a chamois that has been completely soaked in water [5]. This procedure generally requires assistance. By placing the towel or chamois at the bottom of the container, one may lift the ends and use them as a sling to surround and remove the fish from the container. If the procedure is prolonged (approximately longer than 30 seconds), the fish will require branchial perfusion with aerated water.

For many diagnostic techniques used in fish, it may be necessary to use sedation or anesthesia unless the fish is severely compromised. This facilitates handling of the fish and reduces trauma (to both the handler and fish) due to a struggling animal. Several systems for anesthetizing or sedating fish are described in the literature and are not covered here [6–9]. The most commonly used chemical restraint is tricaine methanesulfonate (MS-222, Finquel, Argent Chemical Laboratories, Redmond, Washington). Tricaine is readily available and inexpensive; it has a rapid onset and recovery. For clinics that treat substantial numbers of fish, maintaining a stock solution is suggested. Tricaine is solvent in aqueous solution but is acidic and can cause damage to the gills [10]. The solution should be buffered to neutralize to the pH of the water. Adding sodium bicarbonate, baking soda, at a ratio of one to two parts sodium bicarbonate to one part MS222 is usually sufficient. The level of sedation will depend on water temperature and the concentration of tricaine (Box 2).

To make a stock solution, mix 10 g of tricaine in 1 L of dechlorinated water, 1 teaspoon of sodium bicarbonate and store in a dark bottle (it is light-sensitive). The solution should be discarded if a precipitate develops. Shelf life may be extended by refrigeration or freezing. For recovery, place the fish in well-aerated, nonmedicated water. Stir or gently swish the fish through the water to increase water flow across the gills (branchial perfusion).

Clove oil (active ingredient: eugenol) is an alternative to MS-222 that is available at many pharmacies [11]. Eugenol is not completely soluble in water and should be diluted 1:10 in 95% ethanol to yield a working stock solution of 100 mg/mL. Each milliliter of clove oil contains approximately 1 g of eugenol. Concentrations of 40 to 120 mg/L are effective in freshwater and marine species. Recovery can be more prolonged compared with tricaine.

Box 2. Concentration of tricaine methanesulfonate (MS-222)

Anesthesia induction: 100–200 mg/L
Maintenance: 50–100 mg/L
Sedation: 15–50 mg/L

Support

While diagnostics are being run, the owner can provide support for the remaining community within the aquarium or pond. This type of support may also be provided for a fish that the owner is unable to bring in for examination. Water quality testing to identify any abnormal parameters is of primary importance. Many of these abnormal water quality parameters may easily be corrected with a 30% tank or pond water change.

For freshwater fish under stress, the addition of salt (sodium chloride) at 2 g/L of water will reduce osmotic imbalances. This measure is important in freshwater fish with severe skin ulcerations or gill disease, because they are hypertonic animals in a hypotonic environment. Freshwater fish quickly lose electrolytes and experience disruption of osmotic pressure when there is breaching of the environmental defenses (skin and mucous membranes of the gills). Table salt may be used, although commercial balanced salt mixtures of dry, artificial seawaters are preferred (eg, Instant Ocean, Aquarium Systems, Mentor, Ohio).

In marine species, disruption of the epithelial barrier can result in significant dehydration. Some clinicians have decreased the specific gravity of the tank to levels between 1.019 and 1.024 (typical specific gravity in a marine tank is 1.025) for extended periods in an attempt to minimize the degree of dehydration. Specific gravity is an indirect method of calculating water salinity [12].

The owner should be advised not to add medications or chemicals to the water, because many of these can reduce the water's dissolved oxygen content. Other concerns are the toxicities of the medicants themselves, as well as alteration of tests such as bacterial cultures [13].

Sample collection

Clinical history

One of the most important diagnostic techniques in fish medicine is taking the clinical history. Many disease conditions stem from improper husbandry or water quality. Information should be requested about the tank or pond set-up, filtration system, water changes, and feeding protocols, as well as food storage, other animals in the same community, and any recent additions to the collection. An example of the clinical history is provided in Box 3.

Water quality

Fish are physiologic extensions of their environment, so water quality plays an important part in fish disease. The owner or the veterinarian should test a sample of the water collected when the fish is examined (ie, before the

> **Box 3. Clinical history**
>
> *Tank set-up*
>   How long has the tank(s) been in operation?
>   What is the size of the tank(s) and the number of fish per tank(s)?
>   What type of lighting is used, for how many hours per day?
>   What type of filtration system is used, and how often is it cleaned?
>   What type of bottom substrate is used (eg, commercial aquarium gravel, river sand), and how thick a layer?
>   List all tank decorations and types of plants. When were these introduced to the tank?
>   Is the tank located near an outdoor door or window? Is it in an area of heavy use or activity?
>
> *Water*
>   Temperature
>   Source (aged, dechlorinated, tap water, other)
>   If known: pH, hardness, ammonia, nitrite, nitrate, salinity (if a marine tank)
>   Water changes: how often? how much?
>   Water treatment: ozonizer, protein skimmer, softener, UV, ion exchanger, other
>
> *Feed*
>   Type
>   Quantity
>   Any live food? Source?
>   Frequency
>
> *Fish*
>   Type and number of fish in affected tank?
>   Any recent introductions? (when? what?)
>   Are new introductions quarantined? If so, for how long?
>   Are they medicated before introduction to the main tank?
>   Any previous problems?
>   Please described affected fish.
>   Any deaths?
>   Any treatments? If so, which? Results?

owner does a water change). The common water chemistry tests are for ammonia, nitrites, nitrates, pH, and hardness. Salt-water tanks should be evaluated for levels of copper and salinity, whereas in koi ponds, dissolved oxygen is an important parameter. Several commercial test kits are accurate and inexpensive (Box 4). Temperature is also important, because fish have preferred optimum temperature ranges depending on the species. Testing procedures have been described in detail [14].

Blood collection

Collecting blood from most aquarium fish is a challenge. For survival sampling, particularly in large fish, it is possible to collect blood from the caudal tail vessels. The technique involves advancing the needle at a cranial dorsal angle from the ventral surface of the tail toward the spinal column. The needle is introduced at the ventral midline of the caudal peduncle and caudal to the anal fin. It is also possible to collect blood using a lateral approach [15]. The needle is inserted slightly below and perpendicular to the lateral line and cranial to the caudal peduncle. However, this approach can result in damage to the spinal nerves. Once the needle tip hits bone, one should withdraw the needle slowly with slight pressure on the plunger. Vigorous aspiration can result in a hemolyzed sample. A 1-mL syringe and 25-gauge needle may be used on fish as small as 30 g [5,16]. Pretreating the needle with heparin can help prevent coagulation.

Blood collection from the heart should be reserved as a terminal procedure, because it could result in significant cardiac lacerations. This is a technique that requires skill from practice and a thorough knowledge of fish anatomy should one consider it for survival testing. A blood sample may also be obtained as a terminal procedure by severing the caudal peduncle and collecting from the caudal tail vessels.

The cells of the vascular system are friable, and gentle handling is recommended during collection and making the blood smears. The literature offers interpretation of some blood parameters [5,16]. Useful information that can be obtained immediately from a blood sample includes packed cell volume, presence of blood parasites, and evidence of bacterial septicemias.

Fecal samples

It is possible to run a fecal parasite evaluation in fish. Fecal material may be collected with a fine-mesh net from the water. Often defecation occurs

---

Box 4. Sources of commercial tests for water quality

- Hach Co., P.O. Box 389, Loveland, CO 80539, 1-800-227-4224
- Gilford Instrument Labs, Ovelin, OH 44074, 216-774-1041
- La Motte Chemicals, P.O. Box 329, Chestertown, MD 21260, 301-778-3100
- Orion Research, 840 Memorial Drive, Cambridge, MA 02139, 617-864-5400

when the fish is captured and restrained for examination or other tests. When none is available at examination, the owner may need to provide the sample. It is important to instruct the owner not to take a sample from the bottom of the tank. Contamination by microscopic inhabitants of the tank will result. In larger fish, a swab of the vent (or anus, depending on the species) with the appropriate-sized swab may be used to evaluate for parasites. Both a fecal direct examination and fecal float should be considered, depending on the quantity obtained.

Cytology

One of the more common procedures is the skin scrape for cytology [15]. It should be performed on a fish with manual restraint, because drugs for sedation or anesthesia may alter the population of parasites on the fish. In large fish, keeping the greater part of the body and the gills in the water and the eyes covered will help keep the fish quiet for the procedure. One should have all the equipment ready before catching the fish, including access to a microscope. With a dull blade or a cover slip, collect a sample of the surface mucus. This is the most superficial layer of the skin and is composed of sloughed epithelial cells and mucus produced by the epidermal goblet or mucous cells. Move the blade or coverslip head to tail to avoid descaling the fish. Most parasites tend to concentrate in areas adjacent to the fins or under the mandible, perhaps because of reduced drag in the water along these areas. A variety of microbes may be found in this sample. For erosions or ulcerations, the sample should be collected from the leading edge of the lesion [4]. Do not traumatize the surface, or it will become a portal of entry for infection and may cause osmotic regulation problems.

Place the sample on a slide with a drop of tank water and apply a coverslip. It is important to use tank water on the slide, because chlorinated tap water can cause rapid death of many protozoa parasites. Changing the water osmolality, as by using saline solution for freshwater samples, will result in destruction of any fragile parasites. Evaluate the sample within 10 to 15 minutes, before it dries or the parasites die and stop moving. Small protozoa such as *Ichthyobodo* and *Chilodonella* may die within a few minutes (Helen Roberts, DVM, Orchard Park, NY, personal communication, 2006). Generally the sample will have a few scales, mucus, leukocytes, and bacteria or protozoa ciliates (Fig. 1). For most parasites, especially the protozoa, one should watch for motion. A description of the parasites, including size and motility, is important to identification. Skin cytology also helps identify bacteria and fungal infections. A skin biopsy is suggested when the lesion extends into the deeper layers.

Examining a section of damaged fin is another common procedure. When collecting this sample, clip a small piece in the area of the lesion. Place the fin section on a clean glass slide with a drop or two of tank water and

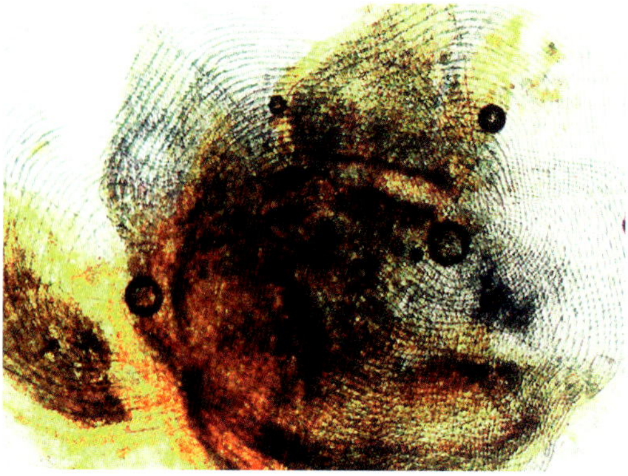

Fig. 1. Photomicrograph of a few normal fish scales from a goldfish. The round black structures are air bubbles (original magnification × 10). (© 2006 Drury R. Reavill, DVM, ABVP, certified in avian practice, Diplomate, ACVP, West Sacramento, CA.)

protect it with a coverslip (Fig. 2). Examine it for mounds or clusters of bacteria or fungus. Parasites may also be visualized. Damaged fins will regenerate, even if the rays have been compromised, once the disease condition is addressed [12].

The gills are another important site for evaluation. These serve the four functions of respiration (exchange of oxygen and carbon dioxide), excretion (ammonia), acid–base balance (chloride cells), and osmoregulation (balance of sodium, potassium, and chloride). The gills are readily subject to any environmental damage, because they are constantly exposed to the water. For examination of the gills, most fish will require some sedation. Gently lift the opercula and, with sharp iris scissors, cut a small sample of gill filaments (Fig. 3). Do not cut so deeply as to take the gill arch. Place the sample on a slide as for a skin scrape and examine immediately (Fig. 4). Many

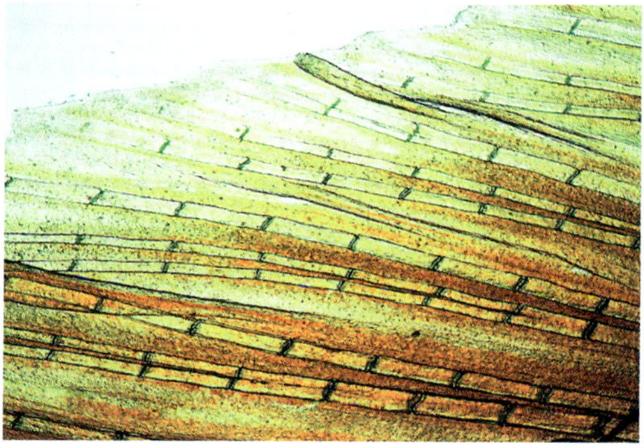

Fig. 2. Photomicrograph of a fin sample from a goldfish. The linear structures are the fin rays (original magnification × 4). (© 2006 Drury R. Reavill, DVM, ABVP, certified in avian practice, Diplomate, ACVP, West Sacramento, CA.)

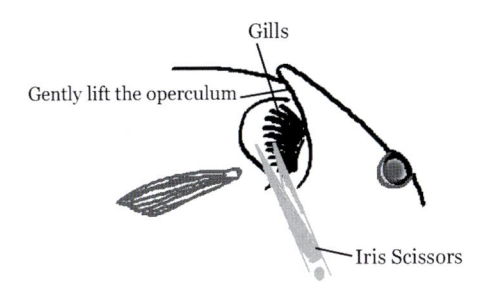

Fig. 3. Collecting a gill biopsy. (© 2006 Drury R. Reavill, DVM, ABVP, certified in avian practice, Diplomate, ACVP, West Sacramento, CA.)

parasitic, bacterial, and fungal disease agents may be identified by gill examination. Water quality insults produce lesions such as excess mucus and epithelial hyperplasia.

Aspiration cytology of fluids within the coelomic cavity or of masses is a useful procedure in fish. For collection of a sample from the coelomic cavity, the fish may need sedation. Generally fluid may be collected with a syringe and needle from a midline ventral tap. The point of entry is cranial to the vent or anus, and the bevel of the needle should be angled toward the body wall to prevent lacerations of the internal organs. Examine any fluid collected, as in any species (ie, for specific gravity, color, cellular components, bacteria), and consider submitting it for bacterial culture and sensitivity. Aspiration of the swim bladder generally requires radiography or ultrasound for centesis location.

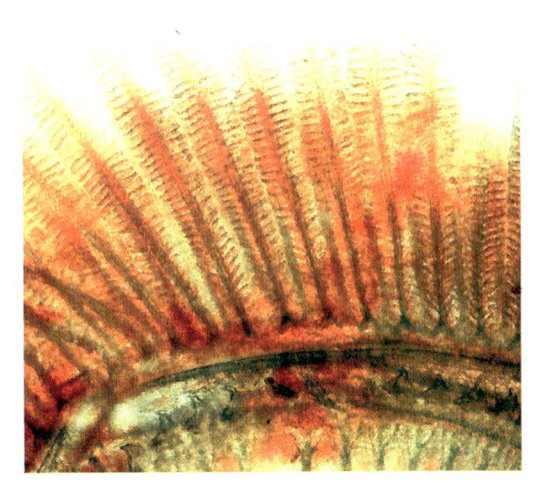

Fig. 4. Photomicrograph of a gill biopsy. A row of primary lamella is attached to the gill arch. The branching secondary lamella are at right angles from the primary lamella (original magnification × 4). (© 2006 Drury R. Reavill, DVM, ABVP, certified in avian practice, Diplomate, ACVP, West Sacramento, CA.)

Radiographs

For radiographs, fish may be placed directly on the cassette or maintained in a plastic bag of water. When they are removed from the water and placed directly on the cassette, it is important to work quickly. Fish become more excitable as they become hypoxic. Some fish may be placed in a plastic bag of water that may then be placed on the cassette. Water decreases the radiographic detail and creates an increased possibility of patient movement. The smallest-sized bag and quantity of water will help reduce this movement. In fish, as in other animal species, it is important to get a lateral and dorsoventral view. On the lateral view, it may be preferable to do this with a horizontal beam so that any fluid accumulation within the swim bladder may be identified.

Supportive care procedures

Enteral support

The stress created by force feeding fish generally outweighs the benefits it provides. Gavage or tube feeding is a method that may be used for unpalatable drugs, although many fish will readily regurgitate gastric contents. Tube feeding involves a syringe and a metal feeding needle or a soft rubber feeding tube. The procedure is stressful for conscious fish; however, sedated fish may regurgitate the material across the gills. Knowledge of the anatomy is important, because not all fish have a stomach to hold even a small quantity of material, and there is a risk for gastrointestinal tract perforation when the tube or needle is placed too vigorously. Some fish have teeth, such as the prominent teeth of many marine fish and the pharyngeal teeth in carp, that complicate the passing of the gavage tube [13,15].

Fluid therapy

Marine fish that are anorexic may also be dehydrated. Sufficiently large fish may be treated with gastric intubations of freshwater or similar physiologic fluid [17].

Medication administration

Most therapies in fish medicine involve adding medications or chemicals to the water. Dips and baths require immersion of the fish in medicated water for various lengths of time ("dips" are shorter than 15 minutes and "baths" are longer). These are administered in smaller containers to spare the display tank the side effects of the treatments. It is important to watch the fish carefully for signs of distress (eg, irregular swimming, gasping or piping at the water surface). After the treatment, place the fish in a clean holding tank for a thorough rinse before replacing it in the display tank.

Indefinite or tank treatment involves medicating the entire display tank and all its inhabitants. This measure may be required for effective treatment of some disease conditions, such as a system-wide parasitic infestation. A drawback is the tendency of some drugs to bind to the substrates and organic debris, to induce changes in biologic filters, or to be toxic to plants and invertebrates. Because of binding, the drug may not reach therapeutic levels, leading to increased bacterial resistance or incomplete destruction of parasites.

It is possible to administer medication by injections. The most common sites are intraperitoneal (IP) and intramuscular (IM). Intravenous injection may be considered for very large, anesthetized specimens. IP may be used with drugs that are nonirritating and capable of crossing endothelial barriers. The technique involves inserting the needle under the scales of the caudal ventral abdomen and then directing it in a cranio-dorsal direction. The intestines will be pushed away from the needle, and the caudal entry point will prevent penetration of the liver, spleen, and kidney.

Recent studies indicate the efficacy of IM injections [18,19]. Inject into the dorsal muscle mass, halfway between the lateral line and the dorsal fin. Direct the needle craniad under the scales. The volume suggested is 1 to 2 µL per gram of body weight. Turning the bevel of the needle as it is withdrawn may help close the injection tract and prevent leaking. In large fish, some clinicians prefer to inject near the base of the caudal aspect of the dorsal fin, along the dorsal midline.

Topical therapy of surface lesions is possible. Carefully elevate the site of the lesion out of the water, apply the medication, rinse the fish, and replace it in the tank. An adhesive waterproof compound may be used to keep topical therapy in contact for longer periods. Orabase (Colgate Orabase Soothe-n-Seal, Colgate-Palmolive Co., New York, New York) is a liquid bandage that may be applied to fish [20].

Oral administration of medications in the food is often useful when the fish are eating. Medicated feed may be used to treat large numbers of fish. A drawback is that fish may refuse to eat the medicated food or to eat their entire portion. If normal feeding intervals are greater than 24 hours, satiated fish may not feed and will effectively end any treatment. Some medications may be given as an oral bolus (gavage). Several recipes for food mixtures used to deliver drugs exist (Box 5). Mazuri makes gelatin diets for delivery of medications (Mazuri Aquatic Gel Diet 5M70, Mazuri Low Fat Aquatic Gel Diet 5ME2, and Mazuri Omnivore Aquatic Gel Diet 5Z94, Mazuri, Richmand, Indiana).

Pain control

It is generally believed that fish feel pain, based on their neuroanatomy, their complement of neurotransmitters, and their behavioral responses to

> **Box 5. General recipe for drug delivery in fish**
>
> Weigh 35 g of a well-balanced flake food; place in blender.
> Add 30 g of finely ground vegetables, such as fresh or frozen peas. Add 5 mL of food-grade cod-liver oil. Add 30 g of cooked oatmeal or wheat germ. Boil water and then add enough warm water to the mixture to make a slurry.
> Add vitamin supplements at this time (after cooling, because heat will inactivate the vitamins), such as 500 mg of B-complex vitamins or 2–3 g of Brewer's yeast, 250 mg of vitamin C, and 50 units of vitamin E. Mix well.
> Also add medicants at this time at 0.25% of the mixture; dissolve in warm water before adding.
> Dissolve 5–10 g of powdered unflavored gelatin in approximately 100 mL of boiling water; stir well until the gelatin is dissolved; allow to cool (but not set) for a few minutes and add to the mixture.
> Place mixture in separate bags and place in refrigerator. Food should be ready within an hour or may be frozen until needed. The food may be broken into bite-sized pieces using a cheese grater or potato peeler. Breaking up the food is important, especially when the food is frozen.
>
> ---
>
> (*From* Groff J. Gel-based diet recipe for fish. Modified by Joe Groff from JB Gratzek. Aquariology: the science of fish health management. Tetra Press; 1992. Online posting. July 29, 1997. Vet-to-Vet Aquatic Animal Medicine. Available at: http://www.vin.com/members/searchdb/boards/b0027500/b0026348.htm. Accessed February 13, 2006; with permission.)

pain stimuli [21]. The question is which types of pain fish experience and which therapeutics might be appropriate for their use. Butorphanol for postoperative analgesia has been reported at dosages of 0.05 to 0.5 mg/kg IM. Reports indicate that koi (*Cyprinus carpio*) given IM butorphanol at a dose of 0.4 mg/kg IM or subcutaneously before recovery from anesthesia return to normal swimming and begin eating sooner than those fish receiving a saline placebo [22]. Ketoprofen at 2 mg/kg IM has also been used for analgesia and has been shown to reduce postoperative increases in creatine kinase, possibly through anti-inflammatory effects [23].

References

[1] Vetrano SJ, Lebowitz JB, Marcus S. Lionfish envenomation. J Emerg Med 2002;23(4): 379–82.

[2] Decostere A, Hermans K, Haesebrouck F. Piscine mycobacteriosis: a literature review covering the agent and the disease it causes in fish and humans. Vet Microbiol 2004;99(3–4): 159–66.
[3] Ghittino PJ. Aquaculture and associated diseases of fish of public health importance. Am Vet Med Assoc 1972;161(11):1476–85.
[4] Groff JM. Cutaneous biology and diseases of fish. Vet Clin North Am Exot Anim Pract 2001; 4(2):321–411.
[5] Groff JM, Zinkl JG. Hematology and clinical chemistry of cyprinid fish. Common carp and goldfish. Vet Clin North Am Exot Anim Pract 1999;2(3):748.
[6] Noga EJ. Fish diseases. Diagnosis and treatment. St. Louis (MO): Mosby; 1996.
[7] Brown LA. Anesthesia in fish. Vet Clin North Am Small Anim Pract 1988;18:317–30.
[8] Brown LA. Anesthesia and restraint. In: Stoskopf MK, editor. Fish medicine. Philadelphia: WB Saunders; 1993. p. 79–90.
[9] Harms CA. Anesthesia in fish. In: Fowler ME, Miller RE, editors. Zoo and wild animal medicine: current therapy. 4th edition. Philadelphia: WB Saunders; 1998. p. 158–63.
[10] Ohr EA. Tricaine methanesulphonate-I. pH and its effects on anesthetic potency. Comp Biochem Physiol 1976;54C:13–7.
[11] Sladky KK, Swanson C, Stoskopf MK, et al. Comparative efficacy of tricaine methanesulfonate and clove oil for use as anesthetics in red pacu (*Piaractus brachypomus*). Am J Vet Res 2001;62(3):337–42.
[12] Fontenot DK, Neiffer DL. Wound management in teleost fish: biology of the healing process, evaluation, and treatment. Vet Clin North Am Exot Anim Pract 2004;7(1):57–86.
[13] Wildgoose WH, Lewbart GA. Therapeutics. In: Wildgoose WH, editor. BSAVA manual of ornamental fish. London: BSAVA; 2001. p. 237–58.
[14] Beleau MH. Evaluating water problems. Vet Clin North Am Small Anim Pract 1988;18(2): 291–302.
[15] Lewbart GA. Emergency and critical care of fish. Vet Clin North Am Exot Anim Pract 1998; 1(1):233–49.
[16] Sakamoto K, Lewbart GA, Smith TM. Blood chemistry values of juvenile red pacu (*Piaractus brachypomus*). Vet Clin Pathol 2001;30(2):50–2.
[17] Francis-Floyd R, Wildgoose WH. Behavioural changes. In: Wildgoose WH, editor. BSAVA manual of ornamental fish. London: BSAVA; 2001. p. 156.
[18] Grondel JL, Nouws JF, Schutte AR, et al. Comparative pharmacokinetics of oxytetracycline in rainbow trout (*Salmo gairdneri*) and African catfish (*Clarias gariepinus*). J Vet Pharmacol Ther 1989;12(2):157–62.
[19] Lewbart GA, Papich MG, Whitt-Smith D. Pharmacokinetics of florfenicol in the red pacu (*Piaractus brachypomus*) after single dose intramuscular administration. J Vet Pharmacol Ther 2005;28(3):317–9.
[20] Harms CA, Wildgoose WH. Surgery. In: Wildgoose WH, editor. BSAVA manual of ornamental fish. London: BSAVA; 2001. p. 259–66.
[21] Gregory N. Do fish feel pain? ANZCCART News 1999;12.4. Available at: http://www.adelaide.edu.au/ANZCCART/news/1999.html. Accessed February 2006.
[22] Harms CA, Lewbart GA, Swanson CR, et al. Behavioral and clinical pathology changes in koi carp (*Cyprinus carpio*) subjected to anesthesia and surgery with and without intraoperative analgesics. Comp Med 2005;55(3):221–6.
[23] Harms CA. Surgery in fish research: common procedures and postoperative care. Lab Animal 2005;34:28–34.

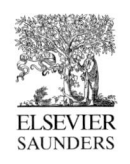

Common Procedures in Reptiles and Amphibians

Byron J.S. de la Navarre, DVM

Animal House of Chicago, Complete Veterinary Care, 2752 West Lawrence Avenue, Chicago, IL 60625, USA

Reptiles and amphibians continue to be popular as pets in the United States and throughout the world. It therefore behooves veterinarians interested in caring for these exotic species to continually gather knowledge concerning both their proper husbandry and the conditions that require medical and/or surgical intervention. To evaluate these animals properly, veterinarians need to be able correctly to examine them. Collecting appropriate laboratory samples to evaluate their health status (based on published hematologic, biochemical, and other relevant data) is also crucial to this endeavor. This article covers husbandry, physical examination, and clinical and diagnostic techniques in an effort to present guidelines for the evaluation of the reptile or amphibian patient. Gathering clinical data will aid veterinarians in arriving at the proper diagnosis, increasing the chances of success with treatment protocols, and educating the clients in proper nutrition and husbandry for their pets.

The information presented here has been collected from various sources: personal experience, personal communication with other veterinarians, texts, journals, bulletins, and the proceedings of past annual meetings of the Association of Reptilian and Amphibian Veterinarians (ARAV). This has been a collaborative effort, and references are provided so that further reading may be pursued.

Review of basic herpetologic herpetoculture and current advances

Veterinarians and herpetoculturalists generally agree that reptiles and amphibians have a "primitive" immune system, that several factors appear to affect the immune system, and that immune system dysfunction is a major

E-mail address: exotxdr@aol.com

problem in many reptile and amphibian pathologic conditions [1–5]. Some of the various factors affecting the immune system are hydration and nutritional status, sex and seasonal variation, stress, age, and environmental temperature [4]. Therefore, supporting the immune system is one of the most important aspects of treating an ill reptile or amphibian. Correcting hydration deficits, poor environmental temperature, and nutritional deficiencies and minimizing stress through correct husbandry practices are essential to maintaining these species in captivity.

Reptile and amphibian husbandry may be subdivided into three general areas, each of which is crucial to the proper maintenance of each species in captivity. These areas have been discussed elsewhere (for environment, see Refs. [6–11]; for nutrition, see Refs. [12–14]), but they may be summarized as follows:

> Environment: This includes the cage, temperature, humidity/water, substrate, other cage accessories, number and type of light or lights, photoperiod (number of hours of light and darkness per day), cagemates, and handling.
> Nutrition: Concern for the proper balance of protein, carbohydrates, fats, fiber, vitamins and minerals, and so on. Ideally, captive reptiles should be provided with the diet that most closely approximates that of the animal in the wild.
> Sanitation: Proper cage cleaning is vital to minimize the number of pathogens present in the environment and lessen environmental stress.

Anamnesis, distribution of educational materials, physical examination, and handling and restraint of reptiles and amphibians

The goal of this section is to present the basics of reptile and amphibian patient physical examination, handling, and restraint [15]. The techniques described should be helpful to veterinarians and veterinary technicians who are new to exotics, while providing a review for the more experienced veterinarians and staff.

Emphasis is placed on (1) the method of asking questions so as to obtain responses that aid in the assessment of the problem and (2) the natural defense mechanisms of the more commonly presented species and how to restrain and handle them properly. Much of this information follows the many presentations and publications of Dr. Teresa Bradley (Belton Animal Clinic, Belton, Missouri).

Anamnesis/History

General questions and ideas
> During the initial contact with clients, the receptionist should encourage them to bring in pictures of the environment and any records

(eg, feeding, weight, shedding) that they may have kept, along with a fresh fecal sample. If this is not possible, one should have the client make a sketch of the cage to show heat, light, humidity sources, and their relative positions to the hide box or boxes, basking site or sites, water bowl, thermometer, and so on.

One should determine the origin of the animal: wild caught or captive bred? Which pet store/breeder/show was involved?

Determine the age, sex, species, and breed of the animal or animals.

How long was the animal owned by the current owner? Past owners? Past history?

Determine the type of collection maintained: number, age, sex, species, and so on. (Some pathogens and parasites are easily spread from one species to another with serious consequences; for instance, amoebiasis in aquatic turtles may be "relatively" benign in that species but can be fatal when contracted by boas.)

Determine the timing of disease: onset, duration, severity?

Have there been changes in the patient's diet, environment, or husbandry in general?

Have there been any recent introductions of new specimens or species into the collection? Specifically, into the patient's cage?

Have any efforts or medications been used by the client to correct or treat the problem?

Determine whether any pesticides or other aerosol sprays or chemicals have been used in the immediate environment (especially when amphibians are involved).

Determine frequency of shedding—complete or partial, evidence of dysecdysis.

How often is the animal eating, drinking, urinating, and defecating? One needs to explain the appearance of normal stool, urine, and urates, because many new owners mistake the production of urates and urine for feces.

Diet questions

What is the diet? What food is being offered, and what is actually eaten?

How frequently are the animals fed, and how long is food left in the enclosure?

Are any supplements being offered, such as vitamins or minerals—names and ages?

When the animal is of an "insect-eating" species—are insects "gut-loaded"? Are insects dusted before being fed?

Which other prey items are offered live or dead (freshly killed or frozen/thawed)?

How long are prey items kept with the animal? Is feeding supervised?

When did the animal last eat? Did it eat well? Did it eat readily?

How is water provided? In what manner, and how often is it cleaned?

Questions about environment: cage and housing

> What type of substrate is used? How frequently and by what method is it cleaned and the cage disinfected?
>
> What is the temperature gradient/range and preferred optimal temperature zone (POTZ) within the enclosure? Each species has its specific POTZ that enables normal metabolism and physiologic homeostasis.
>
> What is the humidity range and source of humidity? (The captive environment should mimic their natural habitat; for most species, 50% to 70% will meet these requirements. Species native to desert or rain forests have different requirements.)
>
> What are the heat and light sources, and how are they arranged to guard against thermal injury?
>
> How are the heat and light sources placed relative to the thermometers?
>
> Is "full spectrum" lighting used? Does the lighting provide UV A and B wavelengths?
>
> How old are the lights? How often are they changed? What is the day/night cycle?
>
> For aquatic species: How is the water cleaned? How often are filters cleaned/changed? Is any type of water testing done? Is the water heated?

Distribution of educational materials and discussion

Educational materials and handouts are a vital aspect of properly caring for exotic species. Presenting and discussing them gives the veterinarian and veterinary technician an excellent opportunity to educate the client and reinforce recommendations made to correct deficiencies determined. The author's hospital provides all clients with general handouts (eg, on husbandry, salmonella) as well as with specific handouts for their particular species and the disease conditions that their animals may be experiencing.

Physical examination: examples of components

Before handling the animal, one should observe its position, posture, color or colors, attitude, locomotor skills and abilities, and so on. Substantial time may be spent initially talking with the owner about the animal, clarifying the history, and asking other pertinent questions, all the while observing the animal and pointing out to the owner the normal and abnormal traits that may be determined from experienced observation alone [15].

Once the actual physical examination begins, the following may be used as a complete checklist and guide [15]:

> Check the entire integument from one end to the other for signs of external parasites, wounds (eg, trauma, burns), dysecdysis or abnormal skin/scales, erythema, petechia or ecchymotic hemorrhage, and so on.

Evaluate each extremity, including the tail, for appearance of the skin or scales, muscles and nails (if present), and the range of motion.

Palpate the coelom to evaluate the internal organs; assess the cavity for the presence of foreign bodies or masses, distension or pain.

Assessment of the cardiovascular and respiratory systems is achieved by means of either auscultation or Doppler flow detector. In most reptiles, auscultation may be aided by the use of a moistened paper towel (to create an offset and lessen the artifactual noise created as the skin rubs against the stethoscope diaphragm).

Assessment of hydration status by evaluating skin turgor, the position of the globe in the orbit, mucous membrane color and wetness, and the presence and consistency of mucus in the oral cavity should also be completed at this time.

Evaluate the ears (if present) and the oral cavity for lesions, exudate, erythema, petecchia, ecchymotic hemorrhage, and the presence of parasites.

Examine the nares for patency, and perform a thorough ophthalmic examination.

Assess neurologic status by evaluating movement during observed locomotion, withdrawal of limbs to painful stimulus, and presence of placing and righting reflex.

Finally, after the examination is finished and all the proper questions have been asked, it is time to take the animal back to an appropriate location in the hospital to collect the necessary laboratory samples and measure the body weight (and compare it with any previously recorded weights). Body weight measurements should be taken for all animals that come into the clinic for any reason; this information is then entered into the patient's medical record.

One potentially difficult aspect of a physical examination (even in a compliant reptile or amphibian patient) is the simple act of ausculting the animal to determine normal heart parameters (heart rate and rhythm). In reptiles and amphibians, it is difficult completely to auscult the cardiac systoli and diastoli, because of their unique cardiovascular system; however, the respiratory system may be evaluated by auscultation in most species. The heart rate may be best evaluated using a Doppler flow probe placed directly over the heart or a major artery. The ultrasonic Doppler flow detector creates an audible representation of the moving red blood cells, allowing one to monitor the heart rate with some accuracy. In lizards, the heart is generally located between the shoulders, cranial to its typical location in mammals. In chelonians, because sound waves do not pass through bone, the Doppler probe is best placed in the thoracic inlet and directed toward midline to pick up cardiac blood flow. The rate of the reptile heartbeat is dependent on a large number of variables, including body size, respiratory rate, metabolic rate, sensory stimulation, and body temperature [16–19].

Other unique characteristics seen in reptiles are aspects of their urogenital anatomy and physiology. Chelonians and some lizards have a urinary bladder, which performs water and electrolyte regulation. The cloaca, colon, and urinary bladder, when present, can reabsorb urinary water, and this may have effects on the pharmacokinetics of drugs excreted through the urinary system [4]. The ureters empty into the neck of the bladder in chelonians, and into the urodeum in lizards. Urine then refluxes from the urodeum into the bladder in lizards with a bladder, or into the colon in those species without a bladder. Because urine is refluxed into the bladder or colon, evaluation of a urine sample as it relates to possible infection or inflammation should be undertaken with the understanding that the sample is not sterile and has probably been contaminated or mixed with colonic material. Crocodilians and chelonians have a single copulatory organ, whereas squamates (lizards and snakes) have paired hemipenes. The urinary system and genital system are completely separate.

Handling and restraint of reptiles and amphibians

Only nonvenomous species are addressed here.

One should never assume that because someone owns an animal he or she knows how to handle it properly. Therefore, only the hospital staff should be involved in the proper restraint of the animal being examined. Experience and preparation facilitate the proper handling of most reptile and amphibian patients. For the most part, this is not difficult, although one should always be prepared for the unexpected [15].

Amphibians

With most amphibians, handling should be kept to a minimum to avoid stress to the animal and potential injury. First evaluate the animal in the enclosure, noting appearance, position, posture, color or colors, and so on. When this is not possible, the patient may be transferred to a clear plastic container (with or without water, depending on the species). Such containers allow for the evaluation of many aspects of the animal (primarily external) without actual handling of the patient. Always use good lighting and magnifying devices to scan the entire amphibian, including transillumination techniques though the clear plastic. Once the patient has been evaluated without restraint (while the veterinarian discusses the visual examination with the client and asks more questions), the patient is ready to be handled (Fig. 1).

Amphibians produce various secretions (ie, mucus) to protect themselves against opportunistic pathogens. Disruption of the skin secretions by abrasions caused by mishandling or desiccation of the skin may allow other infectious agents to gain entry. When handling amphibians, one should always use rubber or latex gloves and rinse the gloves to remove the powder or any other coating on the rubber. When it is difficult to catch the animal, fine

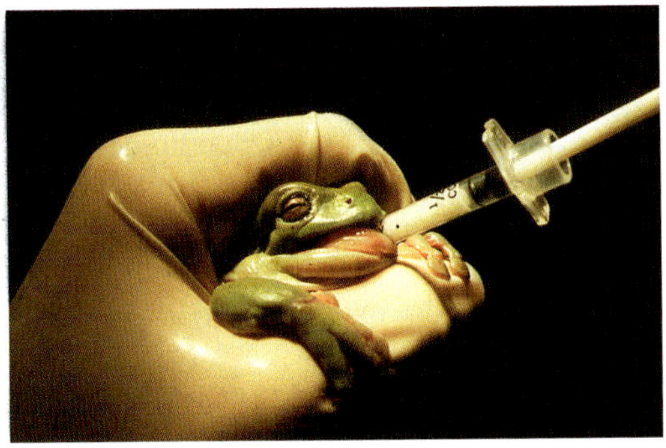

Fig. 1. Proper handling of amphibians using cleaned, powder-free latex gloves to administer oral medications. (© 2006 Byron J.S. de la Navarre, DVM.)

mesh nets may be used. Be careful!—wet amphibians are slippery in rinsed latex gloves. Large toads, giant salamanders, and hellbenders should have their heads properly yet gently restrained, because they may bite; though this is seldom painful, it can be embarrassing. Again, completely survey the exterior of the animal using magnification and transillumination as needed. Palpate the entire animal, assessing all aspects from one end to the other. To evaluate the oral cavity, stimulate the animal to open its mouth by gently pressing on the jaws at the soft tissue of the commissure. When this technique is ineffective, a soft, clean rubber spatula may be used gently to open the mouth to examine the oral pharynx and glottis. At this point, samples may be collected from the posterior naris and nasal passage. Using a minitip, culturette samples for cytology and culture may also be collected from the trachea by passing the small swab through the glottis. After the physical examination in the room has been completed, take the animal back to collect the necessary laboratory samples, as well as to measure the body weight and compare it with previously recorded weights.

Iguanas and other lizards

Use an appropriately sized towel for each animal. In general, lizards are easily restrained, though one does have to be careful with larger species that pose the potential for injury, as well as with smaller specimens that may escape. Small lizards may demonstrate the "fight or flight" response and, if not properly restrained, may be able to get free—possibly injuring themselves in the process, losing their tail (in species that experience tail autotomy), or the worst-case scenario: escaping into the clinic. Several defense mechanisms may be seen in lizards of all sizes but prove most hazardous in larger species. Tail whipping is common in several species (particularly iguanid species and varanid lizards). When a single-holder technique is used, it is a good idea to keep the tail tucked under an arm or immobilized between the holder and the table (or even between the holder's legs). Always use a towel that is long enough to surround not only the animal's body but also the tail. This helps to keep the animal controlled and immobilized. Unwrap areas for evaluation as needed. With two holders, wrap the entire animal and the tail completely in a towel; then, while the animal is properly restrained by the handler, the examiner may unwrap the section to be examined. This arrangement keeps the patient under control throughout the examination, while taking care to avoid injury to any part of the animal (particularly the tail).

Biting is another response that may be seen as both a defensive and an aggressive reaction. Proper control of the head, specifically the mouth, is vital to avoiding possible injuries. The head may be controlled by placing a hand or hands behind the mandible and around the neck. The holder must be careful not to damage the large dorsal spines in species where they are present (eg, adult male iguanas). Using a towel also helps provide a layer of protection between the handler and the lizard, especially in large specimens.

Never reach over or in front of the mouth of a lizard that is not properly restrained: though usually they only feign a bite, there are times when animals can and will inflict serious injury. Clients should also be carefully instructed that they should never come close enough to their pet to risk injury while it is being examined. To evaluate the oral cavity of lizards, stimulate the animal to open its mouth by gently pressing on the jaws at the soft tissue of the commissure or by gently pulling down on the tissue below the mandible. (In some species, this is anatomically called the dewlap.) Slow, gentle pressure on the dewlap often results in the animal's slowly opening its mouth. In lizards and crocodilians, the vagal-vagal response may be used to help the animal "relax." The vagal-vagal response occurs when pressure, often digital, is applied to both eyes for a period of time, as long as a few minutes. It has been shown that some patients respond with a decrease in heart rate and blood pressure, which often results in their becoming more sedate [16]. Even after vagal sedation has been accomplished, one should be vigilant, because the patient may be roused from this state by physical stimulation or noise. When these techniques do not work or do not work completely, a soft, clean rubber spatula may be used gently to open the mouth to examine the oral pharynx and glottis.

Although lizards with long or sharp nails can scratch, the nails are not typically used as a defensive or aggressive mechanism. Nonetheless, ideally the owner/client should clip all the nails before examination. To avoid any possible scratches to handlers, the author's practice commonly provides a complimentary nail trim to lizards being examined. When handling Old World chameleons, which are typically most at rest when all four legs and the tail are securely attached to something—preferably a branch—it may be beneficial to incorporate a suitably sized perch to allow the animal to rest during examination. When directly handling these lizards, one should allow them to hold onto the handler's hand with all their feet and the tail and examine and manipulate one leg at a time while the others remain attached to the handler. In very large lizards that are not cooperating with the physical examination, the best defense is to control head, body, and tail. Again, one may restrain the head by holding firmly behind the mandible and around the neck with the thumb and first finger. To control the front feet and arms, hold them gently yet securely against the body of the lizard. To secure the rear legs, if needed, position and grasp them against the tail, just below the pelvis. The tail should be tucked under the arm or between the holder and the table or wrapped in the appropriately sized towel (Fig. 2).

Crocodilians

The procedure is the same as that described for lizards; however, more handlers may be required, depending on the size and strength of specimens and the procedures to be performed. The head and mouth as well as the tail should always be controlled. The muscles used to open the jaws are weak compared with the biting or jaw-closing muscles, so the mouth can often easily be held closed. It is best for all involved that the mouth of every examined crocodilian be gently though properly taped closed.

Snakes

Approach all snakes slowly and with respect. Most are amenable to handling; so long as the head and body are properly supported, snakes typically do not resist. Snakes that are not correctly supported or are restrained too tightly will struggle. Snakes commonly try to wrap the end of their tails around the examiner or around the table or other furniture. It is best not to let this happen, because it is difficult to get them to release: they often tighten up and can be injured in the untangling process. Some snakes may strike out (ie, those that are ill, threatened, or in a preshedding or shedding

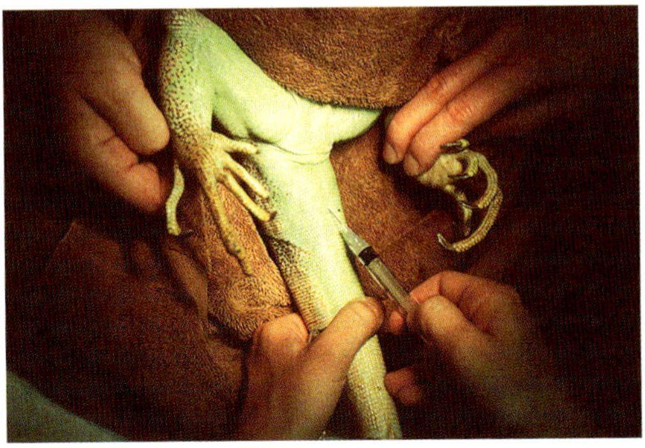

Fig. 2. Demonstration of ventral approach to the ventral coccygeal vein. Towel used for proper handling of lizards to support body, control tail, and to avoid injury to all involved. (© 2006 Byron J.S. de la Navarre, DVM.)

cycle). It is important to locate the head and immobilize it, holding gently but firmly just behind the mandible.

To evaluate the oral cavity of snakes, as in lizards, stimulate the animal to open its mouth by gently pressing on the jaws at the soft tissue of the commissure. Gently pulling down on the tissue below the mandible with slight pressure on this skin often results in the animal's slowly opening its mouth. It is usually a good idea to allow movement of the body with only slight resistance, while maintaining control of the head. When a snake is not threatening at all, the head may not require complete restraint for evaluation of the entire animal. A snake has only one occipital condyle, so dislocation at this joint occurs more easily in snakes than in other species when the head is held too firmly—especially if the snake is fighting to get free.

Concerns about constriction are propagated by bad Hollywood movies, but this is overrated as a defense mechanism. Snakes constrict when they are threatened, when they perceive something as a prey item, or when they feel as if they are not well supported. However, when dealing with very large snakes, one needs to have the required amount of help to restrain the animal properly and securely. To properly examine a snake, one needs to support it well. The snake's head should be held gently but firmly, depending on the temperament of the animal. Properly supporting the snake along its entire body may require multiple handlers. Because the vertebrae extend along the entire body, the weight of the hanging snake could dislocate vertebrae or cause the snake to fight for balance and support. Hold the head gently but firmly behind the mandible and move with the movement of the snake while maintaining control of the head.

Turtles and tortoises

Most tortoises are docile and easy to handle and examine. They do have the capability to bite quite firmly and can be reluctant to let go once they bite. They have no teeth, but the beak is made of keratin and can be strong and sharp. Aquatic chelonians may be more likely to bite and scratch, so additional care should be exercised with these animals. In certain species, especially the male aquatic turtles, the nails can be long and produce scratching. If possible, and with the permission of the owner, these nails may be clipped before too much handling to avert the risk for scratching.

All turtles and tortoises possess strong legs that can be powerful enough to pin or pinch fingers between the shell and their legs; along with being painful, this situation may be quite embarrassing when you cannot free your digits. Care must be taken, because fingers can be easily trapped or pulled up against the spurs and sharp, pointed edges of some shells as one tries to pull out legs for examination, venipuncture, and injections. When attempting to evaluate the oral cavity, one first needs to extend and restrain the head. Typically one person gently immobilizes the exposed and extended forelimbs, either holding them directly or pinning them against the shell of the animal. The head is then gently exposed and held just behind the mandible at about the level of the ears, using the thumb and forefingers. In the case of more resistant turtles, the author has used a pair of closed hemostats placed under the horny upper beak in the area of the premaxilla and carefully levered the head out into a position where it may be restrained. One must be gentle when applying pressure on this premaxilla area, because the beak can break, especially in unhealthy turtles. Though it will most likely grow back completely, this is a temporary abnormality that may bother the turtle and perhaps bother the owner even more.

In certain turtles, and especially the larger tortoises, some form of injectable chemical restraint may be required. Trying to mask or box down a turtle to allow for a complete physical examination may take hours and is typically not advised. To evaluate the oral cavity of turtles, as in snakes, the animal may at times be stimulated to open its mouth by gentle pressure on the jaws at the soft tissue of the commissure. At times, in large enough animals, the tissue below the mandible may be pulled down with gentle pressure; this often results in the animal's slowly opening its mouth. Like lizards, disturbed, frightened turtles or tortoises will often urinate and sometimes defecate as one picks them up and examines them. One must always be ready for this occurrence, both to avoid being the target and to collect possible diagnostic samples. The best defense while examining turtles and tortoises is to hold them midway between the front and rear legs. Keep the animal held away from your body and watch out for urination and defecation. If possible, clip nails before procedures or examination. As in lizards, do not reach across or in front of an unrestrained turtle or tortoise. As with all reptiles and amphibians, sedation or anesthesia may be needed, especially in larger, stronger animals.

Review of clinical and diagnostic techniques in reptiles

Sites for and methods of venipuncture

Amphibians

Blood sampling in amphibians presents unique problems to the veterinary clinician; the most accessible sites are the lingual plexus, ventral midline sinus, and the heart. Unless a blood culture is to be performed on the sample, it is important to heparinize the syringe in venipuncture attempts to avoid coagulation of the sample before it is transferred to the appropriate whole blood tube. When a blood sample is to be obtained for microbial culture, no anticoagulant should be used to pretreat the syringe, needle, or capillary tube, because this may affect the growth of some organisms. Lithium heparin is the anticoagulant of choice for pretreating the syringe and for storage of blood, because it does not affect the values of plasma calcium, sodium, or ammonia. The use of transillumination, possibly along with required sedation, makes cardiac puncture easier and reduces the risks associated with "blind" venipuncture.

Snakes

Cardiocentesis may be used for blood collection in all snakes. The heart is the first palpable mass, located approximately one third of the distance from the head, although its location may vary significantly in certain species. Often cardiac contractions may be visualized when the snake is placed in dorsal recumbency. Using one's index finger and thumb to apply gentle pressure, one may isolate and stabilize the heart's exact location between these fingers. After disinfection of the ventral scutes in this area, one inserts a 22- or 25-gauge needle attached to either a tuberculin or 3-mL syringe slowly at a 45° angle into the ventricle; with gentle aspiration, the blood may be withdrawn. If the aspirant appears transparent, pericardial fluid has probably been collected. The needle should be withdrawn, and another puncture may be performed using a new needle and syringe. In larger snakes, an alternative site for blood collection is the ventral coccygeal (tail) vein. However, when venipuncture is attempted too close to the vent, one runs the risk of puncturing either the hemipenes or musk glands. Other sites have been described but are difficult to access (eg, palatine vein, orbital plexus).

Lizards

The ventral coccygeal (tail) vein is most commonly used in lizards, although care should be exercised in lizard species that undergo tail autotomy. The venipuncture site is approximately one fourth the length of the tail caudal to the vent. As in snakes, when venipuncture is attempted too close to the vent, one runs the risk of puncturing either the hemipenes or musk glands. Care must be taken to use a long enough needle to be able to reach the ventral vertebral processes. The needle is inserted between scales at approximately 90° into the midline on the ventral aspect of the tail until it comes in contact with a ventral vertebral process. Gentle aspiration as the needle is advanced often allows one to collect the sample before the needle reaches the vertebral process. If the needle reaches the process, it is slowly withdrawn 1 to 3 mm and gently aspirated to collect the sample (Fig. 3).

An alternative approach to the ventral coccygeal vein is a lateral one, in which the needle is inserted from the lateral aspect of the tail between scales and between the two large muscle bodies in the middle of the crease of the tail (Fig. 4).

When the ventral tail vein is not productive, the ventral abdominal vein may be used. It is suspended in a broad ligament 1 to 2 mm within the coelomic cavity on the ventral midline between the umbilical scar and the pelvic inlet. Again, caution must be exercised, because this "blind" venipuncture presents the potential for internal or intracoelomic hemorrhage. Less commonly used is the brachial plexus, which is immediately caudal to the shoulder joint. In diminutive lizards, cardiocentesis with the aid of a Doppler may be required.

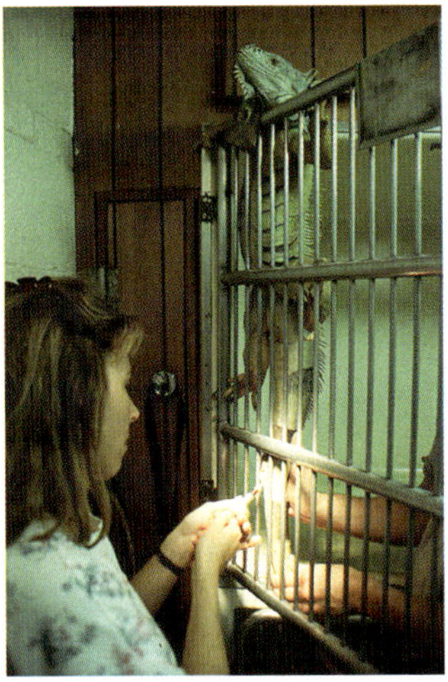

Fig. 3. Blood collection from a ventral approach to the coccygeal vein. (© 2006 Byron J.S. de la Navarre, DVM.)

Chelonians

The preferred place to collect blood from turtles and tortoises is the jugular vein, because these veins have minimal collateral lymphatic vessels. In many specimens the right vein is larger. Each jugular vein typically runs perpendicular and caudal to the ipsilateral tympanum. Sometimes the jugular veins may be visualized when digital pressure is placed on the thoracic inlet. In some chelonians (eg, marine turtles), a postoccipital vein or plexus arises from the right jugular vein and is located between the occipital protuberance and the cranial border of the carapace beneath the ligamenta nuchae (Fig. 5).

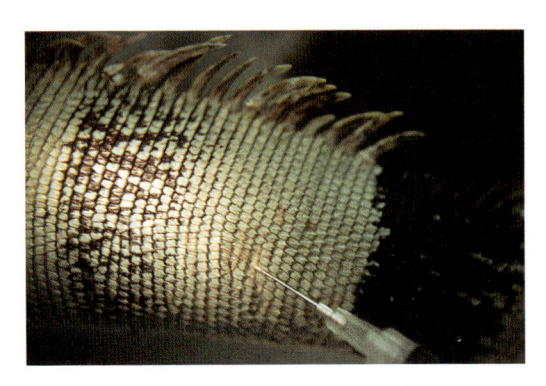

Fig. 4. Lateral approach to the ventral coccygeal vein in lizards. (© 2006 Byron J.S. de la Navarre, DVM.)

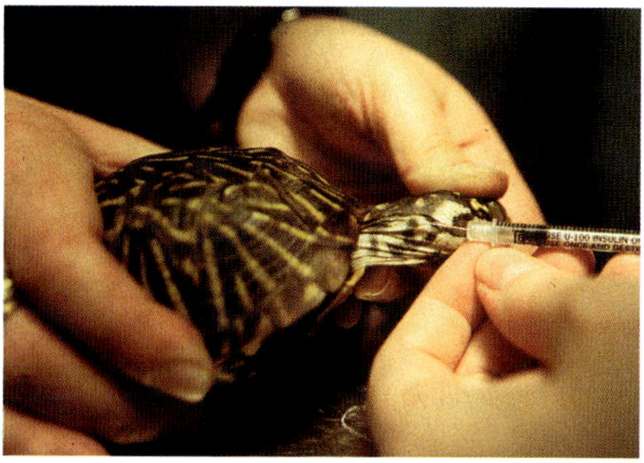

Fig. 5. Site for blood collection from the right jugular vein in turtles. (© 2006 Byron J.S. de la Navarre, DVM.)

A brachial vein or plexus is located behind the elbow joint, under the prominent and palpable tendon of the insertion of the biceps brachii. Access to both these venipuncture sites is "blind," and the samples may be contaminated with lymph, altering the biochemical parameters. When mixed with whole blood, lymph dramatically decreases the white cell count, hematocrit, total solids, sodium, potassium, and chloride values. Chelonians also have a dorsal midline tail vein that is best approached at the base of the tail. Cardiocentesis may be performed, but a hole must be created in the plastron through which a needle may be introduced.

Crocodilians

The most commonly used sites for venipuncture in crocodilians are the caudal (ventral tail) vein, as in larger lizards, and the supravertebral vein, located caudal to the occiput on the midline [4].

Collection of other samples for diagnostic testing

Fecal sample collection

Collecting a fecal sample in a reptile or amphibian can be problematic; most reptiles and amphibians defecate infrequently, especially when they are ill or anorexic. However, evaluation of the feces for protozoal, amoebic, nematode, and other parasites should be considered an essential part of the minimum database. Some species do defecate daily, and a sample may be collected at the next voiding. In some cases, placing the animal in warm water shallow enough for it to keep its head out will stimulate defecation. In sufficiently large patients, a gloved digital cloacal examination is performed, though not usually in the presence of the owner. This procedure may also stimulate the production of cloacal contents. If no sample can be passively collected, then a colonic wash may be performed. The proctodeum, urodeum, and coprodeum are distensible, and the goal is to collect fecal material, so a large-gauge tube is used. The tube is properly lubricated and inserted into the colon area through the vent. In snakes, care must be taken because the colon is located at the most ventral aspect of the cloaca, and, if the tube is directed dorsally, it will enter a blind pocket. Sterile saline at 10 mL/kg is typically injected into the colon, and the coelomic cavity is gently massaged before aspiration of the sample. In some instances, this procedure stimulates voiding, and a larger sample may be obtained. The sample should be evaluated by culture and sensitivity (when indicated), fecal flotation for ova, and a direct wet mount for protozoans.

Urinalysis

Urinalysis [20] can be a useful, economical, and rapid tool for assessing the health status of many reptile and amphibian specimens. Because there are significant differences between reptile and mammalian urine, the interpretation differs as well. In reptiles, uric acid is the principal product of protein catabolism instead of urea. Precipitates of uric acid are normally passed as hard concretions. Reptilian kidneys lack loops of Henle, so reptiles consistently produce isosthenuric urine with a specific gravity of 1.005 to 1.010, regardless of their hydration status. Reptile ureters empty into the cloaca. Urine is subsequently either stored in the cloaca (snakes do not possess urinary bladders) or refluxed into a bladder (in some lizards and all chelonians). Hence microbiologic culturing of urine, even by cystocentesis, can lead to erroneous interpretation.

The color of reptile urine varies from transparent to brown, depending on the diet and the presence of bile pigments. Although renal thresholds for blood glucose have not been evaluated in reptiles, glucosuria is abnormal and has been observed in cases of diabetes mellitus. Hyperglycemia has also been found to be associated with inflammatory diseases of the coelomic cavity, hepatic lipidosis, and severe wasting in chelonians. Some reports indicate that this can be transient, resolving without insulin therapy, although it may also indicate a grave prognosis. When evaluating for glucose in the urine, one must remember that the urine glucose reagent pad may show false-positive results from contamination with substances such as peroxide and hypochlorite. False-negative results may occur when the urine is refrigerated or contains formaldehyde or vitamin C. Ketones do not appear in the urine of hyperglycemic, glucosuric chelonians. Although protein may be present in small amounts in the urine of "healthy" domestic mammals, healthy chelonians appear to have only trace amounts of protein in the urine. However, because the protein assay is sensitive to a variety of other factors, it must be interpreted with care. Contamination with fecal matter, semen, or egg material could introduce proteinaceous materials into the urine, producing a false-positive result. Moreover, a high urine pH can cause a false-positive result by interfering with the buffering mechanism on the test pad. If all these factors have been taken into consideration and ruled out, then elevations in urine protein levels may indicate glomerular damage and plasma protein leakage into the urine.

Repeated retesting is indicated in such cases; consistently high proteinuria, along with other signs of kidney disease, points to the need for further renal evaluation by biochemical testing or biopsies to diagnose the disease process. Urine pH may be influenced by various factors, including diet, mixture with fecal matter, nutritional status, metabolic or respiratory acidosis, and perhaps urinary tract infection with urease-producing bacteria. Herbivorous reptiles normally produce alkaline urine with a pH of 7 to 8. Carnivorous reptiles typically produce urine with a pH of 6 to 7. Anorexic tortoises in a state of metabolic acidosis and those emerging from hibernation can produce acidic urine. Microscopic analysis is one of the most important aspects of the urinalysis. The presence of red and white blood cells is abnormal and may indicate infections of the lower urinary or gastrointestinal tract, or possibly cystic calculi. The presence of parasites in the urine indicates the need for treatment using appropriate parasiticides. Urate crystals have been reported to take many forms and could be confused with cellular casts. However, when a large number of waxy or other cellular casts are found, this is a definite sign that further diagnostic testing is indicated, including plasma biochemical analysis, radiography, and possibly laparoscopy with renal biopsy.

Transtracheal sample collection

Transtracheal collection of material is indicated for optimal evaluation of respiratory disease in reptiles. The sample should be evaluated by aerobic culture and sensitivity testing, direct wet mount, and cytologic examination. Lung worm (order Rhabditida) can be a serious problem in reptiles, and the parasite ova may be observed on a wet mount sample.

The lungs of most reptiles are simple, sac-like structures with ridges for increased gas exchange. They do not have alveoli or bronchioles. Because they have only a trachea and two main stem bronchi that open into the lung, many samples collected from the trachea are actually lung washes. Sedation is infrequently required in debilitated animals. Appropriately sized sterile feeding or urethral catheters work well. Sterile saline at 5 to 10 mL/kg is instilled into the trachea/lung after passage of the catheter through the glottis. In chelonians and lizards with unilateral pulmonary lesions, the tip of the catheter must be bent to ensure that the catheter enters the affected lung. Snakes that have one functional lung may have the catheter passed straight down the trachea into the lung. After the sterile saline has been instilled into the lung, the patient is gently rotated to loosen any exudate. Aspiration is then performed, and harvested material is examined using cytology, parasitology, and bacterial culture and sensitivity.

Concerning culture and sensitivity, the best way to assure a successful culture of pathologic micro-organisms is properly to handle the specimens collected. It is important to contact one's laboratory to determine its specific requirements and recommendations for submitting samples.

Common imaging procedures

Radiography

Radiographs are often indicated as part of a complete work-up and are an invaluable tool for identifying numerous diseases in reptiles. Radiography of specimens may aid in diagnosing "metabolic bone disease," skeletal fractures, osteomyelitis, articular gout, soft tissue mineralization, lower respiratory tract disease, foreign bodies, constipation, gravidity, dystocia, coelomic masses, coelomic effusions, hepato- and renomagaly, and cystic calculi. The exoskeleton of chelonians, the thick dermis of many lizards, and the strong muscle tone of snakes make it challenging to diagnose these and other disorders by palpation during physical examination. The settings for most radiographs are determined on a case-by-case basis. Ideally one should use the high-detail, rare-earth intensifying screens and compatible film for reptile and amphibian radiography. Given the increasing popularity and benefits of digital radiography, the wave of the future, equipment and techniques are bound to change. However, it is important to develop and maintain a proper technique chart for quick reference when taking radiographs of reptiles and amphibians.

If possible, one should use a horizontal beam for lateral and craniocaudal views, especially in chelonians. To produce a horizontal beam x-ray exposure, the x-ray tube must have the capacity to be rotated 90° so that the x-ray beam may be directed horizontally across the table rather than down toward the table. It is still recommended that the distance between the x-ray tube and the x-ray cassette (focal film distance) be 40 in, as is the case for most vertical table top radiographs. Horizontal views permit organs to stay in their normal positions and prevent artifacts. This is especially important when imaging lung fields, because reptiles do not possess a diaphragm to separate the chest cavity from the abdominal viscera. Horizontal viewing allows the visualization of the right and left lung fields as separate structures. In larger snakes and lizards, numbered identification markers should be placed on sections of the body to determine the exact location of lesions and organs. It is recommended that the veterinarian maintain a set of normal radiographs for each species, which may be easily retrieved and compared with those of diseased animals.

Ultrasonography

Ultrasonography is a useful tool in reptile and amphibian medicine. Because of their bony shells, imaging in chelonians may be performed only through the flank and axillary areas. The organs in the coelomic cavity may be visualized and differentiated by their specific ultrasonographic texture. The ultrasound may then be used to image and guide the biopsy of various organs, including the liver, spleen, cystic structures, kidneys, and so on.

As always, it is important to know the normal anatomy of the species when interpreting the image produced by the ultrasound.

Endoscopy

Endoscopy has proved to be a most useful diagnostic tool in veterinary medicine. Specifically, in the field of zoologic medicine, the application of diagnostic endoscopy has shown great promise in a variety of species, and it has been used extensively in avian medicine and surgery [21]. Flexible and rigid endoscopes are used for a number of different applications in reptile and amphibian medicine and surgery, such as coelioscopy, pneumoscopy, gastroscopy, and direct visual biopsy.

CT

CT is an excellent, though not always available, means of evaluating bony lesions. CT scanning produces transverse x-ray slices (tomographs) of tissue and is particularly sensitive to calcium or air-containing structures.

MRI

MRI is an excellent means of evaluating soft tissue lesions, though like CT it is not always available. It uses tissues' magnetic properties and response to radio wave pulses to produce high-detail images of all tissues except bone.

With the continuing advancement and popularity of these last two diagnostic modalities in human medicine, both CT and MRI are becoming increasingly available to veterinarians. The benefits of being able noninvasively to evaluate exquisite detail in multiple dimensions are making these procedures more and more appealing.

Review of therapeutic techniques in reptiles

Sites and techniques for injections and medication administration

Injections may be given intravenously, subcutaneously, intramuscularly, intracoelomically, intracardiacally, or intraosseously. Intravenous injections are administered in the sites described for blood collection. Because of the potential involvement of the renal portal system, some sources recommend that most injections be administered in the cranial half of the body. One exception is intracoelomic injections, which are typically given in lizards in the lateral right caudal quadrant region at a level even with the cranial aspect of the rear leg. Gentle aspiration of the syringe assures that the needle is not in any vital organ. In chelonians, the extremities may be used for intramuscular (IM) injections of small volumes. For larger volumes, the pectoral muscles are the preferred site for IM injection. These large muscles attach the front limbs to the plastron. The injection is given by inserting the needle parallel to the plastron under the arm. Intracoelomic injections are given in the flank near the junction of the skin with the shell, just cranial to the rear leg. Again, gentle aspiration before injection assures that the needle is not in any vital organ. Intracardiac injections are generally reserved for situations where no other vascular access is available.

Transdermal administration of some medications has been found to be useful in amphibians (but not in reptiles). The semipermeable nature of amphibian skin allows for the systemic uptake of medications administered topically. Injectable forms of medications may be locally irritating, and dosing problems can certainly occur in the smaller amphibian patients. Ophthalmic drops (that are pH balanced and can be diluted with saline) may become the most useful transdermal medication in amphibians. Medicated baths may also be of some use in treating certain amphibian conditions [22].

Sites and techniques for catheter placement

Amphibians

Intravenous catheterization is neither easy nor well tolerated in amphibians. However, because of its semipermeable skin, a dehydrated (or electrolyte imbalanced) amphibian may be "fluid supported" by maintenance in a balanced electrolyte solution, such as Normosol (Abbott Laboratories, Chicago, Illinois) or "amphibian Ringer's solution" [22].

Snakes

The jugular veins and the heart are currently the only accepted sites for catheter placement. The right jugular vein is typically larger that the left and is thus the best choice for catheterization. Catheter placement requires that a cut-down incision be made from approximately the fourth to the seventh scute cranial to the heart at the junction of the ventral scutes and the right lateral body scales. The catheter is introduced cranial to caudal (Fig. 6).

Cardiac catheterization is used in snakes for short-term (as long as 24 hours) or emergency procedures. The technique is the same as that used for cardiocentesis. No accessible intraosseous sites exist in snakes.

Lizards

The cephalic veins are the preferred site for intravenous catheterization. The dorsal (anterior) surface of the antebrachium is prepared for a sterile procedure: cut-down and dissection of the vein are required in most cases. The skin incision should extend from the dorsal proximal limit of the antebrachium medially to allow the best visualization of the vein [4]. Intraosseous catheters may be placed in most lizards. The author prefers the proximal tibia. Although insertion of the catheter into the distal femur has been reported, it is currently recommended that this location be

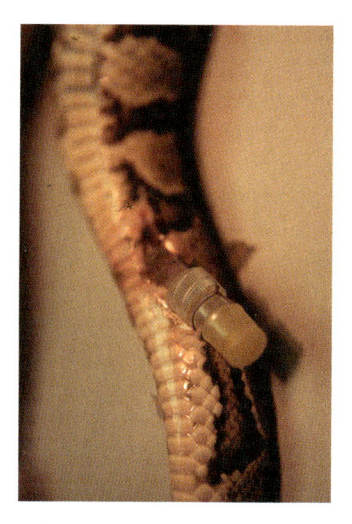

Fig. 6. Location for jugular catheter placement in snakes. (© 2006 Byron J.S. de la Navarre, DVM.)

avoided, because the stifle joint is invaded and the intercondylar cartilage is damaged (Fig. 7) [23].

The proximal tibia is easily accessible, and insertion through the craniomedial aspect of the bone avoids invasion of the joint capsule and articular cartilage. Using a spinal needle (size and length determined by the size of the patient), one drills the needle catheter into the tibia while palpating in the direction of the bone. The placement may be tested by aspirating and obtaining a small flash of blood. When no flash back is observed, a small amount of saline is injected, and the aspiration is attempted again. If the catheter is outside the bone, the muscle will swell with the injection of saline. Ultimately, radiographs may be used to confirm the location of catheter placement (Fig. 8) [23].

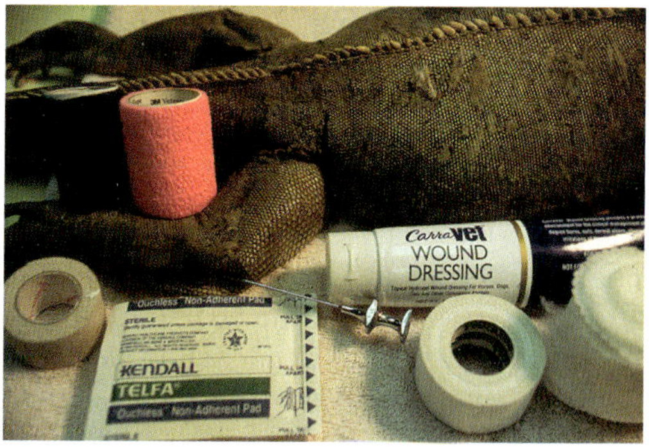

Fig. 7. Materials used and site for intraosseous catheter placement in lizards. (© 2006 Byron J.S. de la Navarre, DVM.)

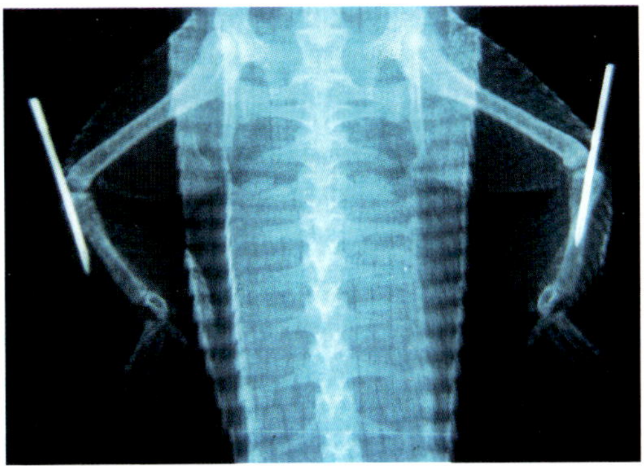

Fig. 8. Radiograph demonstrating proper proximal tibial position of right intramedullary intraosseous catheter and improper/extramedullary catheter placement in lizards. (© 2006 Byron J.S. de la Navarre, DVM.)

Chelonians

As in venipuncture, the right jugular vein is the preferred site for catheter placement in turtles and tortoises, because it is larger than the left in many species. Animals with thick skin over the jugular vein or those with poor peripheral blood pressure may require cut-down and dissection to identify and catheterize the vessel. Discussion is ongoing on the question of whether chelonians have marrow-containing long bones [23]. However, it has been reported that an intraosseous catheter can be placed in the cranial or caudal aspect of the bony bridge—the column of bone between the plastron and carapace [4].

Sites and techniques for fluid therapy

Signs of dehydration in reptiles can be similar to those seen in mammals. Loss of skin elasticity and wrinkled appearance progressing to sunken eyes, dry, tacky mucous membranes, and so forth: all must be interpreted with an understanding of normal appearances for that particular species. Packed cell volume and total solids can also be helpful in evaluating dehydration.

Placing the patient in shallow, warm water usually allows for some absorption of fluids, moisturizes the skin, and in some instances stimulates defecation. Fluid replacement may be done orally in mildly dehydrated, alert patients. Subcutaneous fluids are useful in mildly to moderately dehydrated patients and patients that will not allow oral access. More rapid routes of fluid delivery for patients with severe dehydration or shock-type situations are intracoelomic and intravenous ones. With repeated administration of intracoelomic fluids, it is important to aspirate, not only to ensure the needle is not in a vital organ but to assess that the previously administered fluids have been absorbed. Once again, it may be wise to consider soaking amphibian patients in a balanced electrolyte solution to help provide proper electrolyte and oncotic balance [22].

Significance of thermal support

Reptiles are poikilothermic; therefore, thermal support is vital to the optimal maintenance of these patients. As mentioned earlier, absence of the proper POTZ is often one of the underlying causes for illness. Provision of the POTZ is vital to enable the proper functioning of the immune system, gastrointestinal system, and, potentially, all body functions. One must know the POTZ for each individual species to avoid thermal stress. When this information is not available, most debilitated reptiles will respond to a temperature range of approximately 32.2°C (90°F) until the species-specific information can be obtained. Properly used radiant heat sources tend to be best at providing a safe temperature gradient. Incubators may be used, but they tend to provide a constant temperature, generally adequate only for short-term maintenance. "Hot-rock"–type heat emitters are not recommended, because they can sometimes fail and may thus result in significant thermal injuries.

Nutritional support

Many reptiles that present for medical care are malnourished, either because of dietary deficiencies or improper husbandry that has an adverse effect on the animal's metabolism. It is generally recommended that nutritional support be provided to any patient that has lost 10% of its body weight acutely or 20% chronically. Nutritional support may be provided by a number of means, including syringe or force feeding, orogastric tube feeding, and pharyngostomy feeding-tube placement. At times the greatest challenge is opening the mouth. Once it is open, the glottis, which is typically closed at rest, is located at the base of the tongue in the rostral oral cavity, making it easy to avoid during orogastric intubation.

When continued nutritional support is required for reptiles with mouths that are difficult to open, placement of a pharyngostomy tube is recommended. Tube placement is accomplished in the following manner: The animal is sedated, and a mosquito hemostat is inserted into the pharynx and pointed laterally against the wall of the esophagus. The tip of the hemostat is palpated externally, and a small nick incision is made over the tip (Fig. 9). The tip of the hemostat is then gently, bluntly dissected out through the hole in the skin. Dissection must be cautious, because too large a hole will allow reflux of material from the stoma.

A Sovereign red rubber feeding tube (Sherwood Medical, St. Louis, Missouri; size and length dependent on animal size) is then measured and marked, so as to have the tip end up in the stomach. The hemostat is used to seize the tip/gastric end of the feeding tube, and the tube is pulled through the hole into the esophagus and out the mouth (Fig. 10). At this

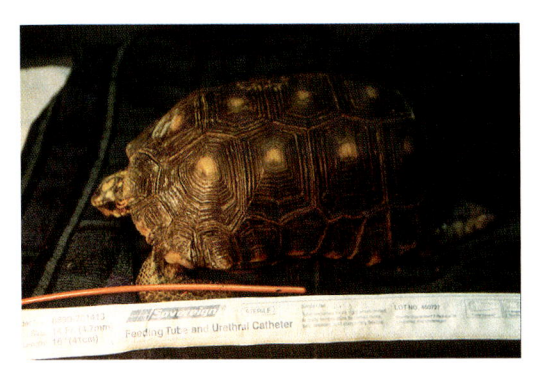

Fig. 9. Measurement of proper location of pharyngostomy tube placement in a sedated red footed tortoise (*Geochelone carbonaria*). (© 2006 Byron J.S. de la Navarre, DVM.)

point, the blunt/solid tip of the feeding tube is trimmed to open the end, and the tube is redirected down the esophagus and into the stomach. The tube is sutured in place using the "Chinese finger-trap" technique (Fig. 11). It is important to flush the tube after feedings and best to place some sort of cap to close the exposed end (Fig. 12).

For herbivorous and omnivorous reptiles, Isocal, Sustacal (Mead Johnson Nutrionals, Evansville, Indiana), Ensure, and Osmolite (Ross Labs, Columbus, Ohio) are appropriate liquid diets. For carnivorous reptiles, Traumacal (Mead Johnson Nutrionals), Pulmocare (Ross Labs), and Feline and Canine Clini-Care Liquid (Pet-AG, Elgin, Illinois) are appropriate liquid diets. Care must be exercised when feeding patients that are suffering from chronic starvation. "Refeeding syndrome," namely a condition of hypophosphatemia and hypokalemia, is seen in patients fed large amounts of calorie-rich foods and can be fatal. The phosphorus and potassium move

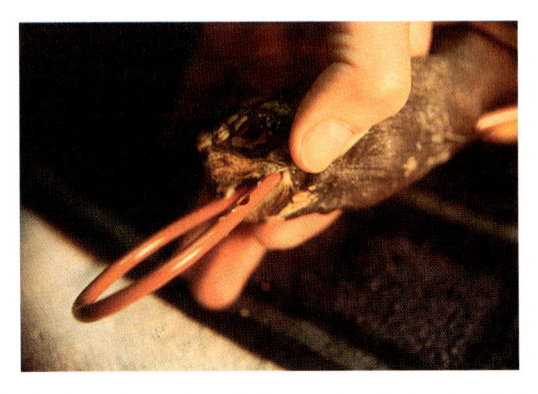

Fig. 10. Pulling the feeding tube out through the mouth and trimming the tip, then redirecting down the pharynx and esophagus into the proper premeasured position. (© 2006 Byron J.S. de la Navarre, DVM.)

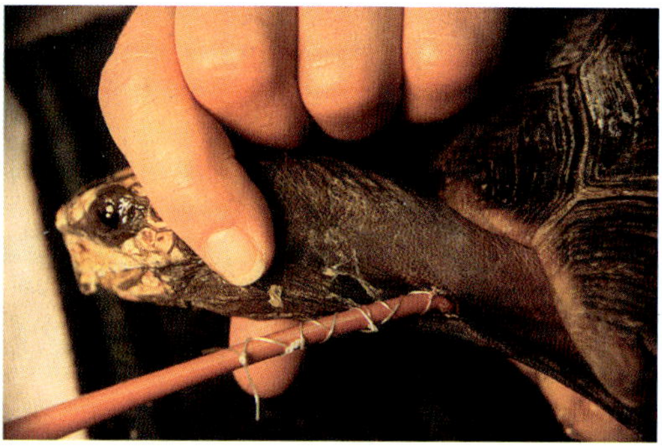

Fig. 11. Proper suturing technique and placement of pharyngostomy feeding tube in turtles. (© 2006 Byron J.S. de la Navarre, DVM.)

into the cells with glucose and thereby deplete circulating levels, resulting in rapid weakness and often coma, which may lead ultimately to death. It is therefore recommended that reptiles that have been chronically starved be fed 50% of their need calculated on the basis of their real, not ideal, weight. This regimen is continued for several days, until the patient's condition improves. The number of calories supplemented is then increased in increments of 10% to 20% until the recommended level of caloric supplementation for that size of animal is reached [23].

For excellent current information on feeding carnivorous, omnivorous, and herbivorous reptiles, please see Ref. [24].

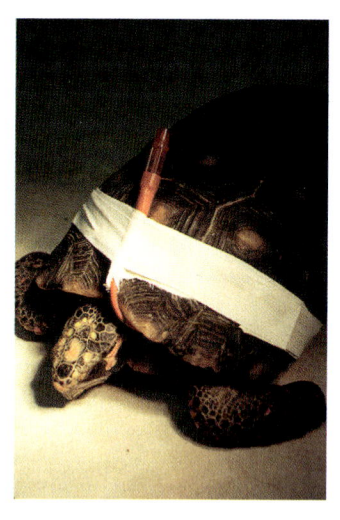

Fig. 12. Technique for securing pharyngostomy tube to carapace: after delivering food or medications, remember to flush tube properly to avoid clogging and cap. (© 2006 Byron J.S. de la Navarre, DVM.)

Other common procedures and concerns in reptiles and amphibians

Problems with shedding (dysecdysis)

In reptiles and amphibians, skin shedding, or ecdysis, is a dynamic process that occurs throughout the life of the animal. As soon as a shedding cycle is completed and the old skin is shed, a new cycle begins.

Healthy amphibians often ingest their shed skin, so it is not observed in the environment. A healthy snake sheds its skin in one piece (like an inverted sock), whereas most lizards normally shed in pieces. Turtles also shed in pieces: scutes from their carapace and plastron and skin from their neck, legs, and tail. Although the actual shedding process differs among species, the physiologic mechanisms involved in causing the shed are similar.

The length of the shedding cycle varies depending on a number of factors, especially the age and nutritional state of the animal (Fig. 13). Improper shedding, or dysecdysis, is not itself a primary problem but rather a symptom. In other words, dysecdysis is not a disease but rather a symptom of a disease. Most often, dysecdysis may be directly associated with problems of proper management or husbandry. Handling reptiles, especially snakes, during the shedding cycle may cause damage and dysecdysis. Low environmental temperature or humidity is also a common cause of shedding problems. Improper nutrition and improper or insufficient cage furniture (eg, rocks, branches, logs) can also have a significant effect on proper shedding. Any reptile or amphibian that is having difficulty shedding should be treated. Usually, the best method of removing the retained skin is to soak the animal in tepid water. The water should be deep enough to cover the animal's body, but obviously not so deep as to pose a danger of drowning. A soaking animal should never be left unattended. Generally nothing needs to be added to the water; however, when there is indication of superficial

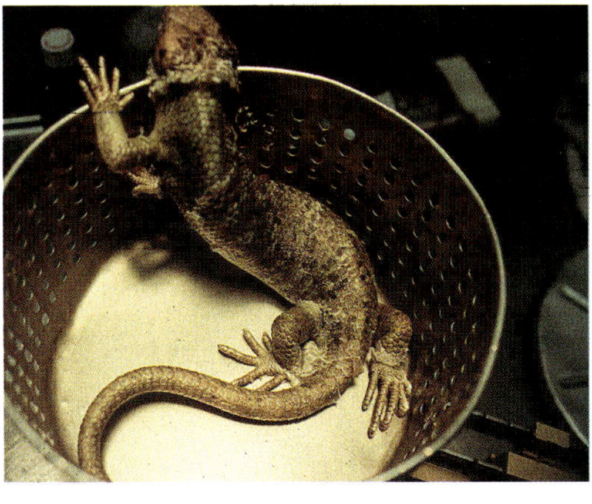

Fig. 13. Example of retained skin and dysecdysis in a prehensile-tailed skink. (© 2006 Byron J.S. de la Navarre, DVM.)

infection or inflammation, diluted chlorhexadine solution (1 part chlorhexadine to 50 parts saline; Nolvasan, Fort Dodge, Iowa) works well. Also, one may place appropriately sized cloth towels in the soaking solution; as the animal moves over the surface of the towels, it will gently remove the retained old skin.

Usually, once the retained skin has been removed and the underlying husbandry factors corrected, the shedding problems should resolve and the shedding should return to normal.

In snakes, one should always make sure that the spectacles, or eye caps, have come off with the shed. If a spectacle is retained, the eye may become affected. Retained eye caps can be difficult to remove, and proper care must be exercised to determine that what is being removed is indeed the retained eye cap and not a normal structure. Removing a retained spectacle is not generally a life or death situation, so when one is unfamiliar with the appearance of a retained eye cap, it is preferable to treat conservatively rather than attempting to remove something and inducing more damage to the patient. One may often delay one full shed cycle before taking any action. Often, treating the eye with sterile ophthalmic lubricants and correcting the underlying husbandry deficiencies will result in the snake's shedding the retained eye caps in the next shed cycle.

If changes in management and husbandry techniques do not rectify the shedding problems, a thorough medical evaluation should be performed, including appropriate laboratory testing. Several medical causes of dysecdysis exist, including fungal or bacterial skin disease, systemic diseases such as septicemia, mites, microfilaria, thermal burns, thyroid gland dysfunction, and old scars. Once the underlying problem has been addressed and resolved, the skin shedding usually returns to normal within two to four cycles [4].

Note on salmonellosis

Salmonellosis is one of the most widely recognized reptilian zoonoses. *Salmonella* is a genus of bacteria of the family Enterobacteriaceae, which also includes such bacteria as *Escherichia coli, Shigella, Citrobacter*, and *Yersinia*. The salmonellae are gram-negative motile rods with peritrichous flagellae, which do not form cysts or spores. More than 2000 serotypes exist within the species *S enteritidis* (eg, *S enteritidis* serotype java), whereas *S typhi*, the causative agent of typhoid fever, and *S choleraesuis* have only one serotype each. They can survive in a wide variety of environmental conditions, from 8°C to 45°C, at a pH of 4 to 9, and as facultative anaerobes they prefer oxygen but can live without it. Salmonella may live for 3 months in tap water, 4 months in pond water, 9 months in soil, and 28 to 30 months in avian or bovine feces. Transovarian infection is documented in poultry, and reptile eggs may be infected within the uterus, while passing through the cloaca, or after being laid in contaminated soil. In reptiles, salmonellae usually are nonclinical infections; apparently virulent strains have been found in clinically healthy animals. The infection rate in reptiles has been estimated at 83% to 94%, depending on the method of testing, and as many as five serotypes have been found in one animal. Thus it is currently believed that most if not all reptiles should be considered carriers of salmonella. It is our obligation as veterinarians to become completely familiar with the status of salmonella in animals so that we may educate, not alarm, our clients concerning the potentially significant health risks associated with keeping reptiles as pets.

There are instances where owners request that their animals be tested for salmonella. These owners should be informed that even repeated negative culture results on fecal, cloacal, and water samples from their pets cannot conclusively identify animals as salmonella-negative, because shedding is intermittent, and many negative results may be false-negatives. If the owner insists, special arrangements will need to be made with the laboratory. With conventional microbiologic techniques, the time required to isolate and confirm the identity of *Salmonella* spp is 72 to 96 hours using the proper media and environment. Even when all the proper techniques are practiced (eg, method, quantity), the reliability of culture may be affected by several uncontrollable factors, including temporal and seasonal variation in shedding. Advances in diagnostic testing have led to the introduction of new technologies, including ELISA and polymerase chain reaction. It is hoped that these newer testing methods will improve the true test characteristics of sensitivity, specificity, positive predictive value, and negative predictive value [25].

Using medications to eliminate the salmonella organism from the reptile patient is difficult, because antibiotics may merely suppress the excretion of detectable organisms without completely eliminating them. This suppression of the excretion of the organisms following antibiotic use may last for periods as long as 8 weeks. Because of the intermittent excretion, it may be difficult to determine whether treatment has been effective and has eliminated the carrier state. Furthermore, treatment failure may promote the development of drug-resistant strains [4].

Therefore, though we must educate ourselves, staff, and clients about the importance of salmonella in reptiles and amphibians, our current inability to resolve salmonella infections means that we must focus our efforts on prevention.

Aural abscesses in turtles

Aural abscesses in turtles are a commonly observed condition. Affected turtles typically present with slowly progressive swellings on one or both sides of the neck, puffiness to both eyes, periodic ocular or nasal discharge from one or both nares, and decreased appetite and activity (Fig. 14).

On physical examination, the turtles typically appear depressed, weak, and lethargic, often with significant bilateral or unilateral aural swellings,

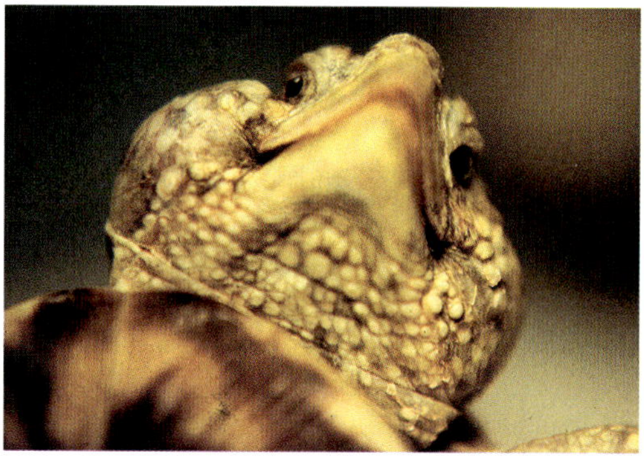

Fig. 14. Location of bilateral aural swellings seen with aural abscesses. (© 2006 Byron J.S. de la Navarre, DVM.)

mild to moderate bilateral blepharoedema, and mild to moderate mucopurulent nasal or ocular discharge or both. Commonly considered differentials for these clinical signs include bilateral aural abscesses, hypovitaminosis A, upper/lower respiratory tract disease, other infectious disease, systemic disease, trauma, and chemical or parasitic inflammation.

Aural abscesses should be treated surgically using appropriate anesthesia. This gives the surgeon the opportunity to perform thorough debridement of the tympanic cavity and alleviates the pain associated with the treatment of the disease process. Typically, the surgical procedure does not take long, and the author has had success using propofol at 10 mg/kg intravenously [26,27]. In the author's experience, propofol provides a quick induction, is short acting, and produces a level plane of anesthesia with a relatively rapid rate of recovery and few side effects. Other anesthetics may also be employed (Fig. 15).

Proper sterile surgical preparation should be employed. This measure is especially important when it is anticipated that specimens will be collected for culture and sensitivity. Each veterinarian may have a different surgical approach to chelonian aural abscesses. The main objective is to effect complete removal of the abscess contents from the tympanic cavity, while avoiding possible damage to the columella (stapes) during debridement and ensuring that fluids or other materials are not aspirated by the patient during or after the procedure [6,8]. The author's technique involves making a full-thickness horizontal incision through the entire tympanum, from the three o'clock position across the center of the tympanum to the nine o'clock position. A second vertical incision is then made from the 12 o'clock position down through the center of the tympanum to the six o'clock position. Together these two incisions form a cross.

The inflammatory debris may then be gently removed using small ear loops or forceps. Again, care must be taken not to damage the columella during the debridement and subsequent flushing. If desired, specimens for

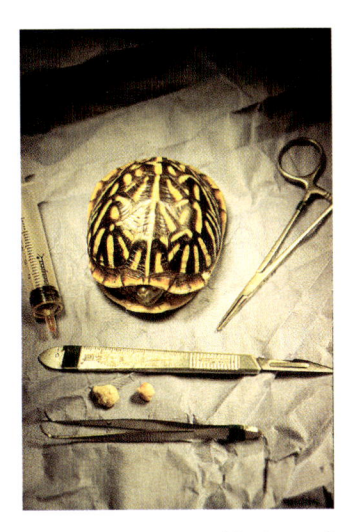

Fig. 15. Some of the instruments and equipment used in the surgical technique of bilateral aural abscesses in turtles. (© 2006 Byron J.S. de la Navarre, DVM.)

culture and sensitivity should be collected at this time. Ideally, the author tries to remove the caseous material in one piece. After removal of all the grossly visible inflammatory debris, all aspects (especially the caudal extent) of the tympanic cavity need to be evaluated, because caseous material may extend quite far, especially in chronic cases.

Once all visible pieces of abscessed material have been removed, the tympanic cavity and the eustachian tube need to be gently but liberally lavaged using an appropriate antimicrobial agent. The author prefers to use diluted chlorhexadine solution (1 part chlorhexadine to 50 parts saline; Nolvasan, Fort Dodge, Iowa) [26,27]. Diluted chlorhexadine solution has a wide spectrum of antimicrobial activity, is relatively nontoxic to tissue, and maintains a sustained residual activity. Although use of diluted povidone-iodine (P-I) solution has been reported, this remains controversial, because in vitro studies have demonstrated that concentrations in excess of 1% P-I solution kill fibroblasts. Also, the active antimicrobial ingredient in P-I, free iodine, is inactivated in the presence of the proteins of serum, which are often present postoperatively within the tympanic cavity [28].

Throughout the procedure, the oral cavity must be examined frequently to prevent aspiration, because debris and liquids may be forced or flushed through the eustachian tube into the oropharynx. While flushing the tympanic cavity and eustachian tube, in an effort to avoid such aspiration, the author typically places the turtle in a head-down position. This measure allows fluid and debris that enter the oropharynx to exit the mouth by means of gravity. After thorough flushing, the surgery site may be filled with an appropriate antibiotic ointment and allowed to heal by secondary intention. The author prefers to use a triple antibiotic ophthalmic ointment

(TriOptic-P, Pfizer, Philadelphia, Pennsylvania). The veterinarian or client should continue to lavage and pack the surgical site on a daily basis until it is healed. The decision to place the patient on systemic antibiotics depends on the results of physical and laboratory evaluations. Typically, when the author has started the animal on presurgical systemic antibiotics, these are continued for a prescribed course of treatment based on the initial physical examination and laboratory work-up.

References

[1] Mader DR. The interrelationship between ambient temperature and reptile health management. In: Proceedings of the Second Annual Symposium on Captive Propagation and Husbandry of Reptiles. Northern California Herpetological Society (special publication) 1985;3:39–48.
[2] Frye FL. Biomedical and surgical aspects of captive reptile husbandry. 2nd edition. Vol. 1. Malabar (FL): Krieger Publishing Co.; 1991.
[3] Jacobsen ER. Exotic animals. In: Jacobsen ER, Kollias GV, editors. Contemporary issues in small animal practice. New York: Churchill Livingstone; 1988. p. 35–48.
[4] Mader DR. Reptile medicine and surgery. 1st edition. Philadelphia: WB Saunders; 1996.
[5] de Vosjoli P. The green iguana manual. Lakeside (CA): Advanced Vivarium Systems; 1993.
[6] Gatten RE. Aspects of the environmental physiology of amphibians and reptiles. In: Frahm MW, editor. Proceedings of the AAZV, Greensboro, NC. Iowa State Press; 1989. p. 104–7.
[7] Vaughn LK, Bernheim HA, Kluger M. Fever in the lizard *Dipsosaurus dorsalis*. Nature 1974; 252:473–4.
[8] Evans EE. Comparative immunology: antibody response in *Dipsosaurus dorsalis* at different temperatures. Proc Soc Exp Biol Med 1963;112:531–3.
[9] Mader DR, Conzelman GM, Baggot JD. Effects of ambient temperature on the half-life and dosage regimen of amikacin in snakes. J Am Vet Med Assoc 1985;187:1134.
[10] Gehrman WH. Reptile lighting: a current perspective. The Vivarium 1996;8(2):44–5.
[11] Swenson MJ, editor. Dukes' physiology of domestic animals. 10th edition. Ithaca (NY): Cornell University Press; 1984.
[12] Rodda G. World commerce in green iguanas. Iguana Times 1993;2:22.
[13] Donoghue S. Nutrition of the green iguana (*Iguana iguana*). In: Frahm MW, editor. Proceedings of the Third ARAV Conference. Tampa (FL); 1996. p. 99–106.
[14] Mitchell MA, Scholl DT, Tully T. Assessing the risk factors for development of metabolic bone disease in juvenile green iguanas (*Iguana iguana*). In: Frahm MW, editor. Proceedings of the Third ARAV Conference, Tampa, FL. Iowa State Press; 1996. p. 111–2.
[15] Bradley T. Anamnesis, physical examination, handling, and restraint of reptiles and amphibians. In: Frahm MW, editor. Proceedings of the Seventh ARAV Conference, Reno, NV. Iowa State Press; 2000. p. 173–6.
[16] Davies PMC. Anatomy and physiology. In: Cooper JE, Jackson OF, editors. Diseases of the reptilia. Vol. 1. New York: Academic Press; 1981. p. 39–45.
[17] Walls GL. The vertebrate eye and its adaptive radiation. Cranbrook Institute of Science Bulletin 1942;19:607.
[18] Lawton MPC. Ophthalmology of exotic species. In: Petersen-Jones SM, Crispin SM, editors. Manual of small animal ophthalmology. Cheltenham (UK): BSAVA; 1993. p. 93–6.
[19] Lawton MPC. Diseases of the spectacle. In: Frahm MW, editor. Proceedings of the Fifth ARAV Conference, Kansas City, MO. Iowa State Press; 1998. p. 119–22.
[20] Gibbons PM, Horton SJ, Brandl S, et al. Urinalysis in box turtles, terrapene spp. In: Frahm MW, editor. Proceedings of the Seventh ARAV Conference, Reno, NV. Iowa State Press; 2000. p. 161–8.

[21] Divers SJ. An introduction to reptile endoscopy. In: Frahm MW, editor. Proceedings of the Fifth ARAV Conference, Kansas City, MO. Iowa State Press; 1998. p. 41–5.
[22] Whitaker BR, Wright KM. Amphibian medicine and captive husbandry. Malabar (FL): Krieger Publishing Co.; 2001.
[23] Bennett RA. Clinical, diagnostic and therapeutic techniques. In: Frahm MW, editor. Proceedings of the Fifth ARAV Conference, Kansas City, MO. Iowa State Press; 1998. p. 35–40.
[24] Stahl S. Feeding carnivorous and omnivorous reptiles. In: Proceedings of the Seventh ARAV Conference. Reno (NV); 2000. p. 177–82.
[25] Mitchell MA. Salmonella testing in the absence of a gold standard. In: Frahm MW, editor. Proceedings of the Seventh ARAV Conference, Reno, NV. Iowa State Press; 2000. p. 143–4.
[26] Swaim SF, Lee AH. Topical wound medications: a review. J Am Vet Med Assoc 1987; 190(12):1588.
[27] Long RD. Self-assessment picture tests in veterinary medicine, small animal practice. Philadelphia: Mosby-Wolfe; 1995.
[28] Nesbitt GH, Ackerman LJ. Dermatology for the small animal practitioner: exotics, felines and canines. Trenton (NJ): Veterinary Learning Systems Co.; 1991.

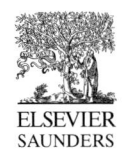

Common Procedures with Venomous Reptiles

Thomas H. Boyer, DVM

Pet Hospital of Penasquitos, 9888-F Carmel Mountain Road, San Diego, CA 92111, USA

Approximately 15% of the 3000 snake species are considered dangerous to humans [1,2]. Currently in the United States, popularity of venomous snakes in private collections is at an all-time high. Zoos and aquaria have always had an interest in venomous reptiles. The purpose of this article is to outline common, safe practices for veterinarians who work with venomous reptiles, although reading it by no means qualifies one to work with these animals. In the author's experience, many clients do not handle venomous reptiles in a safe manner. It is important not to rely on clients' experience when one's own is lacking, because their skill and experience, or lack thereof, may promulgate dangerous handling techniques that could have disastrous results. In this instance, a bad education can be more hazardous than no education, because bad habits die slowly.

If you have no experience handling venomous reptiles, do not work with them until you have gained experience from a knowledgeable, experienced handler. Experience may be gained from reptile departments in many zoos and aquaria, from experienced, conscientious private collectors, through training courses offered by the Association for Reptilian and Amphibian Veterinarians (2001, 2003, 2005), and from the exotic animal departments of some veterinary colleges and zookeeper training colleges [3]. One may practice these techniques on nonvenomous reptiles to become more proficient in treating the venomous, potentially dangerous patients.[1]

Venomous reptiles

It is important accurately to identify the species of venomous reptile that has been presented to the hospital to better appreciate its biology, to know

---

E-mail address: terrapins@san.rr.com

[1] Editor's note: Please refer to Dr. de la Navarre's manuscript in this issue for techniques used in nonvenomous reptiles.

whether it is truly venomous, and to facilitate emergency procedures should envenomation occur [4]. Venomous reptiles are not referred to as poisonous, because poisons are ingested or inhaled, whereas venoms are typically injected. Multiple groups of venomous snakes and one group of venomous lizards exist.

The only venomous lizards are the Helodermatidae, including the Gila monster (*Heloderma suspectum suspectum* and *H suspectum cinctum*) and the beaded lizards (*H horridum horridum, H horridum hexasperatum, H horridum alvarezi,* and *H horridum charlesbogerti*). These are heavy-bodied, medium to large lizards found in the Sonoran desert of the American Southwest, along Mexico's west coast, and in Guatemala. Venom glands are located in the anterior mandible and lead to ducts that empty near the gum line. Enlarged, recurved, grooved teeth in the rear mandible conduct venom into wounds through capillary action and chewing. No commercial antivenom for helodermids exists. Clinical signs of envenomation include pain, edema, erythema, anxiety, nausea, emesis, weakness, hypotension, leukocytosis, and tachycardia [5]. Although these lizards may appear slow-moving, they are capable of quickly inflicting a serious bite with their powerful jaws [4].

Many rear-fanged (opithoglyphic) snakes in the family Colubridae produce mild to serious envenomation in humans. The venom glands are modified salivary glands (Duvernoy's glands). Venom is discharged through a short duct labially, then along enlarged grooved posterior maxillary teeth [4]. Most rear-fanged colubrids are not considered life-threatening, but it is better to handle them with caution than to risk painful local or systemic nonlethal envenomation. Four exceptions have caused fatalities [4]. In Africa, the boomslang (*Dispholidus typus*) and twig or bird snakes (*Thelotornis kirtlandi, T capensis,* and *T usambaricus*) are feared. In Asia, the yamakagashi or Japanese garter snake (*Rhabdophis tigrinus*) and the red-necked keelback (*Rhabdophis subminiatus*) are considered dangerous. Bites from these species may or may not produce swelling, nausea, emesis, colicky abdominal pain, headache, renal failure, and severe, varied coagulopathies [2]. Currently, antivenom is available only for the boomslang. Limited production of some Japanese *Rhabdophis* antivenom has begun (there are 18 venomous *Rhabdophis* species), although these products are not readily available.

Another major group of venomous snakes is the Viperidae, which includes three subfamilies: the pit vipers (Crotalinae), the true vipers (Viperinae), and Fea's viper (Azemiopinae). Viperids have solenoglyphic fangs that function much like hypodermic needles and facilitate deep tissue penetration [4]. The large, hollow fangs are attached to the maxillary bone and folded at rest. Large venom glands ensheathed in muscles of the temporal area give these snakes a pronounced triangular head. During a strike, the maxillary bone rotates 90°, erecting the fangs while muscular contraction of the venom glands forcibly expels venom from the tips of the fangs (all in less time than it takes to blink an eye).

Pit vipers are distinguished from true vipers by the presence of heat-detecting pits between the eyes and nares [4], which allow these snakes to "see" beyond visible wavelengths into the infrared spectrum. Thus the pit vipers can recognize thermal images of prey or victims (even in the dark or from inside a bag). Pit vipers are distributed throughout the Americas, Europe, Asia, and Africa. Pit vipers include the well-known rattlesnakes (*Crotalus* and *Sistrurus* species), cantils, copperheads, water moccasins and their relatives (*Agkistrodon* species), lance-headed pit vipers (*Bothrops* species, such as the fer-de-lance), bushmasters (*Lachesis* species), jumping vipers (*Atropoides* species), palm pit vipers (*Bothriechis* species), forest pit vipers (*Bothriopsis* species), hog-nosed and montane pit vipers (*Porthridium* species), horned pit vipers (*Ophryacus* species), snorkel-nosed vipers (*Deinagkistrodon* species), hump-nosed vipers (*Hypnale* species), Malayan pit vipers (*Calloselasma* species), Asian pit vipers (*Ovophis* and *Trimeresurus* species), and many others. Most viperid bites cause edema, pain, erythema, tissue necrosis, and ecchymoses at the bite site. Systemic signs of pit viper bites include nausea, emesis, unusual tastes (minty, rubbery, or metallic with some species of rattlesnakes), generalized weakness, paresthesias, altered mentation, myokymia, hypotension, shock, respiratory depression or failure (with the neotropical rattlesnake *Crotalus durissus terrificus*), cardiovascular collapse, hemolysis, and defibrination [2].

The true (or Old World) vipers are found in Africa, Europe, and Asia. True vipers include the well-known puff adders (*Bitis* species), bush vipers (*Atheris* species), mole vipers (*Atractaspis* species), saw-scaled vipers (*Echis* species), night adders (*Causus* species), Mid-East vipers (*Daboia* species), horned vipers (*Cerastes* species), false horned vipers (*Pseudocerastes* species), moustache vipers (*Eristocophis* species), Middle Eastern and European vipers and adders (*Vipera* species), Fea's viper (*Azemiops feae*), and many other genera. The local effects of venom are similar to those of the venom of pit vipers; systemic effects include hypotension, shock, arrhythmias, myocardial toxicity, and spontaneous bleeding from the bite site, mucosa, and multiple orifices (incoagulable blood) [2].

Antivenoms for viperids include polyvalent (ie, produced from several species) and monovalent (produced from one species) forms. Monovalent forms are preferred over polyvalent [2,6,7]; however, polyvalent antivenom can be life saving when the species is unknown or when monovalent antivenom is not available. It is often less expensive to stock polyvalent rather than several monovalent antivenoms. Antivenom is not produced for all species but only for species that regularly cause human fatalities. Antivenom is also called antivenin after widely used trade names.

Another major group of venomous snakes is the Elapidae, the cobras, kraits, coral snakes, and their relatives, including all the venomous Australian species. All elapids are front fanged (proteroglyphic). Elapids have rigidly fixed, small, hollow fangs attached to venom glands. The fangs are small because they must fit within the mouth unfolded. Elapids have extremely potent venoms, among the lowest LD_{50} values for venomous reptiles (indicating the smallest amount of venom required for fatality).

In the New World, elapids are represented by coral snakes (*Micrurus, Micruroides,* and *Leptomicrurus* species). Old World elapids include mambas (*Dendroaspis* species), African garter snakes (*Elapsoidea* and *Elaps*), cobras (*Naja, Hemachatus, Aspidelaps, Boulengerina, Ogmodon, Ophiophagus, Paranaja, Walterinnesia,* and *Pseudohaje* species), taipans (*Oxyuranus* species), tiger snakes (*Notechis* species), death adders (*Acanthophis* species), black snakes and their allies (*Pseudechis, Pseudonaja,* and *Austrelaps* species), bandy-bandys (*Vermicella*), whipsnakes (*Demansia* and *Rhinoplocephalus*), Asian coral snakes (*Calliophis, Hemibungaris,* and *Maticora* species), kraits (*Bungarus* species), and many others.

Local signs of elapid envenomation include intense pain, rapid swelling with blistering, and tissue necrosis [2]. Systemic neurotoxic effects give elapids part of their well-deserved bad reputation; respiratory paralysis is a leading cause of death. Other neurotoxin effects include heaviness of eyelids, blurred vision, salivation, abdominal pain, and diarrhea [2]. In addition to their potent venom, elapids are dangerous because they are exceedingly fast, alert, intelligent, and potentially aggressive.

Spitting cobras (*Naja katriensis, N mossambica, N nigricollis, N pallida, N sputatrix, Hemachatus haemachatus*) possess venom that is cytotoxic and not neurotoxic to humans [2]. These snakes use venom defensively and are extremely accurate at spitting venom into the eyes of would-be predators. This venom causes intense ocular pain with blepharospasm, palpebral edema, corneal erosions, and panopthalmitis [2]. Face masks or goggles (not glasses) should be worn when handling spitters. An eyewash station should also be available in case a handler gets venom in his or her eyes [8].

The last groups of venomous snakes are the true sea snakes, Hydrophidae, and sea kraits, Laticaudiae. Sea snakes and kraits are rare in captivity. Sea snakes are nonaggressive, and bites are rare, usually occurring when a snake has been caught in a fishing net [2]. As many as 80% of bites cause few or no systemic effects [2]. Envenomation is usually painless with little or no local reaction. Systemic signs may include myalgia, dizziness, dry throat, nausea, emesis, generalized weakness, pseudotrismus, headache, diaphoresis, swelling of the tongue, myoglobinuria, flaccid paralysis progressing to respiratory paralysis, rhabdomyolysis, and muscle necrosis with renal failure [2]. Myoglobinuria is a hallmark of sea snake envenomation [2].

Viperids and helodermids are much easier to work with than are elapids and arboreal rear-fanged colubrids (*Dispholidus* and *Thelotornis* species). This author tries not to see the latter groups, because they are difficult to manage if not properly contained (ie, loose) in a veterinary hospital.

Venomous snake bite

People often wonder what the outcome of a venomous snake bite will be. The ultimate severity of a venomous snake bite depends on the size and species of snake, the amount and degree of toxicity of the venom, the bite location, the type of first aid provided, the timing of treatment, the presence or absence of underlying medical conditions, and the unique susceptibility of the victim to the venom or antivenom [2,9]. No real generalizations can be made about snake bite [10]. The outcome of venomous snake bite is as unpredictable as that of a car crash [4]. A bite may range in its effects from an insignificant dry bite (approximately 25% to 30% of viperid bites are dry or nonenvenomating) [7,9] or bite from a relatively benign species to a serious, painful, and rapidly lethal bite. One may walk away from the experience with minimal to serious injury or permanent disability or perhaps not walk away at all [4]. Neotropical rattlesnakes (*Crotalus durissus terrificus*) had a case/fatality rate of 72% until antivenom usage decreased it to 12% [7].

Emergency protocol

It is essential to have an emergency bite protocol in place before working with venomous species [3,4,8,11]. Poison control centers and most local zoos maintain lists of physicians experienced in treating snake bite [2,4]. Regional poison control centers (which may be reached through the national hotline at 1-800-222-1222) should be contacted for assistance with snake bite [2]. A written list of ambulance service, antivenom source, hospital and poison control numbers, and 24-hour contact information for personal physicians should be prominently displayed in the hospital [4,8]. See Boyer [4,6], Watt [7], and Gold and colleagues [2] for more information on emergency procedures for snake bite.

When envenomation does occur, immediately move the victim out of striking distance and secure the reptile. The victim should be kept calm, warm, and at rest and should be transported immediately to the nearest medical facility [2,7]. In the United States, telephoning 911 should result in the rapid dispatch of an ambulance. Time is of the essence in snake bite treatment. Even though many patients are initially in denial (concerning the bite), a wait-and-see attitude should never be adopted; one should seek medical care without delay. The injured part of the body should be immobilized in a functional position below the level of the heart [2]. Rings, watches, bracelets, and any other constrictive clothing should be removed immediately [2,4,7]. If antivenom is available, it should be transported with the patient. Use a stretcher, if available, and keep the victim quiet and still. First aid measures that were once recommended, such as tourniquets, incision and suction, cryotherapy, and electric shock therapy, are now strongly discouraged [2,7]. The Sutherland wrap [12] (essentially a tightly fitting Ace bandage [Becton Dickenson, Franklin Lakes, New Jersey] that is wrapped from distal to the bite to proximal of the bite) is recommended for elapid and helodermid bites.

Planning for examination of venomous reptiles

Planning for venomous reptiles should begin before the patient arrives. The author instructs staff and clients that no one, including the owner, is to touch the venomous reptile. This principle appears intuitive, but staff members who are accustomed to handling reptiles may attempt to handle venomous reptiles if not instructed otherwise. The author will never shake the shock of watching a naïve client quickly but calmly reach into a 10-gallon aquarium and scoop up one of two timber rattlesnakes in his wrist-length deerskin glove. Remember that the veterinarian may be held liable if a venomous reptile injures staff or owners while in the hospital [13]. Instruct the owner to bring the reptile properly "bagged" (discussed later) in a solid container. If the owner is unsure how to bag a venomous reptile, this is a clear sign of incompetence or inexperience. Do not let such a keeper assist you.

Safe handling of venomous snakes

Safe handling, both before arrival and in the hospital, is critical to treating venomous reptiles, especially venomous snakes. Aspects of bagging, handling containers, snake hooks, tongs, restraint tubes, shift boxes, and squeeze boxes are detailed in this section.

Bagging

Bagging venomous reptiles is most easily done with a commercial bagging system (Snake Bagger System, Midwest, Greenwood, Missouri; Reptile Bag Stik, Fuhrman Diversified, Seabrook, Texas). The Snake Bagger System (Fig. 1A) includes a long handle attached to a triangular frame that opens the mouth of dual 48-in long, narrow bags that snap onto the frame. This arrangement allows one to hook the snake into the open bag without anyone holding the bag. In addition, the mouth of a commercial bagging system may be placed right in front of the snake on the ground, and many snakes will move into the bag to get out of sight. The bags are long, so that they may be twisted, doubled over, and held closed with the triangular frame (Fig. 1B). The beauty of these systems is immediately apparent to anyone who has ever held open a snake bag as the venomous snake is bagged. Without a commercial bagging system, the bag must be taped to a trash can in two areas and a tong or hook used to create the third corner of a triangular opening through which the snake may be placed. This method is not particularly difficult, but it is certainly inconvenient.

Once the snake is in the bag, the bag must be safely tied off. Never touch a bag with your hands or feet when the snake is in that portion of the bag. Use a hook or a tong. Many people have been bitten through bags, some with fatal consequences. To tie off the bag, place it on a flat surface and put the shaft of a snake hook, tong, or stick across the neck of the bag, being

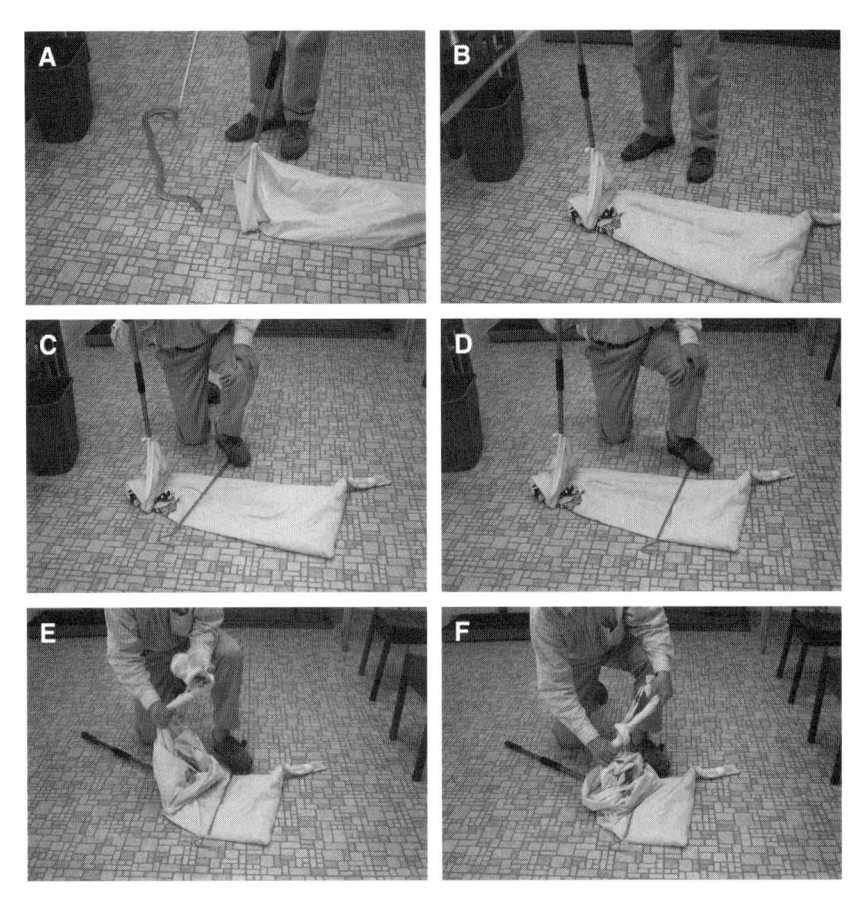

Fig. 1. (*A*) Commercial bagging systems keeps one's hands away from the bag opening, and snakes often retreat into them. (*B*) Once it is in the bag, move the snake down by lifting the bag vertically, then quickly lay the bag down horizontally, twist, and double over the neck while pushing down with the mouth frame to entrap the snake. (*C*) Place the shaft of a snake hook on the upper bag neck while holding it down with your foot. Do not touch the bag with your hands, feet, or any other part of your body. (*D*) Move the hook down the bag to trap the snake at one end. (*E*) With the snake trapped at one end by the downward pressure of the snake hook shaft, one may safely twist the neck of the bag and tie it off. (*F*) Further secure the knot by doubling it over and tying it off with drawstrings or cable ties. Note the double bagging and the corner attachment on the outer bag for tubing.

careful not to crush or pin the snake (Fig. 1C). Coax the snake farther down into the bag by slowly moving the shaft of the hook down the bag (Fig. 1D). Once the snake is at the bottom of the bag, stand on the hook (outside the bag edges) and tie off the neck of the bag (Fig. 1E, F). If the snake is not first secured in the bottom of the bag (with a hook), it is more likely that the snake will be tied in the knot and injured or killed. Failure to secure the snake properly also increases the risk of snake bite. Be sure to keep hands and feet away from the bag edges; remember, pit vipers can "see" a precise infrared image of you from inside the bag. The double bag makes it more difficult for bites to penetrate to the outside but is by no means foolproof. The bag neck may be tied in a knot or twisted, doubled over, and secured with a cable tie. Throughout the bagging process, it is crucial to maintain tight pressure over the snake hook (usually by stepping on the hook). The bag may then be lifted with tongs and placed in a solid container for transport.

To remove the snake from the bag, lay the bag flat, secure the snake in the bottom of the bag with a hook shaft and pressure, then untie the knot. Use tongs to lift the bag into a handling container and elevate the bag, leaving the snake in the container. Under no circumstances should anyone touch the bag, even when wearing gloves.

An additional convenient feature of the Snake Bagger is that the outer bag has a sleeve in one corner (see Fig. 1C–F) that may be taped to a restraining tube, which can simplify tubing if the snake is cooperative (see following discussion).

Handling containers

The best handling containers for venomous reptiles are galvanized metal garbage cans with a handle in the center of the lid and locking mechanisms on the side. Hard plastic or rubber trash cans are less desirable, because the lids are more difficult to place, prone to warping, and dangerous to lock [14]. The handles are often at the edges of the container, which invariably increases the risk for a bite when the lid is placed or removed. Plastic diaper pails with center handles and locking handles work well. Unfortunately, both metal garbage cans and plastic diaper pails are becoming more difficult to find. Five-gallon buckets with screw-in lids are effective when one attaches a handle to the center of the outer lid.

Snake hooks

Snake hooks are used to lift and transport a snake from one area to another (Fig. 2A–C). In the past, snake hooks were used to pin snakes just behind the head; then the snake was quickly grabbed below the head. This method puts both the handler and the patient at risk. Depending on the skill of the handler, it can be relatively safe or downright dangerous. Snakes are adept at turning and stretching to bite anything grabbing them, and snakes pinned behind the head often thrash wildly. Also, if one slips or miscalculates one's grab, or if the snake escapes just before being grabbed, the risk of envenomation becomes serious. Snakes have a single occipital condyle, so intense downward pressure applied at the atlanto-occipital junction while the snake is thrashing carries an increased risk for cervical dislocation. Hence pinning is to be avoided as much as possible. Midwest (Greenwood, Missouri) makes a pinning tool with rubber tubing that is safer for the

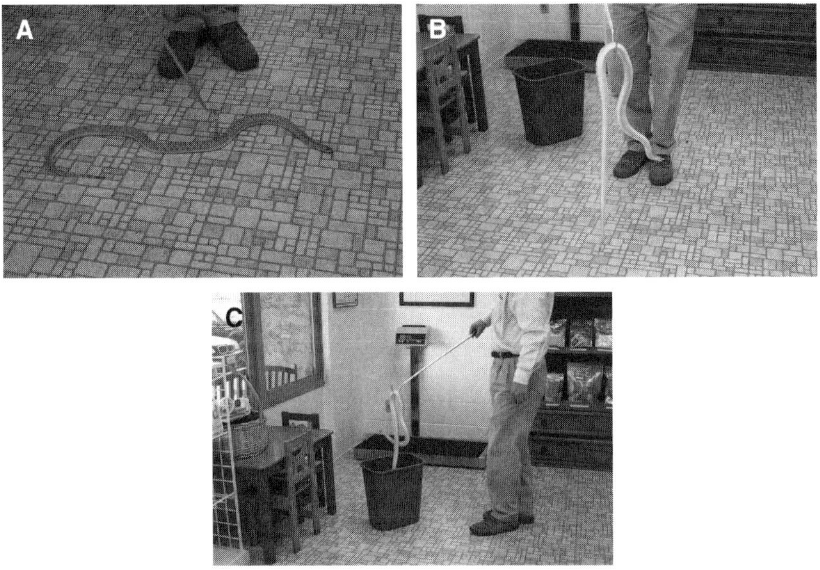

Fig. 2. Snake hooks are for lifting and transporting, not pinning. (*A*) To lift a snake, place the hook slightly forward of midbody and lift the snake off the ground. (*B*) The snake will move forward once hooked and balance near midbody. A gentle shake will keep the snake holding onto the hook. (*C*) The snake may then be moved to another container. Captive snakes balance on hooks or are hook trained; wild snakes require training before they learn to stay on the hook.

snake, but not necessarily safer for the handler. With safer methods of handling available, the author believes pinning is too risky and should not be attempted by novice handlers. Snake hooks are used primarily for lifting and moving, not pinning. However, heloderms are relatively easy to pin and harder to damage, so pinning is an acceptable technique for heloderm handling.

Keep in mind that wild snakes are not hook trained and often do not stay on hooks. Captive snakes are often hook trained. This means that the snake will balance itself on the hook once lifted off the ground. To hook a snake, one should place the blunt-tipped hook beneath the snake, slightly forward of midbody, and lift the snake smoothly off the ground (see Fig. 2A). A gentle shake of the hook once the snake is off the ground usually keeps the snake holding in place. Most snakes move forward when lifted, so hooking forward of midbody ensures the hook will be at the center of the snake when it clears the substrate (see Fig. 2B) [14]. Having several sizes of snake hook is a necessity for different-sized snakes (Fig. 3). The author keeps 12.5-, 24.5-, and 30.5-in hooks in the hospital.

One of the worst mistakes one can make is to use a hook too short for the size of the snake [15]. It is always preferable to overestimate strike distance. Although this distance is subject to debate, one should assume that most

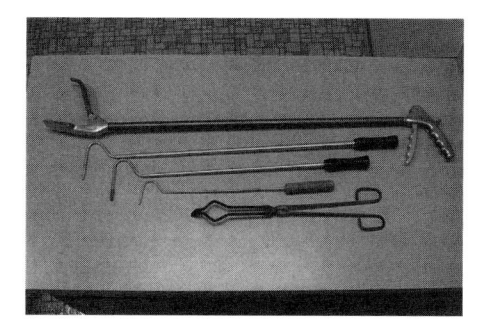

Fig. 3. Essential items for working with venomous snakes. At the bottom are tongs used for offering food to venomous reptiles. Various sizes of snake hook and multiple hooks are needed. Hooks with a grip at one end avert the dangerous mistake of choking up on a snake hook. At the top are Gentle Giant snake tongs (Midwest, Greenwood, Missouri) that grip without crushing and make venomous snake handling easier on all parties.

snakes can strike one half to three quarters their body length [3,14]. Cobras generally will not strike farther than the length of their raised forebody (although they need not raise their body or hood to strike) [14]. Keep in mind that many venomous snakes are exceedingly fast and can lunge forward with incredible speed when striking. It is necessary to have a clear path of retreat in case of need (ie, keep a door behind you). Likewise, keep the floor uncluttered and make sure the room is escape proof (for the snake). Many elapids and arboreal snakes climb hooks readily, so having a second hook within reach is always necessary in case one must release one's initial hook. Have the handling container nearby.

Hooks should be lightweight (hollow aluminum or titanium shafts are currently in vogue), be easily disinfected, and have a grip at one end (see Fig. 3), not extending down the shaft (like a golf club). When the grip extends down the shaft, the handler often chokes up on it and reduces the strike distance inadvertently [3]. Titanium is the strongest hook material, weighs half as much as stainless steel, and is scratch and corrosion resistant, but it is expensive. Aluminum is less expensive and even more lightweight, but it is not as strong as titanium and less scratch resistant. Stainless steel is the heaviest hook material but still works well. Polycarbonate plastic is flexible and lightweight but is restricted in use to snakes weighing less than 500 g and should not be used for pinning. Another disadvantage is that organic solvents can dissolve or slowly crystallize the hook and predispose it to cracking. The lifting section of the hook should be curved (see Fig. 3) rather than L-shaped, to prevent the snake from sliding down the shaft when the hook is lifted higher than the handler's hand [14]. However, the distal portion of the hook should not be lifted above the level of the hand, or the snake may slide down the hook [3]. Flat-bladed hooks (or "python hooks") work well for heavy-bodied snakes such as the puff adder (*Bitis arietans*), Gaboon viper (*Bitis gabonica*), Eastern diamondback rattlesnake (*Crotalus adamanteus*), cottonmouth (*Agkistrodon piscivorous*), and massasauga (*Sistrurus catenatus*) [3,14]. Using two hooks with heavy-bodied or arboreal snakes also makes them more comfortable on the hooks.

Of the many hook manufacturers, two the author has used and recommends are Fuhrman Diversified (2912 Bayport Boulevard, Seabrook, Texas 77586-1501, 281-474-1388, 281-474-1390, fdi@flash.net) and Midwest (14505 South Harris Road, Greenwood, Missouri 64034, 816-537-4444, 816-537-4226, midwestongs.com).

Tongs

In the past tongs were frowned on for handling snakes, because they easily crushed snakes and broke ribs. It is no wonder that snakes thrashed wildly when grabbed with tongs. Midwest has introduced a new tong called the Gentle Giant (Midwest, Greenwood, Missouri) that grips and holds without crushing (see Fig. 3). The best way to appreciate this advance is to grab one's own arm (or that of an unsuspecting colleague) and squeeze as hard as possible. The Gentle Giant tongs do not crush, primarily because of cable spring construction and wide, plastic-coated jaws. Consequently, they are excellent for grabbing and holding snakes. Tongs are also useful for lifting and holding bags.

Restraint tubes

Clear plastic or acrylic tubes (Fig. 4) ranging from 0.375 in to 3 in in diameter, are needed for tubing venomous snakes [16] and are also useful for keeping snakes straight for radiographs. A 13-piece radiolucent combination series is available from Midwest (Plastic Restraining Tubes, Combo, Midwest, Greenwood, Missouri). With tube restraint, it is crucial that the diameter be small enough so that the snake cannot turn around in the tube.

Multiple methods of getting the snake into the tube (ie, "tubing" the snake) exist. The easiest was already discussed in the bagging section (simply allowing the snake to go up the sleeve in a bag corner that has previously

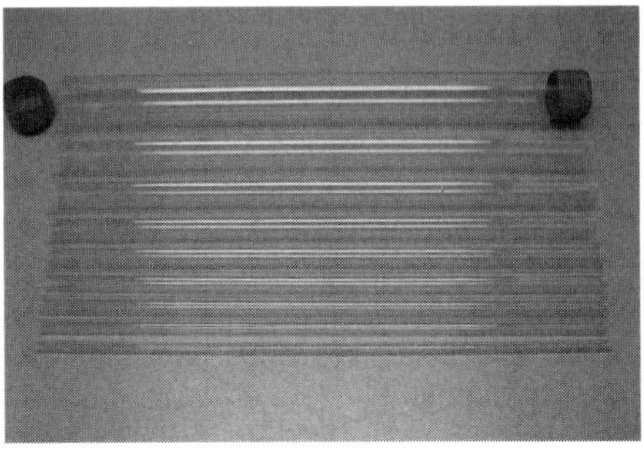

Fig. 4. Clear plastic or acrylic restraint tubes are essential for tubing snakes. Once the snake is in the tube, it is much safer to work with.

been taped to a tube). Once a snake is one third to halfway into the tube, simultaneously grab the snake and the tube with one hand, holding the snake in place. The head is effectively isolated with this technique. For arboreal snakes and elapids, keep a cap on the end (see Fig. 4), or the snake will be out the open tube end and gone before you can react (or worse, turning around to see what is grabbing it!).

Another common method of tubing is to place the snake into a handling container and patiently hold a tube along the inside of the container [16]. As the snake tries to escape the container (Fig. 5A), it will eventually go up the tube (Fig. 5B, C) and may be captured once it is a third to halfway (Fig. 5D). Placing 6 in of lukewarm water at the bottom of the container encourages the snake to go up the tube faster (see Fig. 5A–D) [17].

Another method involves placing the tube (horizontally) along a wall and allowing the snake to enter the tube as it moves along the wall. Tube restraint is convenient in that one may then easily inject the snake or introduce gas anesthesia.

Shift boxes

Zoos use shift boxes for large species that are easily agitated, such as mambas, *Dendroaspis* species, taipans, *Oxyuranus* species, cobras, *Naja*

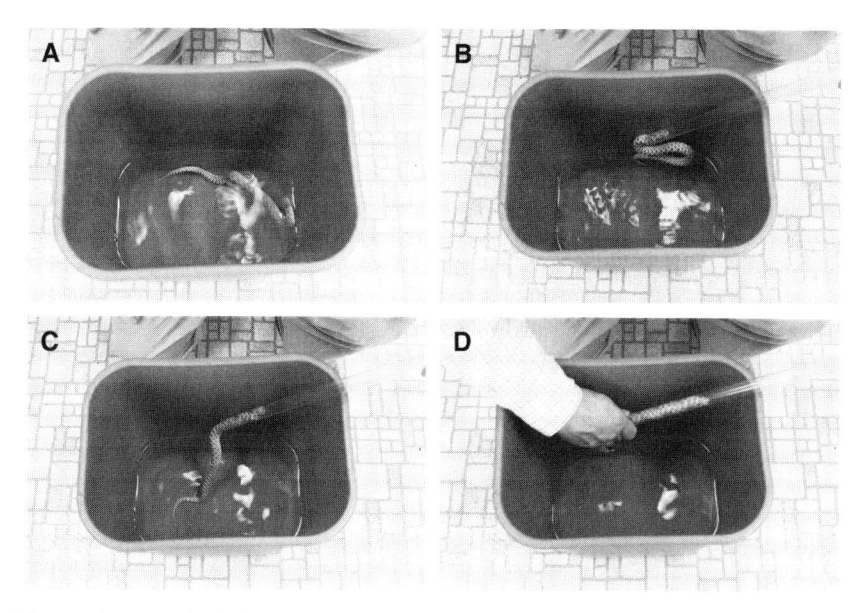

Fig. 5. (*A*) One method of tubing snakes. Place 6 in of lukewarm water in a smooth-sided container. The snake will try to escape up the sides. (Do not leave the snake unsupervised, or it will drown.) (*B*) With patience one may guide the snake into the tube opening. (*C*) Once in the opening, the snake will try to escape the water by climbing the tube. (*D*) One may safely capture the snake once it is a third to halfway up the tube by securing the bottom of the tube and the snake with one hand. Make sure the tube diameter is small enough so the snake cannot turn around.

and *Ophiophagus* species, and many of the Australian elapids [3]. These allow the keeper to service the exhibit without initiating contact with a dangerous animal. Most of these snakes may be taught to move into the shift on command through operant conditioning [3]. Shift boxes may be fitted with squeeze restraints, restraining tubes, or anesthesia ports. Carefully designed shift boxes can greatly simplify restraint.

Squeeze boxes

Squeeze boxes have a bottom fitted with thick foam rubber, four sides, and an open top into which fits the clear plastic, plexiglass, or screen squeeze. The squeeze segment has long handles and slots through which the snake is accessible once squeezed down against the foam rubber [3,8]. When a slot is left open in one side, the front half of the snake may be restrained while the back half is accessible. Squeeze boxes are excellent for ongoing procedures such as antibiotic injections.

Treatment of venomous reptiles

Hospitalization

Venomous reptiles should be treated on an outpatient basis when possible. If they must be hospitalized, warn staff not to clean or service the cage. The cage should be clearly labeled "Venomous, Do Not Handle," with the scientific and common names, the number of animals in the enclosure, and the necessary antivenom type listed on a detachable card [8]. The top of the cage should be double screened or solid with a locking mechanism.

Anesthesia

Anesthetics for venomous reptiles are similar to those for nonvenomous reptiles. This author currently uses propofol intravenously, tiletamine intramuscularly, or isoflurane by inhalation. See Boyer [18] for dosages and more on anesthesia.

Venipuncture

In colubrids and viperids, the ventral coccygeal vein is accessible (as in lizards) and is the preferred site for venipuncture. If ventral coccygeal venipuncture is unsuccessful, cardiac puncture has a low level of mortality (provided that multiple attempts, if necessary, do not excessively traumatize the heart). However, it is prudent to warn clients that, in rare instances, death may result. The heart may be located by palpation or by observing the ventral scales move over the heart as it beats. The heart is usually located within 20% to 40% of the distance between the snout and vent. The heart should be stabilized by pushing anteriorly, with a thumb, at the apex, and by having a second person place a forefinger anterior to the heart base. The second person should also restrain the snake. Anesthesia is recommended, especially in large animals. The heart is then punctured with a 22- to 25-gauge heparinized needle, attached to a 1- to 6-mL syringe, through the apex of the single ventricle. The initial aspiration of clear fluid indicates pericardial fluid contamination, and the needle should be removed and another attempt made.

Paramyxovirus infection

No discussion of veterinary care of venomous snakes would be complete without mentioning paramyxovirus, the most dangerous disease facing large collections of snakes. This virus was discovered after a Swiss outbreak in 1973 killed one quarter of a collection of more than 400 fer-de-lances, *Bothrops atrox*. Since that time there have been numerous fatalities of viperids, especially crotalids, in many large zoologic collections [18]. Although the virus has also been isolated from boids, colubrids, and elapids, these groups are much less commonly affected. Virus transmission may be through the air or through fomites, such as keepers or cage-cleaning utensils. Stressors, such as shipment, hibernation, or ambient temperature fluctuations, may activate latent infections. Outbreaks often follow acquisitions of new animals, resulting from ineffective quarantine.

Clinical signs may be divided into three groups. Acute infections, which constitute the majority of cases, usually result in the death of the animal within 3 to 10 weeks of exposure. Clinical signs can be minimal, such as anorexia or regurgitation, or snakes may be found comatose or dead. In longer infections, as respiratory signs develop, dyspnea and mucous discharge from the glottis may become evident, and serosanguinous fluid may be found in the cage. Neurologic signs such as paresis, ataxia, loss of equilibrium, head tremors, opisthotonus, and slow, infrequent tongue flicking are less commonly observed just before death. The third clinical picture involves chronic "poor-doers," which are often anorexic or hypophagic and may regurgitate. Chronically infected snakes may exhibit lethargy, emaciation, petit mal seizures, decreased muscle tone, and heat seeking. Respiratory signs (as previously discussed), gaseous bowel distention, diarrhea, malodorous stools, and protozoan overgrowth may also be present. Some snakes may remain asymptomatic for as long as 10 months while potentially shedding virus. Eventually most of these animals become chronic "poor-doers," although a few may recover. Paramyxovirus causes a characteristic interstitial pneumonia and pancreatitis when the snake does not die acutely. On necropsy one may find thickened pulmonary tissue and mucoid or caseous exudate supporting secondary gram-negative bacterial infections.

Clinical suspicion of a paramyxovirus outbreak is raised whenever one finds large death tolls in a collection of snakes. Diagnosis may often be made with characteristic histopathology. Hemagglutination inhibition assay for antibody titers can confirm diagnosis and evaluate the spread of paramyxovirus. Hemagglutination assays are available through veterinary schools at the University of Florida (contact Dr. Jacobson; run once a month) and the University of Tennessee (contact the virology laboratory). At the University of Florida, titers less than 1:20 are considered negative (no antibodies to paramyxovirus), titers of 1:40 to 1:80 are suspect (retesting is recommended in 2 to 4 weeks; antibodies could be rising with an active infection), and titers greater than 1:80 are considered positive (active paramyxovirus antibody production). Isolation of affected animals, cage mates, or areas should continue for at least 3 months after the last death. When quarantined animals are healthy and have negative titers after isolation, they are assumed to present little risk to other reptiles. Paramyxovirus is highly contagious. Ethical individuals involved with outbreaks should report any outbreak or positive titer situation to colleagues (who may be interested in sending snakes to or receiving snakes from them). Killed vaccines produced variable transient antibody response in Western diamondback rattlesnakes. Administration of a modified live vaccine induced disease. Neither vaccine is currently in use.

Necropsy

It may come as a surprise that snakes can continue to bite after decapitation. For example, decapitated rattlesnake heads are capable of biting for at least 20 minutes and sometimes as long as an hour [19]. Multiple records of humans bitten by decapitated snakes exist [19]. Be careful with the head of any venomous snake while performing necropsy. Venom remains stable for years with freezing or desiccation or at room temperature. Store the body in such a way that no one becomes envenomated later when handling a frozen reptile [8]. Dead venomous reptiles should be clearly labeled with scientific and common name and handled carefully.

Venomoid surgery

Owners of venomous reptiles may request removal of the venom glands or ligation or transection of the venom duct to make these snakes safer to handle. Such practices should be discouraged for several reasons. First and foremost, so-called "venomoid" snakes encourage irresponsible snake handling. Owners may see other people "free-handling" venomous snakes and want to do the same. Additionally, given the possibility that the procedure was performed incorrectly or the animal "healed" after surgery (eg, reconnected a ligated venom duct), one can never be sure that such an animal is truly nonvenomous. Most of these surgeries are done by laypersons, not veterinarians (there are Web sites to show you how to do this at home!). This author handles "venomoid" snakes as if they were still venomous. Venomoid surgery is painful to the animal, and surgery intended simply to enhance an animal's appeal to the owner appears wrong to the author. The counterargument is that the appeal is enhanced because the snake should be less dangerous. See Jaros [20], Kiel [21,22], Glen and colleagues [23], DeLanglade and colleague [24], and Boomker and colleagues [25] for more information.

Summary

Venomous reptiles should be handled in a safe and consistent manner, even after death. Owners and staff should be warned not to handle the venomous reptile, and one should have emergency protocols in place before the properly bagged and encased reptile is presented. It is important to know what one is treating as well as one's limitations. After being carefully removed from the bag, the venomous reptile may be transferred to a handling container, tubed, or squeezed with the appropriate equipment. The author usually induces injectable or gas anesthesia at this point. During recovery (after sedation or anesthesia), it is imperative for the patient to be in a secure environment. Veterinarians who are inexperienced with venomous reptiles should learn how to handle them through a reputable seminar or class before electing to see them in their practice. Be safe. A bite may be life threatening; recognize this as something to avoid. Professionals take no pride in being bitten.

Acknowledgments

Thanks to Donal M. Boyer, Curator of Reptiles and Amphibians, San Diego Zoo and Wild Animal Park, for constructive criticism.

References

[1] Russell FE. When a snake strikes. Emerg Med 1990;22(12):20–43.
[2] Gold BS, Dart RC, Barish RA. Bites of venomous snakes. N Engl J Med 2002;347(5): 347–56.
[3] Boyer DM, Ettling J, Flanagan JP, et al. Venomous reptile handling: roundtable. J Herp Med Surg 2003;13(1):23–37.
[4] Boyer DM. Venomous reptiles: an overview of families, handling, restraint techniques and emergency protocol. In: Willetts-Fralm M, editor. Proceedings of the Association of Reptilian and Amphibian Veterinarians. Sacramento (CA): Association of Reptilian and Amphibian Veterinarians; 1995. p. 83–95.
[5] Hooker KR, Caravati EM. Gila monster envenomation. Ann Emerg Med 1984;4:731–5.
[6] Boyer DM. Antivenom index. Wheeling (WV): American Zoo and Aquarium Association and American Association of Poison Control Centers; 1994.
[7] Watt G. Snakebite treatment and first aid. In: Campbell JA, Lamar WW, editors. The venomous reptiles of Latin America. Ithaca (NY): Comstock Publishing Associates; 1989. p. 6–13.
[8] Boyer DM. Special considerations for venomous reptiles. In: Girling SJ, Raiti P, editors. BSAVA manual of reptiles. 2nd edition. Gloucester (UK): British Small Animal Veterinary Association; 2004. p. 357–62.

[9] Gold BS, Wingert WA. Snake venom poisoning in the United States: a review of therapeutic practice. South Med J 1994;87:579–89.
[10] Fowler ME. Cobra bite in a keeper. Proceedings of the American Association of Zoo Veterinarians. 1979. p. 8–10.
[11] Johnson-Delaney CA. Reptile zoonoses and threats to public health. In: Mader DR, editor. Reptile medicine and surgery. Philadelphia: WB Saunders; 1996. p. 30–2.
[12] Sutherland SK, Coulter AR, Harris RD. Rationalization of first aid measures for elapid snakebite. Lancet 1979;Jan:183–6.
[13] Funk RS. Treating aggressive, large or dangerous reptiles. Exo Heal 2005;4(1):1–4.
[14] Altimari W. Venomous snakes: a safety guide for reptile keepers. Lawrence (KS): Society for the Study of Amphibians and Reptiles; 1998.
[15] Card W, Roberts DT. Incidence of bites from venomous reptiles in North America. Herpetol Rev 1996;27:15–6.
[16] Murphy JB. A method for immobilizing snakes at the Dallas Zoo. Int Zoo Yearb 1971;11:233.
[17] Walczak JT. A technique for the safe restraint of venomous snakes. Herpetol Rev 1991;22:17–8.
[18] Boyer TH. Essentials of reptiles: a guide for practitioners. Lakewood (CO): AAHA Press; 1998.
[19] Klauber LM. Rattlesnakes. Berkeley (CA): University of California Press; 1972. p. 341–9.
[20] Jaros DB. Occlusion of the venom duct of Crotalidae by electrocoagulation: an innovation in operative technique. Zoological 1940;25:49–51.
[21] Kiel JL. The surgical removal of venom glands from poisonous snakes. SW Vet 1973:283–6.
[22] Kiel JL. Long-term effects of venom gland adenectomy of snakes. Avian/Exotic Practice 1984;1:35–41.
[23] Glenn JL, Straight R, Sayder CC. Surgical technique for isolation of main venom gland of viperid, crotalid and elapid snakes. Toxicon 1973;11:231–3.
[24] DeLanglada FG, Belluomini HE. Contribuicao a technica operatoria de serpents III. Ablacao de gladulas de veneno em serpents do genero Crotalus. Mem Inst Butantan 1972;36:89–100.
[25] Boomker A, Weise A, Bos P, et al. Microsurgical evenomation of the puff adder, *Bitis arietans*. Vivarium 1999;10(3):27–9.

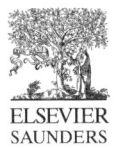

Common Procedures in Psittacines
Lauren V. Powers, DVM, ABVP–Avian

Carolina Veterinary Specialists, 12117 Statesville Road, Huntersville, NC 28078, USA

Psittacines pose interesting and challenging dilemmas for restraint, sample collection, and treatment. Critically ill birds often cannot tolerate prolonged handling or sedation. Although most procedures used in canine and feline patients are easily adapted to the psittacine, anatomic and physiologic differences obligate practitioners to familiarize themselves with the unique features of these patients. Many procedures performed in psittacines are unique to birds owing to these differences. This article reviews procedures commonly used to handle and restrain the psittacine, to collect diagnostic samples, and to deliver therapeutic agents.

Capture and restraint

Before a psittacine is captured, it should be evaluated within its enclosure [1]. Many critically ill birds will panic and may not survive handling [2]. If the bird has either an increased respiratory rate or effort, or if it appears weak and poorly responsive, it should be placed in a heated (85°F to 90°F [29°C to 30°C]), oxygenated cage for at least 20 minutes before handling [2].

Untame or panicky birds are best captured in the pet carrier with a towel. Handcloths are suitable for smaller psittacines, such as budgerigars and cockatiels. Thick bath towels are more appropriate for larger birds such as macaws. The bird may be guided toward an inside wall of the cage and the towel draped around the body [1]. Untame breeder birds in flight cages may be caught in a net and removed in a similar fashion [1,3]. Birds should not be captured while perched on their owners. Capture with bare hands is not recommended, because it increases the chance of receiving bites and may lead to a hand phobia in some birds. One exception is the juvenile pet psittacine, which may often be fully examined without restraint, because it is less prone to biting. Capture with gloves is not recommended, again because

---

E-mail address: wingvet@yahoo.com

1094-9194/06/$ - see front matter © 2006 Elsevier Inc. All rights reserved.
doi:10.1016/j.cvex.2006.03.001   *vetexotic.theclinics.com*

injury is more likely and this method may lead to hand phobia [4]. Many owners of pet psittacines train their birds to become comfortable with being covered by a towel. These birds may be approached from the front with a towel while they are perched, and the towel may be gently wrapped around either side of the body [4,5]. Approaching a bird suddenly from above and behind it is generally not advised, because the back is a vulnerable location for these prey species.

Once removed from the carrier, the bird's neck is grasped with a free hand, the towel is removed, and the feet (not the feathered legs) are grasped with the other hand. Towel restraint allows better control of the wings but increases the risk for hyperthermia, may restrict motion of the keel and ribs, and prevents complete access for examination [1]. The most important factor in determining whether to use a towel for the avian examination is the individual practitioner's experience and comfort level with both toweled and nontoweled examinations. Some situations demand use of a towel; many do not. Guidelines for performing a thorough physical examination have been extensively reviewed elsewhere [1,3,4] and are not described here. All birds should be weighed in grams, ideally at each visit. The examination must be brief and limited in critically ill or dyspneic patients. It may be performed in stages, with initial assessment limited to evaluation of the cardiovascular, respiratory, and neurologic systems. All equipment needed for examination, sample collection, and treatment should be prepared before restraint of the sick psittacine [1].

Sample collection

Venipuncture

The diagnostic value of blood collection is limited by the volume that can be collected and the quality of the sample. Total blood volume of birds is approximately 60 to 120 mL/kg but is generally estimated at about 10% (100 mL/kg) of body weight. As much as 10% of the blood volume (approximately 1% of total body weight) may be safely drawn from healthy-appearing birds for diagnostic testing [6,7]. Smaller samples should be collected in critically ill or anemic birds. The risks of venipuncture must be weighed against the diagnostic value of the blood sample. Critically ill birds may not be stable enough for restraint for sample collection. Coagulopathies may be associated with certain diseases, such as liver failure and aflatoxicosis. The most common site for blood collection in psittacine birds is the right jugular vein. It is the largest peripheral vein in these birds and is easily accessed in a featherless tract on the right side of the neck. Because no soft tissue covers this vein, the right jugular is prone to hematoma, particularly when the vein is inadvertently lacerated. Serious bleeding can have fatal consequences. The risk for laceration is reduced when the bevel of the needle is facing downward during sample collection (D. Harris, personal communication, 2005).[1] The vein should be punctured directly, rather than approached from the side. The smallest practical needle gauge is advised [7]. For birds weighing less than 50 g, this author prefers a 27- or 28-gauge needle (usually that of an insulin syringe). For birds between 50 g and 100 g, a 26- or 27-gauge needle is used. A 25-gauge needle is used for birds heavier than 100 g.

Blood may also be collected from the basilic (wing) vein. Hematoma formation is more common with this vein but is rarely of serious consequence [7]. The medial metatarsal vein may also be used. The skin in this location tends to be thicker, and hematoma formation is less likely. This vein is typically smaller than the basilic, which may reduce the sample volume collected. For small sample volumes, a hypodermic needle may be inserted into the vein and blood collected from the needle hub into capillary tubes. Although a toenail clip is a quick and easy method of collecting minute blood samples for evaluating the hematocrit or blood glucose, it is generally not advised, because it may be more painful than venipuncture and often contains tissue artifacts [7].

Fecal diagnostics

Fecal analysis is commonly performed as part of a comprehensive patient evaluation. The patient does not need to be restrained for sample collection. A small sample of feces, free from urine and urates, may be smeared onto a glass slide for Gram staining. A wet mount of a fresh fecal sample is a useful tool to screen psittacines for protozoal trophyzoites (eg, *Giardia* sp and *Spironucleus* sp) and yeasts such as *Macrorhabdus ornithogaster* (formerly "megabacteria") [8]. Organisms may be more easily identified on the wet mount by adding a drop of Lugol's iodine [9].

Crop cytology

Collection of crop material is indicated in cases of crop stasis, regurgitation, or palpable abnormalities of the ingluvies. A crop swab may be performed with the bird firmly restrained and the neck gently extended as far as possible. A speculum, such as a nylon dog bone, is placed between the upper and lower beaks, and a sterile cotton swab is guided down the esophagus on the right side of the neck into the crop. Washing the crop contents increases cellular recovery and can help to flush out ingested toxins or fetid food material [6]. A feeding tube made of red rubber (Sovereign Feeding Tubes, Sherwood Medical, St. Louis, Missouri) or stainless steel (eg, Ejay International, Glendora, California) is inserted into the crop, and 10 to 20 mL/kg of warm, sterile saline or water are infused, massaged, and

---

[1] Editor's note: This decreased risk has been only anecdotally studied; the safest method is the one that works best for the individual phlebotomist.

aspirated back into the syringe [6,7]. The neck should be palpated before infusion for the presence of two tubes, the feeding tube and the trachea. The oral cavity should be watched during infusion for evidence of regurgitation and the bird immediately set down if this occurs.

Choanal sample collection

The choanal slit communicates between the oropharynx and the upper respiratory tract. Cytology and microbiologic cultures are indicated for birds with gross choanal pathologic conditions, such as blunting or inflammation of the choanal papillae, mucopurulent drainage, and signs of upper respiratory disease [6]. The beaks are held apart with an oral speculum or individually with loops of gauze [6]. A sterile cotton swab is inserted into the rostral choanal sulcus and prepared for microbiologic culture or smeared and stained for cytologic examination.

Nasal flush

The nasal flush is a useful tool for collecting samples of material and fluid found between the external nares and the choanal slit, an area that includes the ventral aspect of the middle nasal concha, the suborbital chamber, and occasionally the preorbital diverticulum of the infraorbital sinus [7]. The bird is firmly restrained with the head tipped downward. One to 10 mL of warm sterile saline is infused into each naris and collected in a sterile container, such as a sterile urine cup, as it exits the oral cavity. The sample may then be submitted for culture, or it may be spun and the sediment examined cytologically. Interpretation must take contamination from oral flora into consideration. The nasal flush may also be used to flush out mucus and debris and instill therapeutics such as antibiotics [6].

Tracheal wash

A tracheal wash is indicated in birds with clinical signs or radiographic evidence of lower airway and lung disease. Birds are generally anesthetized with gas anesthesia. Ideally, the length of the trachea is measured from survey radiographs. A sterile red rubber or other suitable tube is quickly inserted through the glottis or through a sterile endotracheal tube to the tracheal bifurcation at the syrinx. Approximately 1 to 2 mL/kg of sterile saline is infused and immediately aspirated. The bird may be gently rocked or coupaged to increase sample volume. An endoscope with a port for flushing offers the advantage of visualizing areas of interest before saline infusion [7]. An air sac cannula should be placed during endoscope-assisted tracheal washes.

Abdominocentesis/Coelomocentesis

Peritoneal fluid accumulation can occur with certain diseases, such as egg yolk peritonitis (Fig. 1) and neoplasia. Free peritoneal fluid may be collected for cytology, culture, and biochemical analysis. No single potential coelomic pocket in birds exists, owing to the presence of separate coelomic, intestinal-peritoneal, and hepatic-peritoneal cavities [7]. For collection, the bird is firmly restrained in an upright and slightly tipped forward position. The overlying feathers are plucked, if necessary, and aseptically prepared with chlorhexidine gluconate or isopropyl alcohol. A small-gauge needle (21- to 27-gauge) is inserted through the skin and muscle directly into the pocket of fluid, if it is palpable. When an obvious pocket is not palpated, the needle is inserted roughly at the level of the umbilicus to avoid the liver cranially and directed to the right to avoid the ventriculus on the left [7].

Therapeutic delivery

Fluid therapy

Fluid therapy is commonly employed with sick and hospitalized patients. Most critically ill birds are presented with moderate to severe (>7%) dehydration, and they are often in a state of hypovolemic shock. Sick birds are reluctant to eat and drink and are at risk for becoming dehydrated. The route of delivery is indicated by the severity of dehydration, shock, and anemia. Birds that have mild dehydration (<5%) without shock may be hydrated with fluids provided orally or subcutaneously. Daily maintenance fluid requirements are estimated at 50 mL/kg/d [1]. Maintenance plus half the fluid deficit is generally administered during the first 12 to 24 hours,

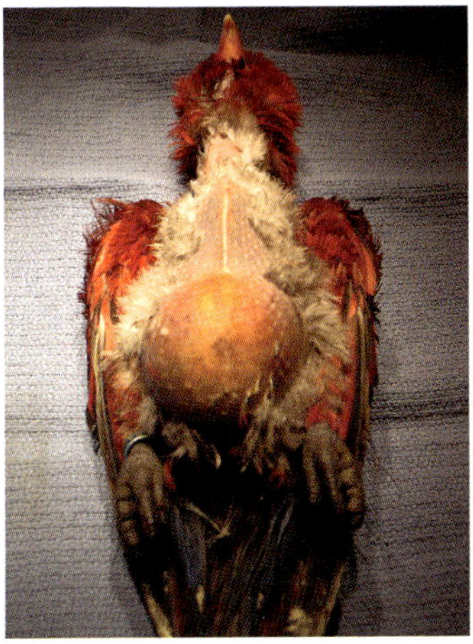

Fig. 1. Red lory (*Eos bornea*) with peritoneal effusion secondary to egg yolk peritonitis.

with the remainder of the deficit replaced over the following 48 hours [1]. Patients with moderate to severe dehydration, shock, or severe blood loss or anemia require intravenous (IV) or intraosseous (IO) fluid support. Fluid type is selected based on results of biochemical analysis, such as evaluation of electrolytes, glucose, and acid-base status. When these values are not known, a balanced isotonic crystalloid solution, such as lactated Ringer's solution, may be used for rehydration and hemodynamic support. For birds with hypotensive shock or hypoproteinemia, a colloidal solution such as hetastarch or Oxyglobin (Biopure, Cambridge, Massachusetts) may be used (at 5 to 15 mL/kg) in combination with crystalloids (at 30 to 40 mL/kg) to restore adequate tissue perfusion rapidly [2,10]. In cases of blood loss or severe anemia, whole blood from a suitable donor (ideally one of the same species) may be administered through an IV or IO catheter fitted with a standard small animal blood filter. IV and IO catheters may be used to administer dextrose solutions and other components of partial or total parenteral nutrition.

Per os fluid administration

Fluids may be administered per os (PO) through a red rubber or stainless steel ball-tipped feeding tube. Using a tube with a diameter greater than that of the trachea reduces the risk for inadvertent tracheal placement. The bird is firmly restrained in an upright position with the neck as extended as possible [1,6,11]. The crop should be palpated before infusion to estimate fluid volume. A speculum, such as a nylon dog bone or plastic syringe case, should always be used with a red rubber tube to prevent biting and severing of the tube. The tube is mildly lubricated, inserted into the left side of the mouth, and guided down the esophagus on the right side of the neck into the crop [6,11]. The neck should be palpated for the presence of both the feeding tube and the trachea, and the oral cavity should be inspected during infusion for the appearance of fluid [6]. Crop capacity may be estimated at roughly 30 to 50 mL/kg, although smaller volumes are often used in sick birds to decrease the risk for regurgitation and aspiration. Fluids should not be administered or should be used cautiously PO in birds with regurgitation, gastrointestinal stasis, neurologic diseases, or orthopedic problems of the legs, because of the risk for aspiration [12]. Fluids administered PO are poorly absorbed in cases of hypovolemic shock as a result of peripheral vasoconstriction.

Subcutaneous fluid administration

Fluids may be administered subcutaneously in the inguinal, interscapular, or axillary regions (Fig. 2). Volumes as great as 20 mL/kg may be administered in one location. The dorsal ventral neck should be avoided, owing to the presence of the cervicocephalic air sac. Fluids administered subcutaneously, like PO fluids, are poorly absorbed during hypovolemic shock.

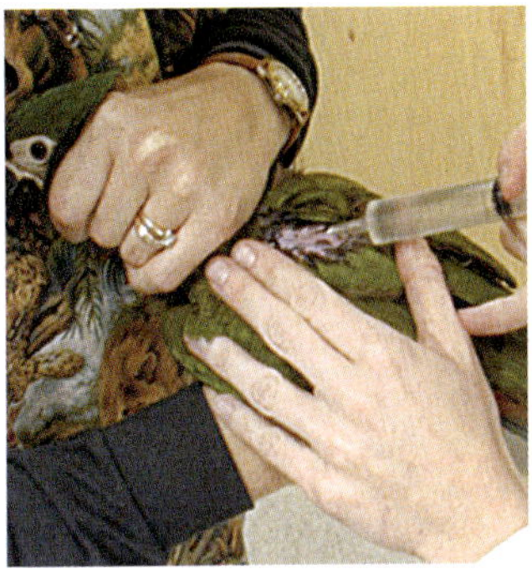

Fig. 2. Interscapular subcutaneous fluid administration in a severe macaw (*Ara severa*).

Intravenous fluid administration

Crystalloid volumes as great as 10 to 15 mL/kg may be safely administered as a single bolus, provided the bird is not critically anemic and repeat administration is not required [1,12]. The right jugular and basilic vein are most commonly used. When slow or ongoing vascular administration of fluid or medications is required, an IV or IO catheter should be placed. IV catheters are difficult to maintain owing to the thin nature of avian skin [6]. Sedation is not usually required but can be helpful to minimize patient movement during placement. The right jugular and basilic veins are most frequently used, although the medial metatarsal vein may be used in larger birds (Fig. 3) [6]. A small (24- to 26-gauge), over-the-needle catheter (eg, 24-gauge, 0.75-in catheter, Terumo Medical Corporation, Elkton, Maryland) is guided into the vein, butterflied with tape, and secured with acrylic glue or sutures to the skin. When one is using the basilic vein, the wing is wrapped in a figure-8 bandage. With a jugular catheter, the neck is lightly wrapped in cotton padding and Vetrap (3M, St. Paul, Minnesota). A fluid pump that can administer small fluid volumes, such as a syringe pump, should be used. Alternatively, a burette or frequent fluid boluses may be used.

Intraosseous fluid administration

Birds are often peripherally vasoconstricted during shock, and vascular access is difficult to impossible. Critically ill birds may not tolerate prolonged restraint or sedation for IV catheter placement. An IO catheter can usually be placed quickly and easily and provides a route for rapid intravascular delivery of fluids and drugs. Sedation reduces pain of insertion and decreases patient movement but may be risky in critically ill birds. The author has experienced several cases in which a profoundly ill bird died during placement of an IO catheter, perhaps partially because of pain and the resultant sympathetic response. A small volume of 2%

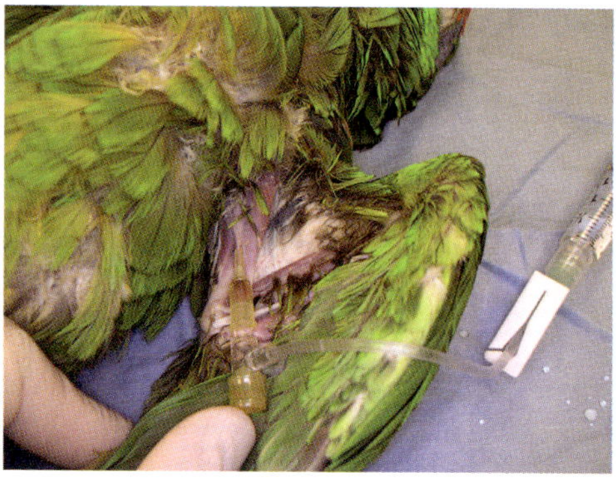

Fig. 3. Placement of an intravenous catheter in the left ulnar vein of a green cheeked Amazon parrot (*Amazona viridigenalis*) using a 24-gauge over-the-needle catheter (Terumo Medical Corporation, Elkton, Maryland).

lidocaine without epinephrine (as much as 4 mg/kg) may be instilled into the skin, subcutaneous tissues, and periosteum before catheter insertion. The author has found that the use of lidocaine has resulted in a reduced number of deaths in critically ill birds during catheter placement.

The distal ulna or proximal tibia is most commonly used [1,6,12]. Potentially pneumatic bones such as the humerus should be avoided. Ideally, a 20- to 25-gauge short spinal needle is used (eg, 22-gauge, 1.5-in spinal needle, Sherwood Medical, St. Louis, Missouri). Spinal needles contain a metal stylet that prevents bone coring and needle occlusion. Alternatively, a 22- to 25-gauge hypodermic needle can be used. The lumen may be occluded with sterile surgical wire before insertion. If the lumen remains open during placement and becomes plugged, the needle may be removed and replaced. However, replacement often enlarges the size of the hole and increases leakage around the catheter. Once inserted, the catheter is flushed to check for patency. It is then connected to a preflushed T-port and fluid line and secured by butterfly taping and acrylic glue or sutures. For the distal ulna (Fig. 4), the distal dorsal condyle is palpated and the surrounding site is plucked and aseptically prepared with chlorhexidine gluconate or isopropyl alcohol. The needle is inserted just ventrally to the condyle and directed proximally toward the elbow along the shaft of the ulna [1,6,12]. The catheter is connected to the flushed fluid line and secured in place; the wing may be wrapped in a figure-8 bandage. Birds will occasionally chew at the bandages, and covering the catheter and bandage with flaps of tape or a syringe case can prevent damage to the catheter [1]. For the proximal tibia, the stifle is flexed and the tibial crest identified. Once the site is plucked and prepared, the needle is advanced through the tibial crest down the shaft of the tibiotarsus toward the hock. The catheter is secured in place and attached to the flushed fluid line, and the leg is lightly padded and bandaged.

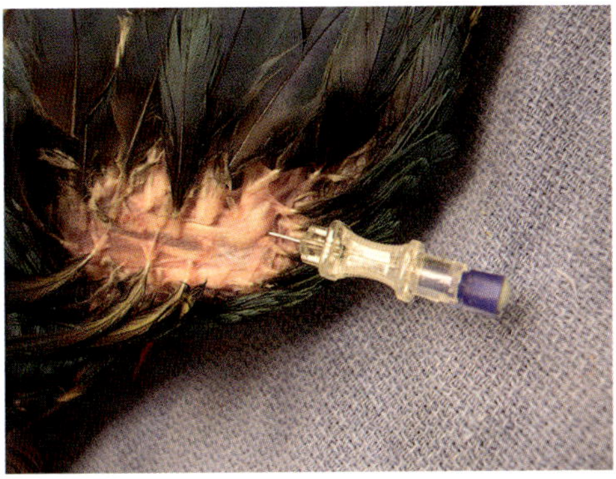

Fig. 4. Placement of an intraosseous catheter in the distal ulna of a blue and gold macaw (*Ara ararauna*) using a 22-gauge, 1.5-in spinal needle (Sherwood Medical, St. Louis, Missouri).

Nutritional support

Crop infusion

Sick birds are reluctant to eat and usually need nutritional support. If the gastrointestinal tract is functioning well, patients may be force fed by crop infusion. A red rubber or stainless steel ball-tipped feeding tube is typically used [12]. The technique is the same as that described for PO fluid administration. A safe starting point for fluid volume per feeding has been reported as 30 to 50 mL/kg [12]; however, the author will usually start with 20 to 30 mL/kg and increase the volume according to what the patient tolerates. The crop should be palpated before infusion, and the residual volume should be considered when determining infusion volume. Enteral nutritional products used include powdered formulas designed for sick birds (eg, Emeraid Critical Care Diet, Lafeber Co., Cornell, Illinois) or growing birds (eg, Exact Hand-Feeding Formula, Kaytee Products, Chilton, Wisconsin) or human enteral products [1,11]. Because powdered, rehydrated formulas occasionally clog the feeding tube, use of the largest-diameter feeding tube that is safely feasible is suggested. All other procedures should be completed before tube feeding, in case the bird regurgitates [1]. Caloric requirements should be calculated for each bird. The basal metabolic rate (BMR) is calculated by the following formula: $BMR(kcal) = 78 \, (W_{kg}^{0.75})$. The maintenance energy requirement (MER) for adult hospitalized birds is approximately 1.5 times the BMR [6,10]. Adjustments are then made to the MER to accommodate specific illnesses; these have been presented in table form elsewhere [6,11].

For example, the BMR of a 500-g African gray parrot is about 46 kcal/d. The MER is 1.5 times this figure, or 69 kcal/d. The adjustment factor to use when this bird has mild trauma is 1.0 to 1.2 times the MER, or approximately 76 kcal/d. The caloric concentration of most enteric formulas ranges from 1.5 to 2.0 kcal/mL [11]. If the formula used on this bird is 1.6 kcal/mL, the total volume will be roughly 47 mL/d. Most hospitalized birds are tube fed two to four times daily [11]. For our example bird, this amounts to 12 mL every 6 hours or 16 mL every 8 hours.

Esophagostomy tube

Esophagostomy tube placement is indicated in cases of severe beak trauma and diseases of the oral cavity or proximal esophagus, such as abscesses and neoplasia [12]. Esophagostomy tubes may be directed down the postcrop esophagus, bypassing the crop in cases of severe crop burn. Silicone or polyurethane catheters (eg, Kendall Argyle Feeding Tube, Kendall Co., Mansfield, Massachusetts) are softer and stiffen less with age than red rubber or polyvinylchloride tubes. The technique is nicely described by Tully [13]. A stab incision is made through the skin and esophageal wall, directed by a hemostat guided into the precrop esophagus at the cranial to midportion of the right side of the neck. The tube is guided through the crop into the proventriculus and secured in place with tape butterflied to the catheter and secured with acrylic glue or sutures. Wrapping of the neck is not always necessary. Tubes should be flushed with water after every feeding and may be left in place for as long as 7 weeks [13]. The tube is removed and the opening allowed to heal by granulation. Surgical closure is not required.

Duodenostomy feeding tube

In cases of severe gastric disease, such as proventricular dilatation disease, the stomach can be bypassed by a duodenostomy tube to provide nutritional support. This technique has been described elsewhere [6,12,13]. To summarize, the bird is placed under general anesthesia and the ventral abdominal area is plucked and aseptically prepared. A ventral midline incision is made through skin and the linea. A stab incision is made into the ascending limb of the duodenum, and a silicone or polyurethane feeding tube or a 17- to 20-gauge over-the-needle jugular catheter is inserted into the lumen. The tube diameter should be no greater than one third the diameter of the duodenum. A second stab incision is made through the body wall, and the tube is fed through this incision and secured in place with a pursestring or Chinese fingertrap pattern [6,12,13]. The tube should remain in place for at least 5 days to ensure that a good seal between the intestine and body wall is formed; this precaution should decrease the chance of peritonitis due to intestinal leakage when the tube is removed [14].

Medication administration

Injectable therapeutics

Injectable therapeutics may be delivered subcutaneously, IV, or IO as described earlier for fluid therapy. Intramuscular injections are typically administered into the pectoral musculature along either side of the midkeel region. The feathers are wiped away from the featherless tract along the ventral midline of the keel with isopropyl alcohol. Small (25- to 28-gauge), short ($\leq$0.625-in) needles are generally advised in psittacines. The needle is inserted at a short ($<30°$) angle into the muscle (Fig. 5).[2]

Nebulization

Direct application of therapeutics into the upper and lower airways by nebulization can increase treatment success for cases of bacterial and fungal sinusitis, tracheitis, bronchopneumonia, and air sacculitis. Many antibiotics, antifungals, and mucolytics have been used in nebulization solutions, although mucolytics may be prohibitively irritating [11]. Ultrasonic nebulizers are capable of emitting a particle size of less than 0.5 to 3 μm, which is believed necessary to penetrate the air capillaries and air sacs for the treatment of air sacculitis, because the diameter of the air capillaries ranges in size from 3 to 10 μm [1,6,11,15]. Compressor nebulizers generally are less expensive but do not emit such a small particle size; they are therefore more useful for the treatment of upper respiratory disease. The nebulizer is typically attached with tubing to an anesthesia induction chamber or similar glass or plastic container. The bird is placed inside the chamber after lubrication of the eyes and nebulized for 10 to 15 minutes, one to two times daily. Concentrations of antimicrobials and other drugs suitable for nebulization have been previously published [16].

Air sac intubation

In cases of severe upper airway obstruction, such as tracheal aspergillosis or a tracheal foreign body, it becomes necessary to provide an alternate route for ventilation by means of an air sac cannula [6,11,12]. Surgical access to the head and neck is easier after placement of an air sac cannula for general anesthesia [11]. The bird can be mask-induced with inhalant anesthesia, although placement may be performed without anesthesia in birds at risk for immediate death [12]. More clinicians are comfortable with a left lateral approach, because this is the same approach used for laparoscopy. The upper leg is flexed and abducted to access the space caudal to the last rib or between the last two ribs. An incision is made through the skin about one third of the way down the length of the femur. A stab incision is made through the abdominal musculature using sterile mosquito hemostats (Fig. 6) [6,11,12].

---

[2] Editor's note: Some practitioners have found that injecting a known irritating drug (such as enrofloxacin) into a subcutaneous fluid pocket (rather than intramuscularly) may decrease local tissue irritation. Initial studies by Flammer (Proceedings of the Association of Avian Veterinarians 2005:4–5) on enrofloxacin indicate that this technique may not decrease the effective level of medication administered.

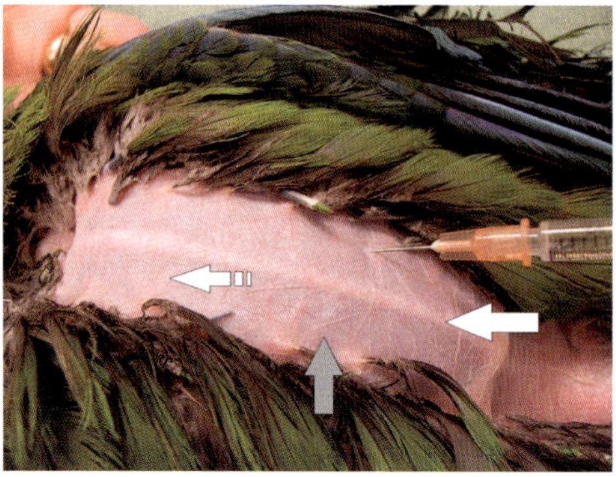

Fig. 5. Intramuscular injection. The feathers are wiped away with isopropyl alcohol, exposing the sternal apterium, or featherless tract of skin (*gray arrow*), and the sternum (*solid white arrow*). Injection into the cranial portion of the muscle (*dashed white arrow*) should be avoided to prevent inadvertent injection into the pectoral vasculature, located in this region.

A red rubber feeding tube or sterile endotracheal tube of similar diameter to the trachea is guided between the halves of the hemostats into the air sac (which will be either the caudal thoracic or abdominal air sac [11]). Air flow is checked with a feather or glass slide held over the opening [6,11,12]. The tube is butterfly-taped and sutured to the skin. The tube may be left in place for at least 3 to 5 days [11]. The tip of the cannula can be cultured on removal. Direct application of antimicrobials or nebulization of drugs may be performed through the air sac cannula [11].

Oxygen therapy

Many birds are presented with dyspnea or profound weakness and appear to improve once placed in an oxygenated enclosure for several minutes

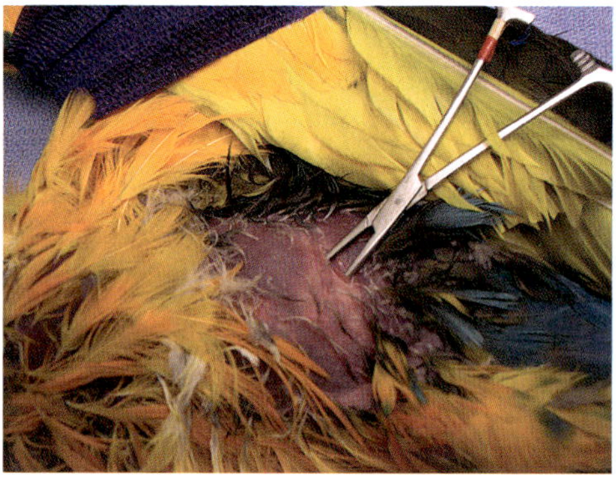

Fig. 6. Surgical approach for placement of an air sac cannula caudal to the last rib on the left lateral flank in a blue and gold macaw (*Ara ararauna*).

[12]. Critically ill birds should be preoxygenated before restraint, sample collection, and administration of therapeutics if time allows. A mask or blow-by oxygen may be used to provide oxygen during restraint [10,12]. Several human cardiac care guidelines suggest oxygen concentrations of 60% to 80% for initial resuscitation in the acute respiratory patient. Cages are inefficient delivery systems for oxygen and may require flow rates of 10 to 15 L/min to achieve oxygen concentrations of more than 50%. However, cages eliminate the need for patient restraint and invasive procedures [17]. Oxygen concentrations of greater than 40% should be limited in duration because of the risk for oxygen toxicosis [10].[3]

Pain management

Birds are inherently adept at hiding signs of illness and pain. Most birds presented for illness or trauma experience some degree of pain or discomfort and may benefit from analgesia. Butorphanol at 0.5 to 1 mg/kg IM has been shown to provide effective analgesia to birds. Buprenorphine does not appear to have analgesic effects in avian patients at the dosages evaluated. A safe and effective dosage of fentanyl has yet to be determined [10]. Meloxicam at 0.1 to 0.5 mg/kg PO every 24 hours or 0.1 to 0.2 mg/kg intramuscularly every 24 hours [18] is also an effective analgesic for birds.

Grooming

Flight reduction (wing feather trimming)

Trimming of the remiges (or "flight feathers") is designed to curtail flight capabilities of psittacine birds. Although the goal of the "wing clip" is not controversial, the many ways to perform it have been disputed [5,12]. It is probably correct to state that there is no single clipping technique that is best for every bird in every situation. Most often, practitioners clip five to eight of the outermost primary feathers (the outer 10 flight feathers). One should consider clipping fewer primaries in clumsy, heavy-bodied birds, such as African grays, and a larger number of primaries in gliding, light-bodied birds, such as cockatiels. Some trim the feathers at the level of the calamus (quill), shorter than the ventral covert feathers so that the clipped ends are not exposed. Some clinicians and many owners clip the primaries a few centimeters longer than the tips of the ventral covert feathers. Some clinicians perform a "cosmetic clip," leaving the outermost one to two primaries (primaries #9 and #10) unclipped for cosmetic purposes and

---

[3] Editor's note: In most incubators and oxygen cages available, oxygen flow rates of less than 5 L/min should provide increased oxygen concentrations without reaching the toxic level of 40%; it is best to monitor these levels whenever possible.

theoretically to protect the distal soft tissues and bone from injury. Some believe that this clip allows the bird to gain height but causes it to lose maneuverability, increasing the risk for injury during flight attempts. Unilateral wing clipping probably more effectively reduces flight than a bilateral clip, but it may cause the bird to spiral during flight attempts and falls, increasing the risk for injury [5,12].

Immature birds are clumsy and tend to fall hard and frequently, particularly African gray parrots (*Psittacus erythacus*) and cockatiels (*Nymphicus hollandicus*). These birds should have fewer feathers clipped until they strengthen their pectoral muscles and become less clumsy. If the clip is inadequate, additional feathers may be trimmed at a later date. Every feather should be checked for blood within its shaft (blood feather) before clipping. The feathers should be clipped with sharp, blunt-tipped, or suture scissors or cat-nail clippers. Cutting with dull scissors tends to shred the feathers, possibly increasing the risks for chewing. Most psittacines molt one to two times a year and need trims as frequently. Owners who wish their birds to remain clipped should be alert for increased flight capabilities or the presence of long flight feathers that cross one another over the lower back.

Birds are often presented with damaged, bleeding blood feathers. During the growth phase of a primary, which can take 3 to 4 weeks or longer, the feather is vulnerable to trauma. A cracked blood feather can continue to ooze blood, requiring extraction. The bird is restrained and the wing held and braced securely to protect it from trauma. Straight hemostats or needle-nosed pliers are used to grasp the calamus. Firm and steady traction is applied to the feather as it is pulled from the follicle in its natural direction. When the feather is broken or sheared within the follicle, sterile hemostats may be guided between the feather and follicle to grasp it. Pressure is applied to the empty follicle for a few seconds to a minute or so, because it often bleeds. Because blood feathers are often broken within the follicle, and there is some risk for injury to the wing, the typical bird owner is not advised to attempt blood feather extraction at home. The extracted feather will immediately be replaced by a new blood feather, which is also at risk for injury.

Nail trimming

Psittacines possess a zygodactyl foot, meaning that digits 1 and 4 face back and digits 2 and 3 face forward [5]. Birds are often presented for nail clipping when the nails become intolerably sharp or long enough to become entrapped. The "quick" of the bird nail is quite long, and clipping often results in pain and bleeding. Hemorrhage after clipping with cat, dog, or human nail clippers can be controlled with application of a styptic powder (eg, ferric subsulfate or silver nitrate). A rotary hobby tool may be used to grind the tips short and blunt, and hemorrhage can usually be stopped by the heat of the tool. Hoop cautery tools simultaneously cut and cauterize the nail and are used by many practitioners [5]. Some owners are able to file nails at home with an Emory board. An appropriate position to clip the nail is at the level where it would form a quarter circle [12].

Beak trimming

The psittacine beak consists of an outer layer of hard keratin covering bone. The beak grows outward from the skin margin to the tomium (cutting edge). The upper and lower beaks keep each other filed to a normal level. Routine beak trimming is not required for most healthy psittacines. Diseases of the beak, such as trauma, infection, neoplasia, and congenital malocclusion, cause the beaks to wear improperly and become overgrown, often necessitating frequent trims. Maxillary beak tip elongation and hyperkeratosis may be associated with liver disease and warrant clinical investigation. The outer layer of keratin can become thick and flaky in some healthy birds, and beak trimming may be done in these birds for cosmetic purposes. The tomium and outer keratin of the beak are typically filed down with a rotary hobby tool fitted with a stone or sandpaper tip. The sandpaper tips are disposable, reducing the risk for disease transmission between birds. The practitioner should be familiar with the normal beak anatomy of each species of psittacine requiring a beak trim. Some species, such as some macaws, normally possess an elongated maxillary beak. If the beak is trimmed too short, the highly vascular deeper tissues can bleed significantly. Hemorrhage may be controlled by direct pressure or application of a styptic gel or liquid, epinephrine, or thrombin.

References

[1] Rupley AE. Manual of avian practice. Philadelphia: Saunders; 1997.
[2] Lichtenberger M. Emergency care of birds. Presented at the Western Veterinary Conference. Las Vegas, NV, February 11–14, 2002.
[3] Romagnano A. Examination and preventative medicine protocols in psittacines. Vet Clin North Am Exot Anim Pract 1999;2:333–55.
[4] Lawton MPC. The physical examination. In: Tully TN, Lawton MPC, Dorrestein GM, editors. Avian medicine. Oxford (UK): Butterworth-Heinemann; 2000. p. 26–42.
[5] Speer BL. Current pet avian disease trends. Presented at the Western Veterinary Conference, Las Vegas, NV, February 11–14, 2002.
[6] Jenkins JR. Hospital techniques and supportive care. In: Altman RB, Clubb SL, Dorrestein GM, et al, editors. Avian medicine and surgery. Philadelphia: Saunders; 1997. p. 232–52.
[7] Echols S. Collecting diagnostic samples in avian patients. Vet Clin North Am Exot Anim Pract 1999;2:621–49.
[8] Antinoff N. Diagnosis and treatment options for megabacteria (*Macrorhabdus ornithogaster*). J Avian Med Surg 2004;18:189–95.
[9] Harris D. Clinical tests. In: Tully TN, Lawton MPC, Dorrestein GM, editors. Avian medicine. Oxford (UK): Butterworth-Heinemann; 2000. p. 43–51.
[10] Wilson H. Avian critical care and stabilization: so much we can do! In: Mazzaferro EM, editor. Proceedings of the International Veterinary Emergency and Critical Care Symposium. Atlanta (GA): 2005. p. 75–9.

[11] Quesenberry KE, Hillyer EV. Supportive care and emergency therapy. In: Ritchie BW, Harrison GJ, Harrison LR, editors. Avian medicine: principles and application. Lake Worth (FL): Wingers Publishing; 1994. p. 382–416.
[12] Harris D. Therapeutic avian techniques. Seminars in Avian and Exotic Pet Medicine 1997;6: 55–62.
[13] Tully TN. Psittacine therapeutics. Vet Clin North Am Exot Anim Pract 2000;3:59–90.
[14] Bennett RA. Soft tissue surgery. In: Ritchie BW, Harrison GJ, Harrison LR, editors. Avian medicine: principles and application. Lake Worth (FL): Wingers Publishing; 1994. p. 1124–5.
[15] deMatos R, Morrisey JK. Emergency and critical care of small psittacines and passerines. Seminars in Avian and Exotic Pet Medicine 2005;14:90–105.
[16] Carpenter JW. Exotic animal formulary. St. Louis (MO): Elsevier; 2001.
[17] Crowe DT. Oxygen therapy: techniques and monitoring. Presented at the International Veterinary Emergency and Critical Care Symposium, September 8–12, 2004. p. 554–6.
[18] Marx KL. Therapeutic agents. In: Harrison GJ, Lightfoot TL, editors. Clinical avian medicine. Palm Beach (FL): Spix Publishing; 2006. p. 293.

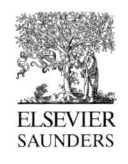

Common Procedures in Other Avian Species

Angela M. Lennox, DVM, DABVP–Avian

Avian and Exotic Animal Clinic of Indianapolis, 9330 Waldemar Road, Indianapolis, IN 46268, USA

Although psittacine species represent the majority of avian patients seen in most exotic animal practices, nonpsittacine species such as passerines and galliformes may be presented as pets, as members of zoo collections, or as injured or ill wildlife. Many features of handling, restraint, sample collection, medicine, and surgery are similar in psittacine and nonpsittacine species. In many cases, the equipment required will be similar as well, with a few modifications.

Handling and restraint

Size and temperament differences among these species can be extreme, ranging from the relatively defenseless finch, dove, and pigeon species and pet poultry to powerful and potentially aggressive large waterfowl. Handling and restraint of waterfowl are discussed elsewhere in this issue.

Restraint of psittacine species is well described. Various-sized towels are used to grasp the bird firmly around the neck and help prevent wing thrashing. Restriction of the coelomic cavity and consequent potentially dangerous impairment of respiratory effort must be carefully avoided. (For further illustration of this risk, it should be remembered that at one time "thoracic compression" was listed as an acceptable euthanasia technique for birds.)

Most nonpsittacine birds may be restrained using the same method (Fig. 1). In some cases, for example very small birds, towels and cloths may actually hamper examination, and restraint may be accomplished with a single-hand technique (Fig. 2). Pet poultry are generally calm and easy to handle. One may restrain them by manually holding the wings to the body as the bird stands on the examination table or by grasping the

E-mail address: birddr@aol.com

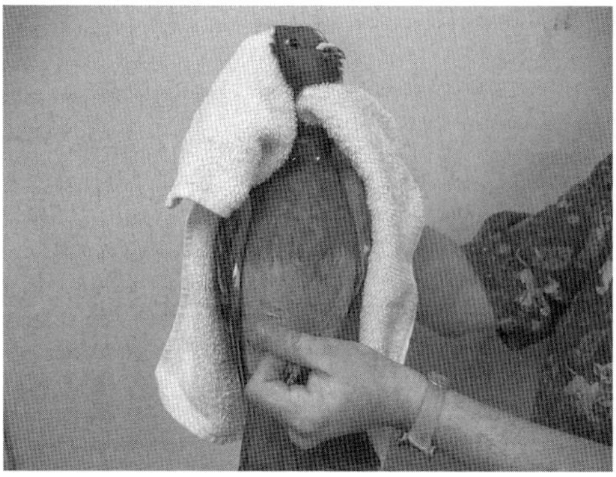

Fig. 1. Safe towel restraint of a pigeon.

wings at the proximal humeri (Fig. 3). Heavy poultry should not be lifted by the humeri because of the risk for damage to bones or soft tissue.

Although some nonpsittacine birds are acclimated to frequent human contact and handling—for example, birds used for exhibition and very tame or hand-reared birds—others experience greater levels of handling stress. Therefore, capture and restraint should be accomplished as efficiently and carefully as possible, and handling time should be minimized.

All birds should be examined and palpated thoroughly and carefully, from oral cavity to vent, to avoid missing subtle abnormalities, especially in areas covered with feathers. Physical examination of passerines and gallinaceous birds is described in detail elsewhere [1,2]. Initial evaluation should be performed before restraining the bird. Mental attitude, gait, and respiratory rate and effort give important clues to the overall condition of the patient. Severely depressed patients or those exhibiting signs of

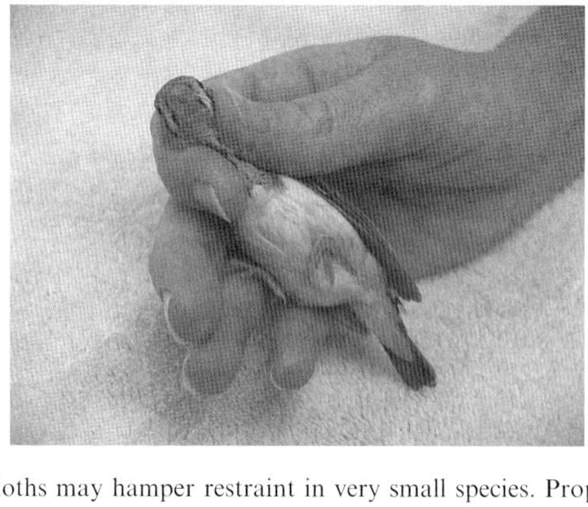

Fig. 2. Towels or cloths may hamper restraint in very small species. Proper hand restraint of a zebra finch.

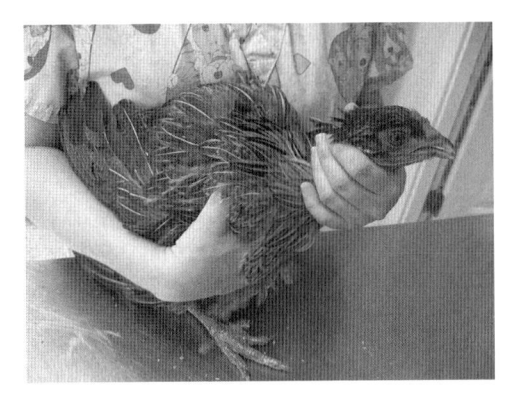

Fig. 3. Calm pet poultry may be restrained by grasping both humeri in one hand. Heavy poultry should not be lifted off the table in this manner.

respiratory distress often benefit from stabilization before the thorough physical examination begins (see section on Supportive Care).

An accurate weight in grams must be obtained for all patients. Therefore, scales must be able to accommodate species weighing from less than 20 g to several kilograms. Small flighted birds may be weighed in small closed containers placed directly on the scale, with adjustments made for the weight of the container (Fig. 4).

Sample collection

Collection of blood samples for diagnostic testing requires appropriately sized needles and syringes. In birds in general, blood may be safely collected from the right jugular, ulnar, or medial tibiotarsal veins (Figs. 5 and 6).

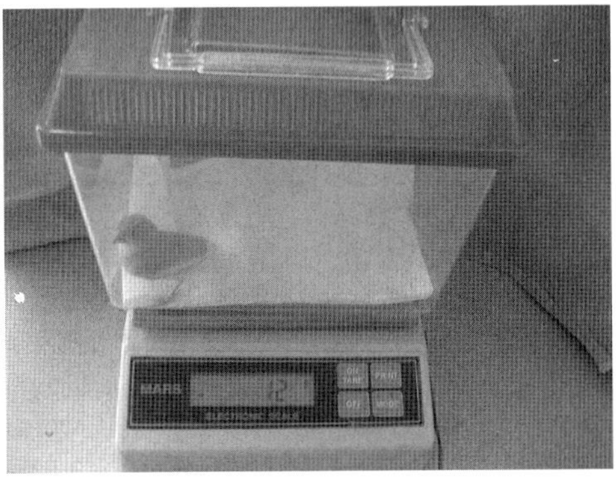

Fig. 4. Accurate weight must be obtained in all avian patients. The scale has been tared for the weight of the container.

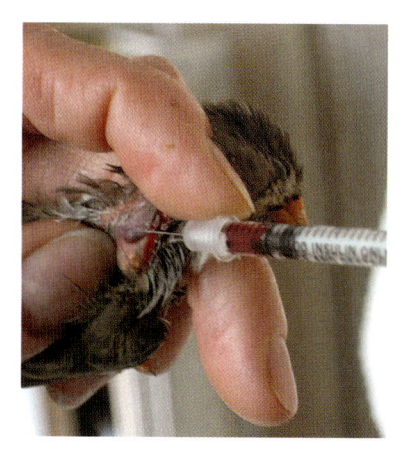

Fig. 5. Collection of blood from the jugular vein of a zebra finch. Care must be taken not to exceed the maximum volume of blood that may be safely collected, especially in very small patients.

However, a few anatomic variations can complicate phlebotomy, for example, feathered feet and legs, horny keratin epidermis in certain galliform species, and presence of a plexus of veins instead of a discrete jugular vein in pigeons [3].

Determination of appropriate volume to collect follows the same guideline as for other avian species: roughly 1% of body weight. For a 20-g finch, this means 0.02 mL at the maximum, whereas a 2-kg goose could easily contribute 20 mL of whole blood [4].

Although blood collection may appear daunting in smaller species, its value should not be underestimated. A single drop of blood collected in a hematocrit tube is more than adequate for in-house complete blood count in

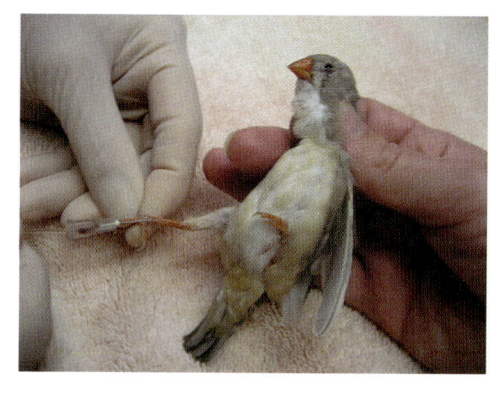

Fig. 6. The medial tarsal vein may be used to collect small samples. Drops of blood collected into a hematocrit are enough for determination of a complete blood count in even the smallest avian species.

even the smallest avian species (see Fig. 6). White blood cells are counted manually with a hemocytometer, and remaining blood is spun for determination of packed cell volume and total serum solids. Even when a hemocytometer is unavailable, an estimated white blood cell count may be obtained from a well-prepared blood film. Techniques for avian complete blood count are described in detail elsewhere [4]. Most avian reference laboratories will also evaluate on request a well-prepared blood film submitted alone.

Other diagnostic samples include specimens such as feces for culture and sensitivity, cytology, and parasite evaluation and cytology and histopathology of various tissues.

Treatment and supportive care

Oral medications for psittacines are often administered in liquid form, because the likelihood of safely dosing and administering medication in tablet form is negligible. However, tablet administration to larger passerines, galliformes, and other "softbill" species is relatively easy. Using the same principle as for pill administration in dogs, one uses the finger to guide the tablet gently over the rim of the glottis, located at the base of the tongue, and into the esophagus. Regurgitation of medication is uncommon. The glottis of many birds is large; hence it is possible inadvertently to introduce medications directly into the trachea. Medications in liquid form should be given by syringe in small boluses to prevent aspiration.

Intramuscular (IM) injection sites are chosen depending on patient size and available muscle mass. The pectoral muscle mass is the preferred site for IM injection, because studies in chickens show that a percentage of blood flow of vasculature of the legs is directed to organs such as the kidneys [5,6]. Some species, in particular certain galliformes, may have reduced pectoral muscle mass with better-developed muscles of the leg. Drug distribution and pharmacokinetics should be kept in mind when choosing injection sites in avian species.

Subcutaneous injection of fluids is relatively easy to perform in most birds. The most common site for injection is the web of skin between the leg and the body wall, but subscapular and axillary routes have also been described [7].

Feasibility of intravenous (IV) injection depends on the size of the patient and access to available veins. In all but the smallest birds, IV administration into the ulnar vein is ideal. The vein is easily visible, and correct needle placement and administration are readily apparent (Fig. 7). Jugular or tarsal veins may also be used for this purpose, depending on patient size, tractability, and ease of restraint [7].

IV or intraosseous (IO) catheterization is possible even in smaller patients. Common sites for IV catheterization in smaller birds include jugular, tarsal, and ulnar veins, and sites for IO catheterization include the proximal

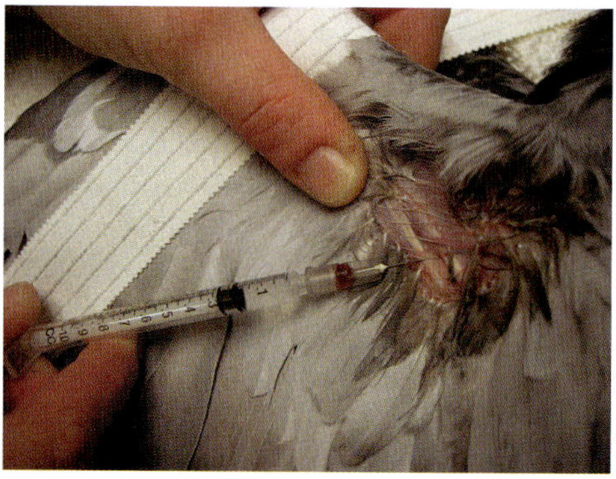

Fig. 7. IV injection into the ulnar vein of a pigeon.

tibia and ulna (Fig. 8) [7]. Sites are chosen based on the size of the patient and likelihood of being able adequately to secure the catheter in position. In the author's experience, IO catheterization of the tibiotarsus is easy to perform and maintain.

Anorexic patients may require force-feeding. The ideal hand-feeding product should match the natural diet of the bird in question and be able to pass through a syringe and feeding tube or needle (Table 1). Keep in mind that, although many of the suggested foods are excellent as a part of short-term medical care, in some species they may be inadequate for longer-term care and rehabilitation. Commercial metal ball-tipped syringes are available for hand feeding reptiles and psittacines, and these are excellent for use in smaller, parrot-sized birds (Figs. 9 and 10). Waterfowl and other larger softbill birds incapable of lacerating a rubber tube may be fed with various-sized red rubber catheters. Both tubes and needles are introduced

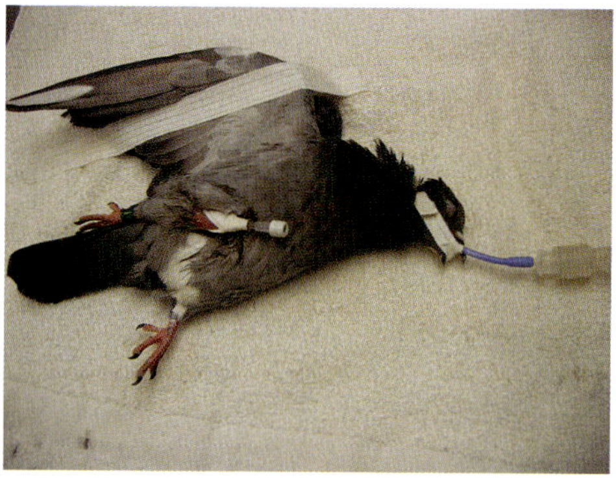

Fig. 8. Proper placement of an intraosseous catheter into the tibiotarsus of a pigeon. The catheter (in this case a 22-gauge injection needle) is secured with tape and fitted with a standard catheter injection cap.

Table 1
Suggested tube feeding products for various nonpsittacine birds

Species	Product
Granivorous birds: Some songbirds, poultry, granivorous waterfowl (many ducks, swans, geese)	Commercial parrot hand-feeding formula for unweaned chicks
Carnivorous/Piscivorous birds: Herons, cranes, other fish-eaters	Carnivore care diet, Oxbow Pet Products, Murdock, Nebraska Canned high-protein, convalescent dog/cat products, such as Hill's A/D (Hill's Pet Nutrition, Topeka, Kansas), Commercial trout chow reduced to powder with a food processor
Insectivorous birds: Many songbirds	Commercial insectivore diet reduced to powder with a food processor Canned high-protein convalescent dog/cat products, such as Hill's A/D

Powdered formulations are reconstituted with water in a dilution to allow passage through the feeding tube.

past the glottis and into the distal esophagus or crop. Care must be taken not to enter the trachea. An easy technique to determine proper feeding tube or needle placement is to palpate the neck after introducing the tube. The presence of two separate firm structures (trachea and tube) indicates that the tube or needle cannot have been introduced into the trachea.

Occasionally medications may be administered topically. The most common topically administered drug in the author's practice is ivermectin. All medications must be dosed carefully based on an accurate measurement of patient weight, and in some cases they may require careful dilution. Even apparently innocuous topical ointments may reach toxic levels in smaller birds that ingest large amounts during preening [8].

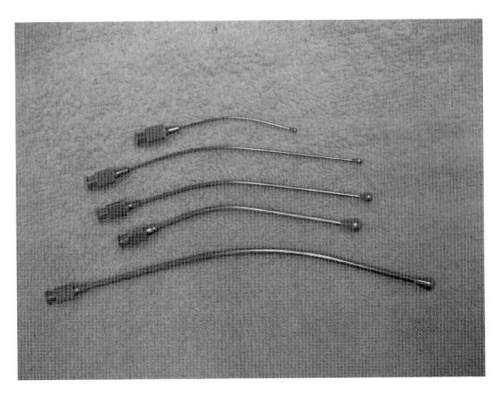

Fig. 9. Various sizes of ball-tipped metal gavage feeding needles are useful for administration of oral fluids and hand-feeding formulas. The relatively large ball of the needle helps prevent inadvertent introduction of the needle into the trachea.

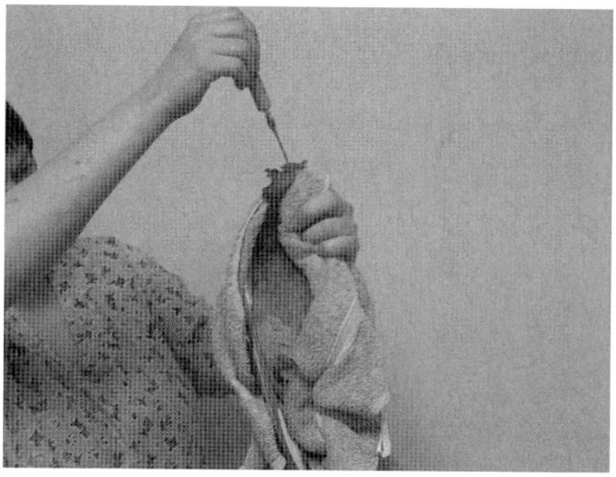

Fig. 10. Hand feeding a pigeon with a curved metal ball-tipped gavage needle and commercial psittacine hand-feeding formula.

Hospitalization of all birds is avoided unless necessary, because of the stress of an unfamiliar environment. In cases where hospitalization represents the patient's best interest, the hospital must include safe, quiet enclosures out of visual and auditory range of other animals, especially predator species such as dogs, cats, and ferrets. The ideal hospital cage is climate controlled and can accommodate administration of oxygen or medication administered by nebulization. A number of commercial incubators are manufactured specifically for small exotic pets (Fig. 11).

Anesthesia

Patient evaluation before anesthesia includes history, careful examination, and, ideally, preanesthetic blood work, which often may be safely collected in all but the smallest patients (see Sample Collection).

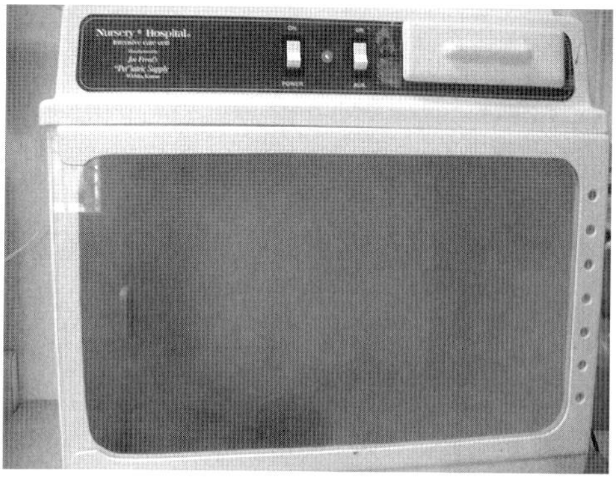

Fig. 11. Temperature-controlled commercial incubator, useful for smaller exotic patients.

Preanesthetic fasting length varies with the size, metabolic rate, and condition of the bird. Many references recommend no more than 4 to 6 hours for smaller birds and 8 to 12 hours for larger birds [9]. In debilitated patients, anesthetic procedures may need to be delayed or fasting times reduced. In the author's experience, the highest rates of complications due to aspiration are in birds that have diseases or conditions producing delayed gastrointestinal transit times. When anesthesia is necessary in birds with delayed transit time or food or liquid in the crop, risk for aspiration may be reduced by careful handling, maintenance in an upright position for as long as possible, placement of an endotracheal tube, and placement of a strip of flexible bandage material securely around the neck to prevent or reduce reflux of crop material.

Isoflurane or sevoflurane induced by means of a facemask and maintained with a mask or endotracheal tube remains the anesthetic of choice in all birds in which manual restraint is feasible and safe for both bird and anesthetist. The use of parenteral anesthetic agents such as ketamine hydrochloride has decreased significantly in avian practice [9]. Intubation is possible in birds as small as finches. The benefits of endotracheal intubation during anesthetic procedures in any species are well understood. Anecdotally, however, the author finds that occlusion of small endotracheal tubes with respiratory secretions may occur more commonly in smaller avian patients. Size differences and head and beak structure modifications necessitate modifications in anesthetic cones and endotracheal tubes. Commercial anesthetic cones for birds with extremely long beaks (such as toucans) may not be available. In these cases, basic ingenuity may provide acceptable alternatives. Materials described for homemade anesthetic cones include liter soft drink bottles (Fig. 12).

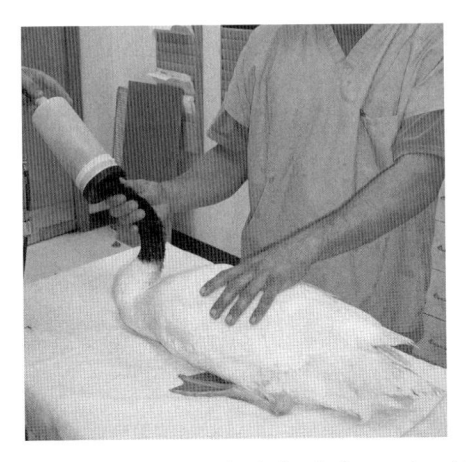

Fig. 12. Modified mask constructed from a plastic bottle for use in a bird with an extremely long beak. These types of masks are useful for induction of toucan species as well. (*Courtesy of* M. Kramer.)

Conversely, tiny patients require accordingly sized cones. Although smaller cones and tubes specifically for exotic patients are commercially available, these may still not be adequate for extremely small patients (Fig. 13). Induction of anesthesia in very small patients may be accomplished using a standard canine/feline anesthetic cone as a miniature induction chamber (Fig. 14). Modified syringe cases of various sizes are described (Fig. 15).

Anesthetic monitoring in avian species is well described. Critical attention must be given to thermoregulation, because drops in body temperature can be associated with cardiac instability [9]. A study comparing the capability of various heat sources to maintain body temperature in the anesthetized avian patient showed radiant sources, such as heat bulbs and ceramic heaters, to be most effective [10]. Other heat sources include heating pads, warm-water heating pads, and forced air heaters. Very small patients may be positioned on a warm water–filled examination glove (Fig. 16). An accurate measurement of body temperature trends may be obtained using a flexible temperature probe. Veterinary Specialty Products (Mission, Kansas) provides a constant read-out probe that may be gently placed into the crop of all but the smallest avian patients (Fig. 17).

Some standard monitoring equipment can be adapted to even very small patients. Although monitoring equipment is important, the most crucial component is the experienced and attentive veterinary anesthetist, who evaluates standard parameters such as reaction to painful stimuli, cardiac and respiratory rate and character, and mucous membrane color. The most versatile monitoring tool is the Doppler flow detector evaluation of the cardiovascular system (Parks Medical Electronics, Aloha, Oregon). The Doppler probe may be adapted to many patient body types and locations. The most useful location in the smallest avian patients is the ulnar artery (see Fig. 16). EKG and pulse oximetry are also described [11]. Other anesthetic

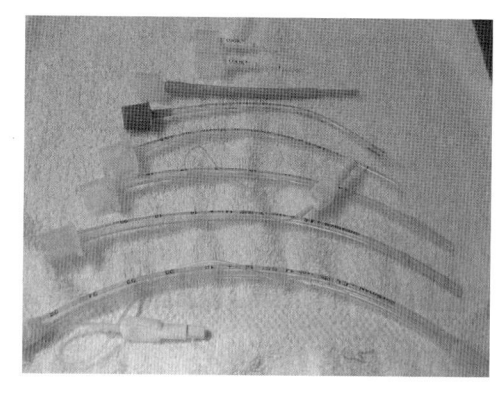

Fig. 13. Several manufacturers produce very small endotracheal tubes specifically designed for avian and exotic animal use (SurgiVet [formerly Cook], Waukesha, Wisconsin).

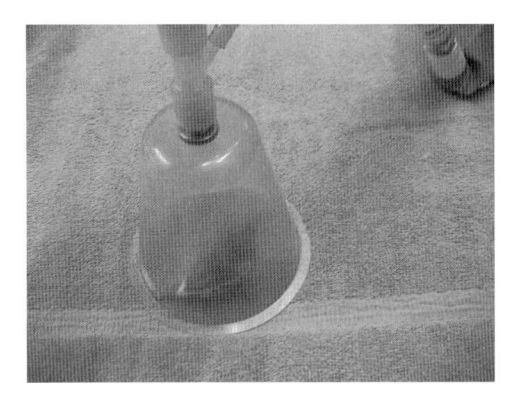

Fig. 14. Smaller dog/cat anesthetic cone used as a mini–anesthetic chamber for induction of smaller avian patients.

monitoring modalities, such as indirect measurement of blood pressure, can be useful in larger species but are increasingly difficult in smaller patients (Fig. 18) [12].

Many indications for surgery exist in nonpsittacine avian species, and procedures such as endoscopic biopsy, celiotomy, mass removal, and wound and fracture repair are well described [13]. Basic principles of sterility and tissue handling apply to all avian patients, despite increasing difficulty as patient size decreases. Patient preparation includes careful removal of feathers from the surgical site and use of warmed surgical scrub and sterile saline rinse. Alcohol may significantly cool smaller patients. Transparent drapes are valuable in all surgical patients but are ideal for smaller patients, where a standard drape would completely obscure the anesthetist's view of the patient. A number of retractors greatly aid surgery in small patients. The Lonestar retractor (Jorgensen Laboratories, Loveland, Colorado) is a plastic

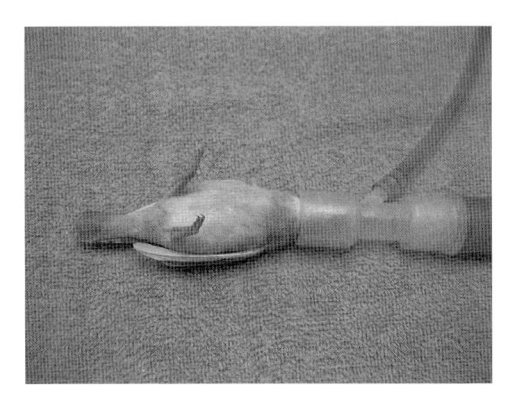

Fig. 15. Modification for "mask" anesthetic maintenance of a very small avian patient.

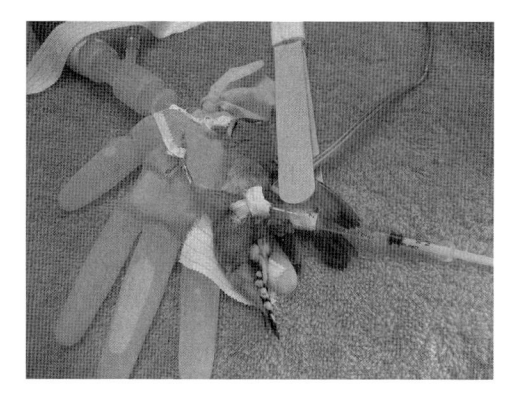

Fig. 16. A zebra finch prepared for surgical hysterectomy. Note the 2.0 endotracheal tube secured with white tape, a tongue depressor splint to hold the Doppler in place over the ulnar artery, placement of the intraosseous catheter, and a warm, water-filled glove for prevention of excessive loss of body heat during surgery. An overhead ceramic heat bulb is not pictured.

device with flexible hooks that can be adapted for use in birds as small as finches (Figs. 19 and 20).

Medications

In general, exotic animal veterinarians enjoy the privilege of off-label drug use in avian patients. A few medications have been approved for use in commercial poultry, but these have limited applications to individual pet animals. Dosages for most drugs used in poultry and other birds are anecdotal and do not have the benefit of trials to evaluate efficacy or toxicity. Another complication is the use of drugs without established withdrawal times in any animal whose flesh or other products might be used for human

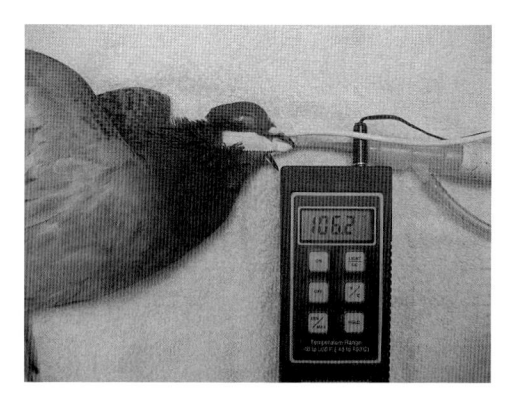

Fig. 17. Anesthetized and intubated pigeon with a flexible temperature probe inserted into the crop (Veterinary Specialty Products, Mission, Kansas).

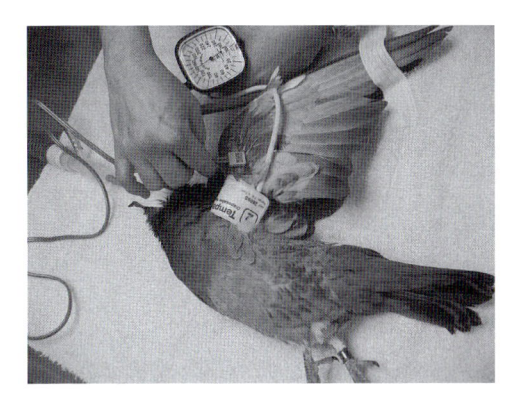

Fig. 18. Determination of indirect blood pressure in an anesthetized, intubated pigeon.

food—for example, the eggs of pet or backyard poultry. Veterinarians are responsible for ensuring that drugs prescribed for patients do not enter the human food chain [14]. Withdrawal times for some drugs have been well established, whereas others are specifically forbidden under any circumstances [14].

As of September 12, 2005, the US Food and Drug Administration announced that fluoroquinolones approved for use in poultry will be withdrawn from the market and "may no longer be sold, distributed or administered to chickens or turkeys." This ruling was made after determination that fluoroquinolone use in poultry was a leading cause of resistant *Campylobacter* infection in humans. The Food Animal Residue Avoidance Databank (FARAD) specifically states that off-label use of fluoroquinolones in turkeys and chickens is forbidden, eliminating drugs such as enrofloxacin from use. Practitioners may obtain complete guidelines for use of

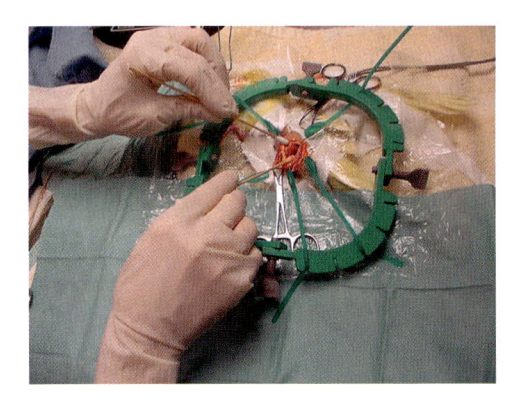

Fig. 19. The Lonestar retractor (Jorgensen Laboratories, Loveland, CO) to facilitate hysterectomy in a small avian patient.

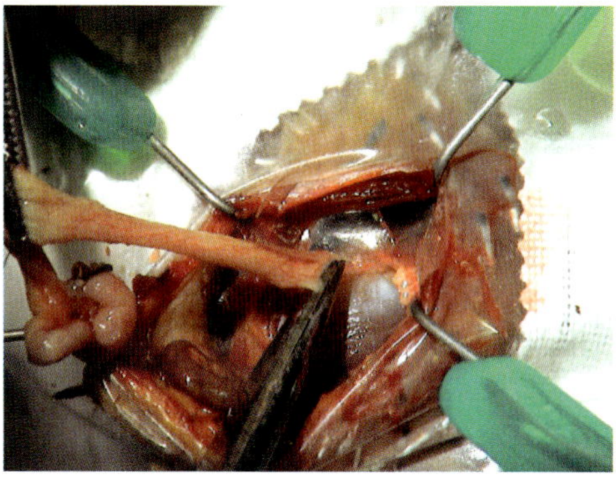

Fig. 20. The Lonestar retractor (Jorgensen Laboratories, Loveland, CO) to facilitate hysterectomy in a small avian patient.

drugs in potentially food-producing animals from the FARAD at www.farad.org [15].

Nutrition, preventive medicine, and vaccinations

As in all species, prevention of disease relies heavily on good husbandry, including appropriate diet. Commercial diets are readily available for many nonpsittacine pet birds, including various species of pet galliformes, pigeons, doves, and finches. Owners of pet poultry should take advantage of the many years of nutritional research behind inexpensive, complete rations designed for growing and egg-producing chickens, turkeys, waterfowl, pheasants, quail, and other ornamental fowl. Many feed companies provide instructions for use of one or more feeds in combination for different species of growing or adult birds, pet birds or birds intended for eggs or meat, and birds fed in confinement or with free-range access to natural foods. Commercial foods designed to maximize muscle growth in meat birds may produce disease in birds kept as long-term pets. Cracked corn, so-called "scratch grains," and seeds fed alone are not appropriate for any species [16].

Although most passerines, such as finches and canaries, are primarily seed eaters, traditional, commercially available seeds are often inadequate for optimum health [17]. Obesity is not uncommon in clinical practice, especially in canaries. Although much nutritional research remains to be completed, formulated diets and supplementation with so-called "egg foods," vegetables, and fruits may be beneficial [17].

Some nonpsittacine pet birds have more complex nutritional requirements. Certain species of birds are susceptible to iron storage disease (ISD), which is the accumulation of iron in various tissues, particularly the liver. Commonly affected birds include mynahs, starlings, and toucans.

Although ISD is certainly linked to iron levels in excess of the bird's ability to metabolize, other combinations of nutritional imbalances have been implicated, including the presence of vitamin C and excessive vitamin A. Factors such as concurrent disease, stress, and heredity may be important as well. Owners of these species are advised to choose diets low in iron and to avoid excessive vitamins C and A [17].

This diverse group of birds benefits from excellent husbandry, and careful attention should be paid to adequate cage size, provision of roosts, shelters, nesting sites, and enrichment activities, and cleanliness. Many owners of pet poultry and similar birds house them outdoors. Additional care must then be taken to prevent predation and stress due to inclement weather. Owners of birds permitted to range freely must be willing to accept increased risk for injury and death from predators such as raptors, wild carnivores, and domestic dogs and cats, as well as vehicular trauma.

Vaccinations are available for a number of nonpsittacine species. Vaccines for salmonella, poxvirus, and paramyxovirus-1 are commercially available for pigeons and can be valuable in flocks experiencing disease outbreaks or stress—for example, racing pigeons [18].

Commercial poultry producers have a number of vaccines available for prevention of a variety of viral and bacterial diseases. However, these vaccines are generally not available in small enough quantities to make vaccination of small backyard flocks practical [16]. Many large commercial breeders of birds for the backyard or pet market sell birds already vaccinated against Merek's disease. Vaccination might be considered in cases of extremely valuable birds in areas where particular diseases are especially virulent or endemic [16].

Poxvirus vaccine is available for canaries and may be valuable in endemic areas, especially where birds are raised outdoors and exposed to mosquitos. Although canaries and finches are susceptible to polyomavirus, a commercially available vaccine was not found to offer protection in these species [19].

Common disease conditions

It is impossible to list in detail all disease conditions encountered in nonpsittacine birds, but a general list includes infectious, traumatic, neoplastic, toxic, and metabolic conditions. Birds housed outdoors are more susceptible to trauma, in particular predator trauma and toxin exposure.

Highly pathogenic avian influenza subtype H5N1 has received enormous attention as increasing numbers of cases are reported in poultry and wild birds. As of November 2005, the World Health Organization logged 62 confirmed human deaths, mostly in poultry workers. Eighty percent of confirmed human cases involved exposure to live poultry [20]. The disease is well-established in wild bird populations in Asia and is spreading into

Europe, as asymptomatic wild birds travel established migratory routes. Poultry and birds in zoologic collections are most likely infected by exposure to wild birds. As of November 2005, more than 150 million birds have died or been destroyed in culling efforts [20].

Avian veterinarians in the United States are asked to answer questions about the significance of this disease for pet bird populations. Although predictions are difficult, most experts agree that highly pathogenic forms of avian flu will at some time or may already be present in United States wild bird populations. The most effective prevention strategy will most likely be protection of pet poultry and other pet birds from exposure to wild birds, which is often difficult for owners of backyard free-ranging poultry. Anecdotal reports of vaccine trials for protection of valuable zoo collections may represent another future management tool (Derek Spielman, Ocean Park Co., Hong Kong, personal communication, 2005).

References

[1] Massey JG. Physical examination of passerines. Vet Clin North Am Exot Anim Pract 1999; 2(2):357–82.
[2] Morshita TY. Clinical assessment of gallinaceous birds and waterfowl in backyard flocks. Vet Clin North Am Exot Anim Pract 1999;2(2):383–404.
[3] Echols S. Collecting diagnostic samples in avian patients. Vet Clin North Am Exot Anim Pract 1999;2(3):621–49.
[4] Fudge A. Avian laboratory medicine. In: Fudge A, editor. Laboratory medicine: avian and exotic pets. Philadelphia: WB Saunders; 2000. p. 1–18.
[5] Sturkie PD. Heart and circulation: anatomy, hemodynamic, blood pressure, blood flow. In: Sturkie PD, editor. Avian physiology. 4th edition. New York: Springer-Verlag; 1986. p. 130–66.
[6] King AS, McLelland J. Cardiovascular system. In: Birds: their structure and function. 2nd edition. East Sussex (UK): Bailliere Tindall; 1984. p. 214–28.
[7] Tully TN. Psittacine therapeutics. Vet Clin North Am Exot Anim Pract 2000;3(1):59–90.
[8] Dorrestein GM. Passerine and softbill therapeutics. Vet Clin North Am Exot Anim Pract 2000;3(1):35–57.
[9] Abu-Madi N. Avian anesthesia. Vet Clin North Am Exot Anim Pract 2001;4(1):147–67.
[10] Phalen DN, Mitchel ME, Cavazos-Mertinez ML. Evaluation of three heat sources for their ability to maintain core body temperature in the anesthetized avian patient. J Avian Med Surg 1996;10:174–8.
[11] Bennet A. Preparation and equipment useful for surgery in small exotic pets. Vet Clin North Am Exot Anim Pract 2000;3(3):563–86.
[12] Lichtenberg M. Avian shock, fluids and cardiopulmonary/cerebral resuscitation. Proceedings of the International Conference on Exotics, Supplement. 2005. p. 23–27.
[13] Jenkins JR. Surgery of the avian reproductive and gastrointestinal systems. Vet Clin North Am Exot Anim Pract 2000;3(3):673–92.
[14] Spenser E. Compounding, extralabel drug use, and other pharmaceutical quagmires in avian and exotics practice. Vet Clin North Am Exot Anim Pract 2000;13(1):16–24.
[15] US Department of Agriculture. Food Animal Residue Avoidance Database (FARAD). Available at: http://www.farad.org. Accessed November 15, 2005.
[16] Butcher G. Management of galliformes. In: Harrison G, Lightfoot T, editors. Clinical avian medicine. Palm Beach (FL): Spix Publishing; 2006. p. 861–77.

[17] Harrison G, McDonald D. Nutritional considerations. Section II. In: Harrison G, Lightfoot T, editors. Clinical avian medicine. Palm Beach (FL): Spix Publishing; 2006. p. 108–40.
[18] Greenacre CB. Viral diseases of companion birds. Vet Clin North Am Exot Anim Pract 2005;8(1):85–105.
[19] Sandmeier P, Coutteel P. Canaries, finches and mynahs. In: Harrison G, Lightfoot T, editors. Clinical avian medicine. Palm Beach (FL): Spix Publishing; 2006. p. 879–913.
[20] Beigel JH, Farrar J, Han AM, et al. Writing Committee of the World Health Organization (WHO) consultation of human influenza A/H5, avian influenza A (H5N1) infection in humans. N Engl J Med 2005;353:1374–85.

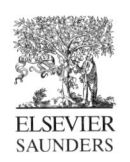

Raptor Medicine: An Approach to Wild, Falconry, and Educational Birds of Prey

Victoria Joseph, DVM, DABVP–Avian

Bird and Pet Clinic of Roseville, 3985 Foothills Boulevard, Roseville, CA 95747, USA

A veterinarian receiving birds of prey (raptors) will often be presented with wild, educational, or falconry raptors. Raptors trained for the sport of falconry and educational raptors are handled in a precise manner, often differently from the wild raptors. It is imperative for veterinarians treating raptors to be familiar with the equipment and terminology used by the individuals caring for these birds. The hospital staff must also be educated to handle the raptors properly, both wild and tame, because differences do exist between the approaches. Although there are a few distinct features in the types of injuries and medical conditions with which this category of raptors presents, the approach to the diagnostic work-up and therapeutic plan will be similar to that in other raptors. Raptor medicine requires a thorough diagnostic work-up and aggressive therapeutic plan to help ensure a fast and complete recovery.

Terminology

The individuals caring for raptors often use terms to describe certain conditions, objects, or animal behavior. Although not inclusive of all terms, the following list gives the reader a sound basis on which to build [1].

Austringer: An individual who trains and flies short-winged hawks.
Aylmeri jess: A jess in two parts: a leather cuff or anklet attached to the tarsometatarsus by a rivet or grommet and a slender piece of leather with a button at one end. The slender piece may be removed.
Bate: To fly from the perch or fist (toward food or the falconer's fist or away from a fearful situation).

A portion of the text was previously published in: Joseph V. Raptor hematology and chemistry evaluation. Vet Clin North Am Exot Anim Pract 1999;2(3):689–99; with permission.
  E-mail address: gosridge@foothill.net

Bewit: A small leather strap that allows attachment of a bell to the leg.

Block: A wooden or concrete perch with a padded top. It may taper toward the bottom and end on a spike that may be driven into the ground.

Bow-perch: A semicircular bar or piece of wood, padded in the center and provided with a ring.

Brace: The drawstrings of a hood.

Brancher: A young raptor that has left the nest but not the immediate area.

Cast: Two falcons or hawks flown together. To hold a raptor for examination or treatment. To cough up or expel a casting.

Casting: The indigestible portion of the meal fed to a raptor. Referred to by some as a pellet.

Cope: To trim the beak or talons.

Cramp: A vitamin or calcium imbalance resulting in muscle cramps.

Creance: A long, light line hooked to the jesses of a raptor being flight trained.

Deck feathers: The two middle and dorsal feathers of the tail.

Eyass: A young raptor removed from the nest.

Falcon: A long, winged raptor of the genus Falco. A female peregrine.

Falconer: One who trains and flies raptors.

Falconry: The sport of flying a trained raptor.

Foot: To grab quarry or to be grabbed by the talons.

Frounce: A disease of the upper digestive tract caused by Trichomonas gallinae. Usually contracted by eating infected pigeons and doves.

Hack: A newly fledged eyass freed from an enclosure, returning to the site for food.

Haggard: A raptor in adult plumage.

Hood: A leather cap for a raptor.

Hunger-streak or stress marks: A weakness in a feather shown as a transverse clear area (stress bars). Cause may be nutritional, metabolic, or behavioral.

Imp: To repair a broken feather by splicing onto a good section of a previously molted feather.

Intermewed: A raptor that has completed a molt.

Jess: A leather strap with a button at one end. Placed through the cuff.

Leash: A piece of strong leather or braided nylon used to attach the raptor to the perch.

Lure: A padded weight (often in the shape of a bird) covered with bits of food, from which a raptor is fed.

Mantle: A raptor spreading the wings and tail to cover or hide its food.

Mews: The housing or chambers of a raptor.

Mute: To defecate.

Mutes: The fecal material of a raptor.

Passage: A raptor trapped while in immature plumage, usually during migration.

Ring perch: A circular padded perch.
Rouse: To raise the feathers, shake them vigorously, and slowly let them return to a normal position.
Screen perch: A long, horizontal perch with a coarse fabric hanging vertically and weighted at the bottom.
Sharp set: Hungry and eager to hunt.
Shelf perch: A type of indoor perch.
Slice: To defecate (short-winged hawk).
Swivel: A double-ringed metal device that is used to attach the leash and jesses.
Tiercel: A male raptor.
Weather: To place a raptor outdoors so that it is exposed to the fresh air, sun, people, and animals. Legally a raptor may only be weathered in a protective yard so that wild animals and birds cannot attack it.

Equipment

The veterinary hospital and staff must be properly prepared to examine and hospitalize a raptor. Falconry birds and educational birds are often brought into the clinic on the fist of the falconer or the handler, respectively. Tethered to the glove, these birds usually have their jesses, swivel, leash, and hood in place (Fig. 1). If the waiting room is large enough, a corner may be used to house a block or shelf perch. Away from the center of activity, the raptor can perch undisturbed while waiting for its appointment. Most wild raptors presenting to the clinic arrive in a box or pet carrier. A darkened environment, either a hood or a covered pet carrier, will help to keep the bird calm.

A variety of perches should be available to accommodate the different species of raptors. Most often in hospital situations, block perches are used. A plastic weighted bucket with heavy Astroturf (Monsanto Solutia, St. Louis, Missouri) on the dorsal surface is adequate for most raptors (Fig. 2). For small raptors with delicate feet, the heavy Astroturf may be

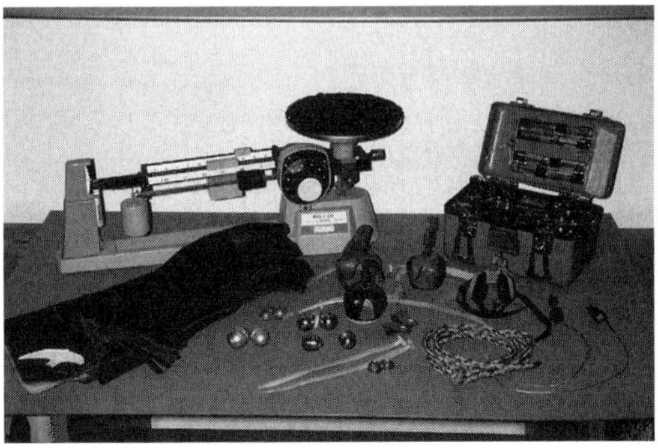

Fig. 1. Examples of gloves, hoods, and equipment used by the falconer or handler. Note the triple-beam balance flat-top gram scale.

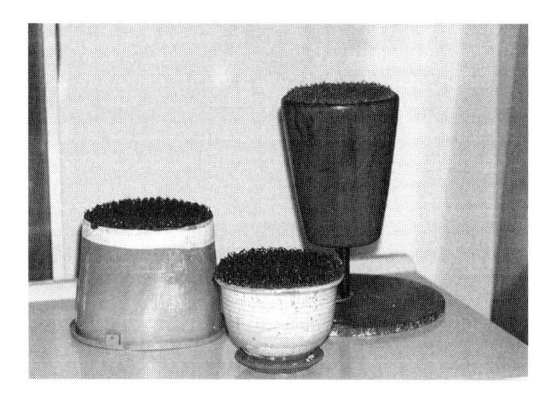

Fig. 2. Various perches made from buckets, planters, or wood.

too rough. Placing a small towel over the top of the perch and securing it at the base with tape gives a small raptor like the kestrel (*Falco sparverius*) a comfortable perch. Wooden block perches with a flat steel base and metal shaft are excellent for perching raptors. These perches have a steel ring at the bottom of the shaft that allows the raptor to be tethered and helps prevent it from becoming tangled in the leash. The perch to the far right in Fig. 2 is an example of a traditional block perch. Perches are disinfected following their use by spraying the entire perch with the disinfectant and letting it set for 20 minutes, then rinsing well with water. It is beneficial to have on hand a limited supply of leashes, swivels, and aylmeri jesses for raptors needing hospitalization. Most falconers and handlers provide this equipment, but it is best to be prepared.

A variety of hoods should be available for use on the raptors. A raptor hood keeps the bird quiet and makes handling easier. The hood must fit properly so as to cover the eyes and sit on the back of the head. Most falconers have personal hoods for each raptor they fly and will bring in a bird that is already hooded. Always check with the falconer before placing a hood on the raptor. An improperly fitted hood may rub the cornea, damage the cere, or bruise the corners of the mouth, resulting in a bird that is more difficult to manage than it would have been if left unhooded. A stockinet made of stretch cotton and tied at one end with umbilical tape or gauze is sufficient to use as a hood on the wild raptors. These may be washed between uses. Some raptors are hood shy and will be uncontrollable after the placement of any hood. These birds may be transported in a giant hood: a large box made of lightweight material and fitted with a perch and door, allowing easy access to the perched raptor.

To weigh a raptor properly, one must have a flat-top scale covered with Astroturf. The larger raptors will not perch on the typical dowel-type perch often used for psittacines. Exceptions are the little kestrels, merlins (*Falco columbarius*), and owls used as falconry or educational birds. Most falconry and educational raptors will step on the scale to be weighed. This is not true of the wild raptors, which must be weighed in a secured position. A rectangular piece of cloth with Velcro edges may be wrapped gently around the body of the raptor to secure the bird in position. The feet must be protected so that no one will get taloned. Adjustments should be made for the weight of the hood, jesses, swivel, and leash. Gloves are required for casting the raptors and protecting the handler. Welders' gloves are adequate for most of the medium to large raptor species. They are too large for the proper handling of the small raptors, for which padded garden gloves are adequate. Specialty gloves, such as those required for handling an eagle, may be ordered through falconry equipment companies. Experienced raptor handlers may use a towel instead of the gloves, but this is not recommended for the inexperienced, given the possibility of being taloned or footed.

Caging

The stainless steel caging that most veterinarians have in the clinic is sufficient to house the raptors temporarily. Perch size may be adjusted to fit in the cage and allow the raptor to perch comfortably if it is able. For those raptors not able to stand, a padded towel is used to place them on their sides and slightly propped up. It is not advisable to let the raptor lie on its chest or on its back with feet in the air. The former position may result in impairment of respiration; the latter in the aspiration of crop fluids. A dog run may be used for the eagles; however, be sure the top is enclosed. Eagles have the ability to jump and possibly reach the top of the kennel. The most important point to remember is that one should be able to keep the enclosure dark and quiet. Lights, barking dogs, and many voices will make the housed raptor jumpy and add to its stress level. A towel partially covering the cage door but allowing air circulation may help to keep the raptor quiet. For those veterinarians who cannot properly house the raptor, it is best, if possible, to treat the bird as an outpatient twice daily. Handler or owner assistance is usually required to make this process effective. In the author's clinic, there is a separate raptor ward where only raptors are housed. The area is away from all other animals, quiet, and easily darkened. This approach maximizes the ability of the raptor to rest and recover.

Technical support

Training the technical staff is the most time-consuming and difficult part of preparing a veterinary practice to see raptors. No matter how thorough one's examination and diagnostic work-up is, a raptor showing frayed or broken feathers after being handled will leave the falconer in dismay. Falconers work hard to keep their birds in feather-perfect condition and expect to have them returned that way. It is just as important to protect the wild raptors' feather condition, because injury to their feathers may delay their rehabilitation and release. Raptors requiring several days of hospitalization may benefit from a tail guard being placed on the tail. In general, a lightweight, stiff material (eg, envelope, radiography film) encompasses the tail and is taped in place. The tail guard may be cut and adjusted to create a form fit. This guard will help protect the tail feathers in raptors that are nervous and jumpy in the hospital setting. For long, overseas transport of a falcon, tail and wing guards are placed on the bird (Fig. 3).

Training must involve raptor handling to prevent injury to the bird and, just as important, prevent injury to the handler. In the clinic, two people must be present when raptors are handled. The buddy system helps prevent problems or situations that may endanger the bird or handler. In a veterinary practice that treats raptors, the injured wildlife raptors provide opportunities for the necessary training of technicians. These birds often require extensive handling and diagnostic work-ups. Once technicians are comfortable with casting the wild raptor for diagnostic procedures and treatment regimens, they may apply these techniques to the falconry birds. The great difference between wild raptors and falconry birds is temperament. Many wild raptors "freeze" when being handled, whereas most falconry birds are not used to being casted or held and try aggressively to get free of the restrainer. Biting and footing are common occurrences when casting falconry birds. It is absolutely necessary that the technician be alert at all times.

Some raptors require the use of gloves and a towel for restraint. Falconry or educational raptors are often casted off the glove of the handler. Whether a towel or gloves are used, the technician approaches the bird from behind and firmly but gently secures it over the shoulder area, preventing the wings from flapping. The feet are held away from the technician until the legs and feet are secured. The bird is held up against the technician, with the technician's arms cradling its body and his or her gloved hands securing the distal

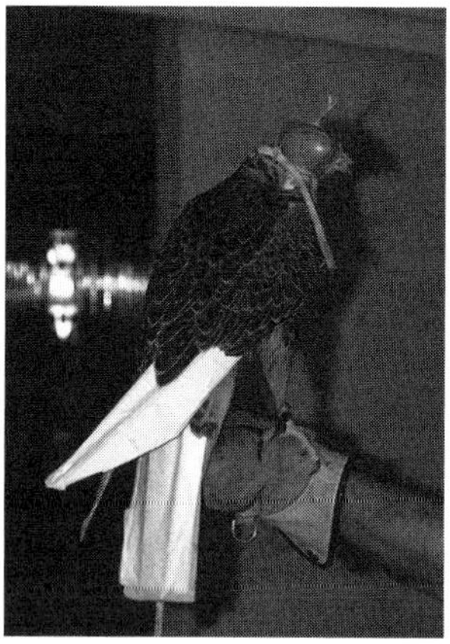

Fig. 3. Falcon with wing and tail guards in place. This bird is being prepared for shipment overseas. Nervous raptors in the hospital will benefit from a tail guard.

portion of the raptor's legs with the feet pointing away from the technician. The falconer or handler then removes the glove from the raptor, or removes his or her hand from the glove if the raptor is gripping the glove, so that the physical examination may be conducted. For those birds that are not hooded, the approach to casting is the same, except that the lights must be turned off so the raptor cannot see what is going on. In a darkened room, a penlight will give you enough light to secure the bird without frightening it. Once it is secured, the lights come back on. Wild raptors often require both a towel and gloves. The towel helps to turn the bird away from you, so that the handler may secure the bird over the shoulder area and point the talons away from him or her. Once the raptor is secured, the technician may remove the towel, allowing for easier and less cumbersome restraint. All of this is accomplished with minimal restraint and protection of the feathers from damage. With inexperienced technical staff, it may be wise to tape the foot of the raptor closed with masking tape or vet wrap to help prevent the occurrence of someone's being footed. When the physical examination is performed, one should stand to the side of the raptor and not directly in front of it. Raptors, even with the legs held, have the ability to strike out and talon. All wild raptors are routinely dusted with a poultry dust containing 0.25% permethrin on arrival in the clinic.

Physical examination

All raptors are carnivores and have developed specialized characteristics that reflect their lifestyle and mode of hunting. All raptors have large, sensitive eyes, with the nocturnal raptors, such as the owls, having larger eyes than the diurnal raptors. The owls in general also have large ear openings that are asymmetric in position. This aids in sound detection, an important ability for hunting in total darkness. The feathers and plumage also reflect each raptor's specialization. The accipiters (goshawks [*Accipiter gentiles*], sharp-shinned hawks [*Accipiter striatus*], and cooper's hawks [*Accipiter cooperii*]) have short, rounded wings and long tails to increase their maneuverability and aid them in short, fast flight through heavily wooded areas. Falcons have long, tapered, pointed wings that assist them in climbing to great heights and stooping their prey in flight at great speeds. Buteos (red-tailed hawk [*Buteo jamaicensis*], red-shoulder hawk [*Buteo lineatus*], broad-winged hawk [*Buteo platypterus*]) have broad, rounded wings and tails, facilitating their soaring and riding the thermals (currents of warm air). Owls in general have flight feathers with serrated leading edges, giving the bird soundless flight and aiding them in hunting in the darkness. The feet of the raptor vary greatly among the species. All raptors have strong toes with curved talons, capable of inflicting damage on the prey or quarry they hold. Buteos have thick, strong toes, whereas falcons and the accipiters have long, slender toes and a longer tarsus. This difference reflects the different sizes of prey taken, such as squirrels, rabbits, and large rodents versus the smaller rodents and birds, respectively.

Osprey (*Pandion haliaetus*) have specialized pads with spicules on the ventral surface, enabling them to grab and hold onto fish. Osprey and owls are semi-zygodactylous, with some ability to rotate the fourth digit to the rear, increasing their dexterity in capturing and holding onto the prey item. Falconry and wild raptors require their talons to be needle-sharp for proper hunting. Educational raptors should have the ends of the talons blunted to protect against self-inflicted injuries [2].

Variations in the gastrointestinal tract need to be noted for the physical examination. Raptors (except for the owls) have crops. The crop acts as a food storage organ. A raptor presented with an injury or medical issue may have a crop full of sour food and be unable to digest properly and move the food through. This situation can be life threatening and must be addressed immediately. The food contents may have to be removed as part of the initial triage while one addresses dehydration and septic issues. Owls often swallow their prey whole, filling the proventriculus and lower esophagus. After several minutes, the food enters the ventriculus. Owls are not capable of digesting the bones of their prey completely, whereas the rest of the raptors are. Owls produce a pellet with each meal, whereas hawks may eat more than one meal before regurgitating a pellet [2,3].

The overall skeletal anatomy varies slightly among the raptor species. These variations are minor and will not affect the physical examination and approach to the diagnostic work-up.

When performing the physical examination, one needs to make several observations:

Posture—is the raptor standing erect and alert, or is it hunched with wings drooped or leaning to one side? Is a muscular twitch or seizure activity present? (Rule out poisonings, hypoglycemia, or hypocalcemia.)

Respiration—is the raptor breathing quietly, with little or no evidence of respiratory effort, or is it tail bobbing with exaggerated respiratory movements or abdominal respiratory effort? Is there movement of the wings in the shoulder region with each breath or open-mouth breathing? Is coughing or a respiratory click present?

Eyes—are they open, bright, and clear, or are they closed, squinted, or showing discharge?

Sinuses—are they distended or bulging with each breath?

Ears—are the openings clear, is discharge present, or do bots (insect larvae) inhabit the ear canal?

Feathers—are they clean and in good condition, or do they show evidence of being soiled, broken, or damaged?

Cere and beak—is the cere damaged or the beak cracked? Is the falcon tooth (ie, a notch- or V-shaped portion of the maxilla forming a tooth-like projection in the falcon species, enabling them to sever the neck of the vertebrate prey) present or damaged (Fig. 4)? Are nodules suggestive of pox present on the face?

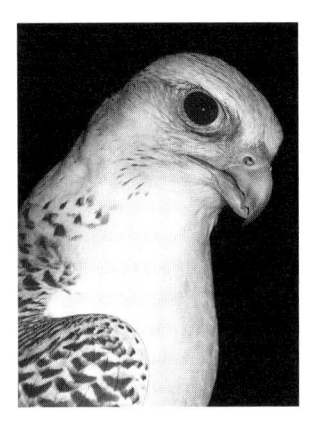

Fig. 4. A gyrfalcon with the "toothed" beak on the maxilla.

Oral cavity—is it clear and colored, or are white plaques present? (Rule out trichomonas, fungal or yeast, capillaria, pox, or bacterial infections.)

Body—check for lacerations or wounds. (Rule out traumatic injuries or gun shot wounds.)

Extremities—check for edema or necrotic areas suggestive of electrocution. Rule out fractures and dislocations. Note drooping wings or asymmetric appearance to the wings. Check the patagium for lacerations and tendon damage. Check all joints for swellings and range of motion.

Legs and talons—is there damage to the feet or talons? Are the talons too long or curved? Are they twisted or missing? Check for abnormal position of the digits suggestive of tendon injuries. Look for bumble foot lesions.

Mutes—should be composed of the urates (white) and the feces (dark black). The fecal material may be tan with a diet of day-old chicks or have a bright green center in a fasted raptor. The urates may have an occasional reddish pigment. Yellow or lime-green staining to the feces or urates and flecks of blood in the mutes are abnormal [2,4].

Approach to diagnostic procedures

Before any work is begun on the raptors, all necessary equipment is prepared and set out. The goal is to minimize the number of times and length of time a raptor is restrained. All laboratory supplies should be set out so samples may be quickly taken. Even when the plan is to run a preliminary test or tests (eg, complete blood count, Gram stain, or fecal), it is wise to take enough blood initially for a complete panel, protein electrophoresis, aspergillosis titer, metal screens, or other specialized testing that may be indicated later. Microbiology samples and cytology samples, if necessary, should be obtained at this time for further use, to avoid another casting. Depending on the temperament of the raptor, some buteos, small accipiters, and small falcons may have their blood drawn or be radiographed awake. The majority, however, need to be anesthetized with a gas anesthetic such as isoflurane or sevoflurane. Supportive care supplies, such as intravenous catheters, injections, and fluid therapy, should also be prepared in advance with the intention of having all sampling and supportive care done at the same time. Advance planning will minimize the time during which the bird must be restrained or under anesthesia. Recommendations for examination and diagnostic procedures are as follows:

- In those raptors not requiring anesthesia, the physical examination, diagnostic procedures, and supportive care may be done in stages. Initially, a limited physical examination is performed with the bird hooded and on the fist of the falconer or handler. Heart rate and rhythm, respiratory evaluation and auscultation, muscle condition, and hydration status may be easily assessed.
- Docile raptors may now be casted to complete the physical examination. The hood is removed to allow examination of the face, oral cavity, eyes, and ears. Swabs of the mouth may also be taken at this time. Once this part of the examination is done, the hood is replaced. Palpation of the wings, body, and feet is completed. Auscultation of the heart, lungs, and air sacs may once again be performed. If the raptor remains calm, diagnostic sampling and supportive care may be initiated. If necessary, these procedures may be performed in stepwise fashion, depending on the behavior and perceived stress level of the bird.
- Raptors requiring anesthesia are masked with a gas anesthetic. After the preliminary examination, the bird is either kept on the falconer's glove or a block perch. The hood is kept in place. The technician will cast the bird from behind, keeping the bird on the fist or the perch. The mask is placed over the face and hood. Once the bird is relaxed and partially anesthetized, the hood is removed and the mask repositioned. All procedures are done quickly and efficiently. The hood is replaced on the bird before the bird awakes. Once again, the raptor is gently casted by the technician until it is awake enough to stand on the falconer's fist or perch. The raptor never sees who casted it, a measure that helps curtail any traumatic reactions toward its owner (Fig. 5). (Note that the vet wrap is used to replace the hard rubber cover of the face masks. The vet wrap makes possible a softer, form-fitting mask and may be replaced after each use.)
- Blood collection is performed in the same manner as in all birds with a few exceptions. The jugular vein is rarely used on the awake falconry or educational bird. It may be difficult to secure the talons and hold the bird in the proper position for this type of blood draw. More than likely it would also be visually upsetting to the falconer or handler. A better choice is the medial metatarsal vein. This vein is easier to

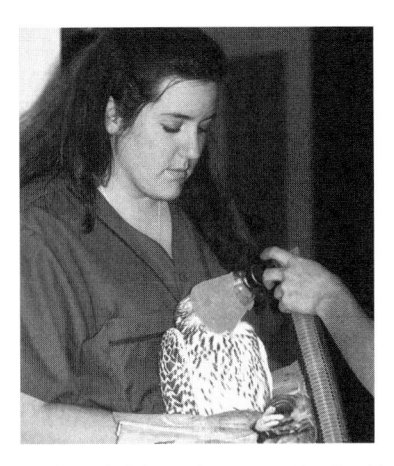

Fig. 5. The falcon is casted by the technician, who secures the distal legs with the talons pointed away from her. This falcon is being anesthetized with gas anesthetic.

approach and less likely to develop a hematoma than the ulnar vein. In larger docile hawks and eagles, the ulnar vein is easy to use. As the technician cradles the bird's body with his or her arms, the wing is slightly unfolded to expose the vein. The bird may be maintained in the upright position for the blood draw. Many red-tailed and Harris's hawks are docile enough to be positioned on their backs for a blood draw. Eyasses are a challenge when it comes to obtaining a blood sample. Care must be taken if the raptor is casted. The feathers may just be starting to emerge and are vulnerable to damage at this stage. Many eyasses will sit comfortably on a towel with the handler cupping the bird for support. The blood sample is then drawn from the medial metatarsal vein as the baby raptor sits in its normal position (Fig. 6).

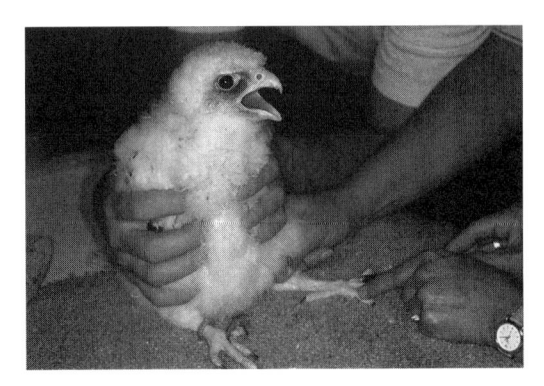

Fig. 6. An eyass being restrained for a blood draw. Minimal restraint is used, with care to avoid injury to the feathers.

The minimal database for any raptor should include a complete blood count and fecal examination. Full chemistry panels and specialized testing are often necessary properly to evaluate the raptor. Radiographs are often required to complete the diagnostic work-up. Even when a raptor is presented with a fractured wing, whole body radiographs are recommended to rule out other complicating factors, such as fractured shoulders or legs, internal trauma to the organs, additional trauma such as gunshot wounds, and smoldering fungal infections. Trauma cases may require surgical intervention once the patient is stabilized. Fractures are not immediately repaired; the overall health of the raptor and the response to supportive care must first be established. Medical cases may become involved, requiring contrast radiography, endoscopy, or histopathology. Two areas of concern that must be addressed for any raptor presented in ill health are the supportive care administered and the preventive fungal program instituted for sensitive species.

Supportive care procedures

Raptors presented for illness or injury usually suffer from some degree of dehydration. Wild raptors may have gone days without eating or drinking, depending on their ability (when healthy) to obtain food. Many raptors presented in an emergency situation are in some degree of shock. Three categories of the shock syndrome exist. Hypovolemic shock is the result of decreased circulating blood volume secondary to hemorrhage or fluid loss. Cardiogenic shock is the result of cardiovascular compromise (iatrogenic dysrhythmias, arrhythmias, or pericardial effusion seen with electrocution). Vasogenic shock is the result of end-stage disease, including sepsis, endotoxemia, or toxins. With any form of shock, the goal of therapy is to restore the effective blood volume, improve oxygenation of the tissues, and maintain adequate perfusion to the vital organs [5–8]. Guidelines for determining the degree of dehydration, such as tenting of the skin, appearance of the eyes, humidity of the mucous membranes, and coolness of the lower extremities, may be difficult to follow in the raptor. The veterinarian can safely assume that a raptor is 10% dehydrated as a result of trauma or chronic disease and treat accordingly. Fluid recommendations are as follows:

Maintenance fluid requirements = 40 to 60 mL/kg/d
Estimated deficit in milliliters = normal body weight (grams) × the decimal value of dehydration

The goal of fluid therapy is to replace the estimated deficit over 48 to 72 hours while providing maintenance daily. Fluids must always be warmed to body temperature to avoid hypothermia. The total volume of daily fluids is divided into at least three doses to avoid overwhelming the cardiovascular system or creating tissue edema. Pediatric raptors may require as much as

50% more fluids than the adult. Some of this requirement may be obtained with tube feedings or hydration of the meats fed. Sufficient fluids are required by the pediatric raptor to aid in proper digestion. The fluids may be delivered via the intraosseous (IO), intravenous (IV), subcutaneous (SQ), or oral route.

Thus a 1-kg raptor presented with an assumed dehydration percentage of 10% would require 50 mL per day for maintenance, plus an additional 100 mL for 2 or 3 days. This would result in three daily doses of 28 mL each for 3 days or three daily doses of 33 mL each for 2 days.

IO catheters should be reserved for the severely sick or shocked patient that has a predilection for vascular collapse. Sterile techniques for catheter placement and maintenance of the catheter must be cautiously maintained to prevent introduction of infection. The distal ulna or the proximal tibiotarsus is the standard site for catheter placement. The pneumatic properties of the humerus and the femur prohibit their use for this procedure. This technique is good for small raptors (<150 g) in which placing an IV catheter may be difficult [5]. When a falconry or educational raptor is presented, permission from the falconer or handler to pluck feathers and place an IO catheter should be obtained. Osteomyelitis, subcutaneous extravasations of fluids, iatrogenic fractures, and fat or bone marrow emboli to the lungs are all possible complications of IO catheterization and should be addressed with the owner.

IV catheters are best placed in the medial metatarsal vein; this is acceptable for the falconry or educational raptor. Minimal plucking of feathers is required. The catheter is placed below the tarsometatarsal joint, in the medial metatarsal vein. It is taped in place and an injection cap screwed on. Often the cuff of leather on the leg of the falconry bird rests over the catheter and does not need to be cut away (Fig. 7). The falconry and educational raptors tolerate this well: they do not pick at the catheter, and they do not require restraint for administration of fluid therapy. When fluid therapy is required, the raptor is hooded, placed on a block perch, and administered the fluids through

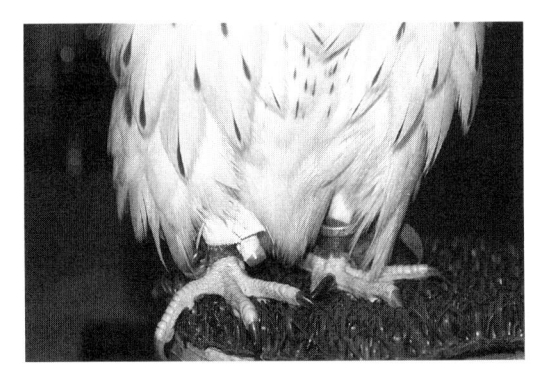

Fig. 7. IV catheter placement in the medial metatarsal vein.

the catheter by means of a 25-gauge needle attached to the fluid line (Fig. 8). Catheters placed in the ulnar vein are reserved for those raptors that may not tolerate a hood or stand on a block perch. The wing must be taped in a figure-eight fashion after catheter placement to help secure the catheter. The disadvantage of this technique is the lack of the visualization required to be sure the catheter remains in place. Jugular catheters may be placed in the right jugular vein. A tape butterfly technique to secure the catheter to the neck is required, followed by a light neck wrap. When properly placed, most birds tolerate this catheter and can eat without difficulty. Restraint of the raptor during fluid administration is often required for wild raptors or raptors not used to being hooded and placed on a block perch. This problem may decrease the feasibility of giving wild raptors continuous IV fluid administration, unless they are severely debilitated.

SQ fluid therapy is a convenient and acceptable mode of fluid administration in the mildly ill raptor. The best site to deliver a bolus of fluid is the inguinal region where the leg and the body wall meet. Fluids given over the midback area may be inappropriate, because of the possibility of injecting fluids into the clavicular air sacs. The patagium area of the wing does not lend itself to ease of administration or volume loading and is usually avoided. Hyaluronidase enzyme added to the lactated Ringer's solution at 1 mL/L appears to increase the rate of SQ fluid absorption. Most fluids administered in this fashion are absorbed within 10 to 15 minutes. No toxicity reaction occurs if this treated fluid goes intravenously. Oral administration of fluids to ill or injured raptors is not routine. In the debilitated raptor, absorption of fluid from the gastrointestinal tract appears to be minimal. Oral fluids should never be given to a raptor that is vomiting or that has crop stasis, ileus, or gastrointestinal impaction. The risk for aspiration pneumonia is high in a severely ill raptor [5].

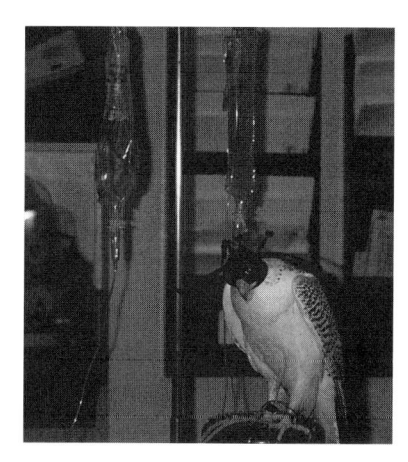

Fig. 8. A falconry falcon receiving IV fluids. The bird is hooded twice daily to receive IV fluid therapy.

While the raptor is receiving fluids, one should monitor daily changes in weight, estimated daily fluid intake versus output (urine and feces), and changes in the packed cell volume or total protein. These values are important in the anemic or hypoproteinemic patient. Aggressive fluid therapy may cause cardiovascular collapse or pulmonary edema. The following are guidelines for shock therapy in the raptor:

- Raptors presented for illness or injury are considered 10% dehydrated. Calculate fluid requirements for this degree of dehydration.
- Preoxygenate the raptor in respiratory distress or anesthetize the fractious raptor with isoflurane/sevoflurane to administer supportive care and take laboratory samples.
- If possible, take baseline blood samples for hematology and chemistries before treatment is initiated. However, in critical cases always do supportive care first.
- Insert an IO or IV catheter.
- Calculate the maintenance and deficit fluid requirements and administer over a 24- to 48-hour period.
- Give steroids, antibiotics, vitamins, or analgesics if the situation warrants.
- For head trauma, add mannitol if the neurologic condition deteriorates.
- Monitor the packed cell volume (PCV), total protein, and urine output daily during fluid therapy.
- Provide a heat source.
- Begin oral nutritional support once the raptor is stable.

Nutritional support

Severe debilitation due to inadequate nutritional intake is a complicating factor for most disease presentations and is an emergency situation on its own. A raptor from the wild may have gone without food for several days to 1 or 2 weeks before presentation. Falconry birds actively flying are kept in a state of lean body mass and may not have the nutritional reserves to maintain themselves during an illness. Correcting the underlying dehydration and withholding food for the first 12 to 24 hours is often required in the critically ill patient. It is important to understand some basic nutritional facts of the raptor to outline a proper nutritional plan. Carnivorous birds, such as raptors, eat two to five times more protein per kilogram of body weight and have higher nitrogen excretion than do granivorous birds [9]. In a normal situation, raptors have little glucose in their diets, and, when fed large proportions of glucose, they may not thrive. When they are in a severely debilitated state, large quantities of glucose may hasten death. The natural diet of a raptor is low in carbohydrates (2%) and high in fat (2% to 28%) and protein (17% to 20%). Three factors to consider when evaluating the caloric requirements of the raptor are the species of raptor presented, the weight of the raptor, and the metabolic state of the raptor. An injured raptor or a young, growing raptor uses more energy per kilogram of body weight than a healthy raptor. The following are recommendations for developing a nutritional plan for convalescing raptors:

Replacement fluid therapy is the first step.

Oral supplementation may be initiated after the initial period of rehydration. Raptors with moderate to severe starvation are started on an isotonic tube-feeding formula such as Ultracal (Mead Johnson, Princeton, New Jersey) or Isocal (Mead Johnson) at a dosage of 55 mL/kg/d divided into multiple feedings. A new formulation, Raptor Critical Care (Lafeber Co., Cornell, Illinois) is easy to use and well balanced for the convalescing raptor.

Coutornix quail, minus the feet, feathers, and gastrointestinal tract, may be ground with a meat grinder into a hamburger consistency. This balanced diet is an excellent nutritional source that is easily digestible for the convalescing raptor. The ground meat can be prepared in advance and frozen into flattened meat patties for convenient rations and storage.

Breast meat of the coutornix quail, cut into small pieces and soaked in an oral electrolyte solution, is an easily digested food for raptors. However, the meat alone is not balanced in the vitamin and mineral content and should be used with caution in the long term. It is best to feed this type of food only for the first 2 to 5 days of convalescence. Once the raptor is responding to treatment and showing normal food behavior and proper digestion, a more natural diet may be fed, such as whole mice, rats, jackrabbit, and so on. Proper nutritional support enhances and speeds the recovery of any injured or ill raptor. It is important to know the specific nutritional requirements of the raptor presented for evaluation. Merlins need the rich red meat of a wild passerine or pigeon. They do not thrive well on a diet of quail or chicken. In a pinch, they can be fed mice. Pigeon is usually not recommended as a food source for most raptors, because of the possibility of infecting the raptor with trichomoniasis (frounce). A golden eagle (*Aquila chrysaetos*) does well on a diet of small mammals, rodents, rabbits, or birds but does not eat fish. Bald eagles (*Haliaeetus leucocephalus*) eat everything a golden eagle will eat with the addition of fish. Ospreys are strictly fish eaters. When feeding fish to raptors, it is important to remember that frozen fish are devoid of vitamin B, and this can produce a central nervous system disorder with prolonged feeding. It is best to feed fresh fish. Day-old chicks, a common food source for raptor rehabilitators, are low in protein and have an imbalance in the calcium/phosphorus ratio. This food is not adequate for the convalescing raptor. Domesticated rabbits and poultry are not recommended as a food source. Their nutritional value is inadequate for raptors compared with that of wild game or coutornix quail.

Interpretation of hematology and chemistry values for raptors

Understanding how the raptor species may respond to disease is necessary for proper medical evaluation and treatment. Multiple disease entities are often present when raptors are presented to the veterinarian. Interpretation of the hematology and chemistry panel of raptors may be challenging and vary among species [10–14].

Aspartate aminotransferase

Activity of aspartate aminotransferase is found in the liver, skeletal muscle, heart, brain, and kidney. Elevations may be seen in liver disease, soft tissue injury, bumble foot, and septicemia and after surgery. Young raptors have a lower value than adults.

Alanine aminotransferase

Alanine aminotransferase has little diagnostic value, because this enzyme is found in many different tissues. Seasonal variations are found in the raptors and are independent of reproductive activity. However, the significance of this variation is not well understood.

Creatinine kinase

Activity of creatinine kinase (CK) is found primarily in the skeletal muscle, heart muscle, and brain tissue. CK is often used as a diagnostic indicator of muscle damage. However, research has shown that rehabilitated raptors trained for free flight and ready for release have a greater resting CK level than does the sedentary, disabled raptor. It is not unusual for the flight-trained raptor to have a CK value of 1000 mg/dL and be considered normal.

Lactate dehydrogenase

The sites where lactate dehydrogenase (LDH) may be found are skeletal muscle, cardiac muscle, liver, kidney, bone, and red blood cells. Although not specific for organ disease, LDH in raptors may be used to evaluate muscle fitness. LDH increases immediately after exercise and peaks in 24 hours. The resting and post-exercise plasma levels decrease with endurance and training. A flight-trained raptor ready for release has a low resting level of LDH.

Alkaline phosphatase

Activity of alkaline phosphatase is found in the duodenum, kidney, liver, and bone. Osteoplastic activity causes elevated levels of this enzyme. Juvenile raptors have higher levels, as do those raptors with a nutritional or secondary nutritional hyperparathyroidism disorder.

Bile acid

This enzyme may be difficult to interpret in the raptor species. Pre- and post-meal bile acid samples were evaluated in the red-tailed hawk, with the preprandial samples ranging from less than 1 to 30 µmol/L and the postprandial samples ranging from less than 1 to 117 µmol/L. Increases in the bile acid sample may occur with severe liver dysfunction.

Cholesterol

Carnivorous birds have higher cholesterol values than do psittacines. Diagnostic interpretation may be difficult, however, because elevated cholesterol values may be seen in birds with fatty liver degeneration, hypothyroidism, bile duct obstruction, starvation, or high-fat diets.

Calcium

Levels of calcium do not vary widely among species. Diet-induced hyperparathyroidism and hypervitaminosis D result in hypercalcemia. Decreased values in raptors have been associated with hypoalbuminemia, fat necrosis, deficiency of calcium in the diet, and end-stage renal disease.

Phosphorus and glucose

Increased levels of phosphorus are seen in severe renal failure. Hypoglycemia is a noted problem, especially in flight-trained raptors. Hypoglycemic convulsions occur in raptors at glucose levels of 60 to 80 mg/dL. This condition is usually accompanied by a history of starvation or restricted food intake for training and continued hard exercise. The smaller raptors, such as the kestrel, cooper's hawk, sharp-shinned hawk, and merlin, may be prone to this problem.

Uric acid

Levels of uric acid are higher in carnivorous birds. When the level is greater than 20 mg/dL, there is cause for concern. Elevations may be caused by renal disease, shock, or starvation. Falconry birds entering their training period are often fed small amounts of food to regulate their body weight. These birds may show an elevated uric acid level until their weight is brought back up to a more normal level. After a meat meal, postprandial elevations of the plasma uric acid concentrations are evident. These elevations may approach the levels of other avians suffering from hyperuricemia and gout (>30 mg/dL). Although it is not clearly understood why this physiologic condition occurs in raptors, this transient hyperuricemia for at least 12 hours after a meal does not result in uric acid deposition in the tissues. To rule out disease associated with elevated uric acid levels, a blood sample taken on a 24-hour fast is recommended. Hypouricemia (<2.1 mg/dL) may indicate severe liver dysfunction.

Blood urea nitrogen

This enzyme has limited value in the avian species. It may be used to evaluate prerenal causes of renal failure (ie, dehydration).

Total plasma protein

Values of total plasma protein (TPP) are more accurate than the total serum solid levels measured with the refractometer. Considerable variation in TPP is found among raptor species. Generally speaking, the larger the raptor species, the greater the TPP. It has been documented that some of the smaller owls have a TPP of 0.5 g/dL and are considered normal. A low TPP value may indicate malnutrition, acute hemorrhage, or chronic intestinal parasitism. High values may reflect dehydration, chronic disease, acute inflammation, or infection. Artifactual elevations occur with lipemia or hemolyzed sample.

Hematology

Interpretation of the hemogram of raptors may be confusing, owing to the blood parasites seen, the stress response, and the multidisease syndromes reflected. Tables 1 and 2 summarize the changes the veterinarian may see in the hemogram in response to disease.

Selected medical topics in raptors

Although it is not the intent of this article to elaborate on the medical issues plaguing raptors, the term raptor medicine often stimulates one thought—trauma. Although broken bones, laceration, and impact injuries do contribute to the overall caseload, the majority of raptors require intensive medical diagnostics and stabilization. Certain medical conditions are addressed here to help the practitioner outline a diagnostic and treatment plan that will help secure a rapid and complete recovery [5,15].

Respiratory emergencies

Respiratory emergencies encompass bacterial or fungal infections, foreign body inhalation, trauma, and parasitic infections. In most situations the diagnostic work-up follows the same course to rule out all the possibilities of respiratory disease. Full hematology and chemistry panels are recommended to rule out a metabolic cause for the respiratory distress and to help categorize the type of respiratory infection present. All respiratory cases should be evaluated radiographically and with microbiology of the

Table 1
Summarized changes in total plasma protein, packed cell volume, red blood cells, and anemia in response to disease

Differential diagnosis	TPP	PCV	Anemia	Polychromatic red blood cells
Dehydration	+	+	+/−	+/−
Starvation	−	−	nonregen	+/−
Hemorrhage	−	−	regen	+
Infections	n/+	−	regen/nonregen	+/−
Fungal/TB	+	n/−	nonregen	+/−
Viral	n/−	−	regen/nonregen	+/−
Parasites	−	−	regen	++ (hematozoa)
Lead toxicity	n/−	−	regen	++ (ballooning or basophilic stippling may be present)
Stress response	n	n	None	+

Abbreviations: +, increase; − decrease; n, normal; nonregen, nonregeneration; regen regeneration; TB, tuberculosis.

From Joseph V. Raptor hematology and chemistry evaluation. Vet Clin North Am Exot Anim Pract 1999;2(3):689–99; with permission.

affected sites. Specialized tests, such as aspergillosis antigen and antibody testing, chlamydiophila testing, acid-fast stains, bronchoscopy, and endoscopy to obtain direct visualization and biopsy of the affected tissues, may be needed to evaluate the raptor fully.

Raptors presented in respiratory distress may benefit from oxygenation and general anesthesia with isoflurane to minimize the stress of restraint, to provide oxygen support and control of ventilation, to aid in collection of diagnostic samples, and to facilitate administration of supportive care. Air-sac cannulation is reserved for those patients that have upper airway obstruction. Supplemental oxygen is beneficial to the raptor with lower

Table 2
Summarized changes in the white blood cell in response to disease

Differential diagnosis	WBCt	Lymphs	Heterophils	Eosinophils	Monos	Basos
Dehydration	n	n	n	n	n	n
Starvation	−	−	+	n/−	n	n
Hemorrhage	n/+	n	n/+	n/+	n	n
Infection	+/−	n/−	+/−	n/+	n/+	+
Fungal/TB	++	n/−	+	n	+	n
Viral	−	+	−	n	n	n
Parasites	+/n	+	n/+	n/+	n	n/+
Lead toxicity	n/+	n/−	n/+	n	n	n/+
Stress response	+	n/−	n/+	n	n	n

With hemorrhage and tissue trauma, the eosinophil count may be elevated. With overwhelming septicemia, the WBCt and the heterophil count may decrease. Toxic changes in the heterophils and bands may also be present.

Abbreviations: + increase; − decrease; basos, basophils; lymphs, lymphocytes; monos, monocytes; n, normal; WBCt, white blood cell count.

From Joseph V. Raptor hematology and chemistry evaluation. Vet Clin North Am Exot Anim Pract 1999;2(3):689–99; with permission.

respiratory tract disease. Humidification of inspired air and maintenance of the raptor's hydration status with systemic fluid therapy are essential to aiding in the removal of secretions from the trachea and bronchi. Nebulization is an adjunct therapy with tremendously beneficial results. It delivers moisture and medications to the respiratory mucous membranes. Nebulizers should deliver a particle size of less than 5 ppm to reach the lower respiratory tract adequately. In cases of severe respiratory disease, such as a fungal infection, nebulization therapy may be performed for several months. Nebulized agents may include antibiotics and antifungals with saline or sterile water as the diluent. Oxygen may be used as the delivery vehicle, but it is not required unless hypoxemia is a problem. Nebulizations should be performed two to four times daily for 20 to 30 minutes each time. This author uses the DeVillbis Pulmoaide nebulizer (Sunrise Medical, Somerset, Pennsylvania) with the LC Plus disposable administration vial (Pan, Midlothian, Virginia) to achieve the proper micrometer particle size. This arrangement allows the owner to administer nebulization treatments at home. Most often, antibiotics or antifungals are used either parenterally or orally to fight the bacterial or fungal infection, respectively. Thorough examination of the ears will rule out bacterial and fungal otitis as a complicating factor of chronic respiratory disease or parasitic infiltration (myiasis), especially in raptors from the wild.

Respiratory fungal infections predominate in the raptor species. *Aspergillus* sp is the causal agent seen most often in raptor fungal infections. Certain species of raptors are considered at high risk for fungal infections. They are the gyrfalcon (*Falco rusticolus*), golden eagle (*Aquila chrysaetos*), osprey (*Pandion haliaetus*), goshawk (*Accipiter gentiles*), rough-legged hawk (*Buteo lagopus*), and red-tailed hawk (*Buteo jamaicensis*). Raptors in good health and clean environments are not candidates for fungal infection. Predisposing factors for infection include malnutrition, pre-existing bacterial, viral, or parasitic disease, unsanitary environmental conditions, stress, and immunosuppression. Nesting material with organic debris that becomes moist enhances mold growth and contaminates incubating eggs or nestlings. All raptors presenting to the veterinarian should be evaluated for a smoldering subclinical fungal infection. Treatment of a respiratory fungal infection is involved and expensive. A preventive program of itraconazole or fluconazole for 2 weeks and possibly nebulization with an antifungal should be considered for any raptor presenting for medical or traumatic problems, especially high-risk raptors.

Trauma-induced respiratory distress is a frequent occurrence in the raptor species. A raptor may hit a fence, auto, or prey species in its pursuit. Impact injuries may cause ruptured air sacs or lung contusions with devastating results. Aggressive therapy should be administered for the first 24 to 36 hours. It is during this time that the lung functions may begin to deteriorate. Steroids, fluid support, oxygenation, and antibiotics are needed to help sustain the pulmonary hemorrhage and oxygenation deficits that may follow impact injuries. Diuretics may be necessary if pulmonary edema is forming. Foreign body inhalation is not uncommon in the raptor species. Raptors eat their prey items fast and furiously. Plucking feathers or fur, taking bites, and gulping their food may lead to aspiration of food particles. When a small piece is aspirated, death may not be immediate; however, a chronic bacterial or fungal infection may persist in the trachea, lungs, or air sacs. A granuloma may form at the site of the aspiration.

Parasitic respiratory infections are uncommon in the raptor species, except for the air-sac worm *Serratospiculum amaculata*. This nematode inhabits the air sacs mainly of falcons—predominantly the prairie falcon (*Falco mexicanus*). Infected air sacs become thickened, white, and fibrous. Treatment is accomplished with ivermectin or fenbendazole. As the worms die and begin to disintegrate, damage to the air sacs and thromboembolism are possible. The raptor is to be kept quiet for 1 to 2 weeks after treatment.

Traumatic injuries

Traumatic injuries are well represented in the raptor literature. Soft tissue injuries or broken bones from barbed wire fences, predator–prey interactions, territorial conflicts, or impact injuries often result in blood loss and visceral damage. Ocular trauma may result in a raptor's becoming visually compromised. Many of these birds become nonreleasable or end their falconry careers. Much debate focuses on the ability of the raptor to adjust to uniocular vision and be successful in obtaining prey species and avoiding predators.

Cardiac arrest from ventricular fibrillation, pericardial effusion, thermal burns, muscle or generalized convulsions, fractured bones, skull or brain damage, and spinal trauma with paresis are all possible results of an electrocution. Often the consequences of electrocution are of a chronic nature and take several days to appear. Serious tissue damage and necrosis of the extremities from electrocution may take days to become visibly evident. Whole-body radiographs are highly recommended to evaluate the bony skeleton and rule out hidden fractures of the shoulders and spine that may have resulted from the fall.

Head trauma is usually the result of an impact injury. Those raptors not responding in 48 hours to supportive care carry a guarded prognosis for full recovery. A common occurrence in head trauma cases is difficulty in getting raptors to eat on their own. Often this simple task takes 1 to 2 weeks, even when the raptor appears to have recovered from the head trauma. Long-term medical and supportive care is usually required in head trauma cases.

Toxins

Exposure to toxins, such as lead, mercury, and pesticides, is a common occurrence in raptors. The signs of lead toxicity are variable and may include regurgitation, weight loss, depression, and green, sticky feces. As the disease progresses, head tremors, paresis, or paralysis of the lower extremities may appear. Radiographs may be misleading, because the lead particles have usually moved out of the gastrointestinal tract by the time the bird is showing symptoms. Blood-lead levels are usually needed to make a definitive diagnosis of lead toxicity. Mercury poisoning can occur in the bald eagle or osprey that eats contaminated fish from lakes and streams. (These fish are migratory and may not reflect the lake or stream from which they were caught.) Clinical signs include weakness, incoordination, and weight loss. Pesticide intoxications in raptors result from exposure to the many environmental toxins and from secondary exposures when they eat contaminated prey. Anticholinesterase (carbamates and organophosphates) and organochlorine (dichlorodiphenyl-trichloroethane [DDT] dieldrin) intoxication produce tremors or convulsions in raptors. Strychnine results in tetanic convulsions. Raptors eating rodents poisoned with rodenticides may become secondarily poisoned. The coagulation factors II, VII, IX, and X are affected, and hemorrhage occurs.

Miscellaneous problems such as hypocalcemia and hypoglycemia are not uncommon in the raptors. When sufficiently severe, either problem can result in seizure activity. A condition termed by the falconer "cramps" (in a rapidly growing, downy chick) results from a complex set of factors, including calcium deficiency, chilling, and a poor diet. These chicks often present in distress and discomfort, with intermittent muscle spasms that distort the bone growth. This is a difficult situation to address and always carries a guarded prognosis. Hypoglycemia results in seizure activity. Lethargy, weakness, or the inability to stand may precede a seizure. Although hypoglycemia is common in accipiters, any raptor that is kept too sharp for hunting or that is starving because of the inability to hunt is susceptible to developing this condition. Cold-weather anemia is a condition seen in flying raptors during the winter months. This anemia is usually brought on by poor food quality, inadequate food intake, and exposure to low temperatures. Falconry birds maintained at flying weights and housed outdoors in a cold climate are most susceptible. If not treated, this condition may be fatal within 24 hours of presentation. Raptors with inappetence, lethargy, unwillingness to fly, minor tremors or shaking, glassy-eyed appearance, and sudden weight loss with a prominent keel should be evaluated for this condition. Aggressive supportive care is necessary. A blood transfusion may be needed to stabilize the patient. No casting material should be given for several days, only easily digestible food. Recovery may take as long as 3 weeks. Frostbite may occur in some raptor species subject to extreme cold. The Harris's hawk (*Parabuteo unicinctus*) is a desert-type species found in the Southwest that cannot tolerate cold weather. When supplemental heat is not supplied to these raptors housed outdoors in a cold climate, frostbite of the extremities occurs.

The blood parasites most likely to affect the raptors are parasites of the family Hemoproteidae [10]. Hemoproteus, Plasmodium, and Leucocytozoon represent this family of parasites. Little is known about the effects of a hemoptroteus infection in the raptor. Clinical signs may include anorexia, depression, and hemolytic anemia. Most infections appear to be subclinical; however, severe infections in the stressed or immunocompromised raptor may result in clinical disease. *Plasmodium* spp and *Leucocytozoon* spp are more likely to cause clinical disease in the raptors. *Plasmodium* is responsible for the disease avian malaria, common in the falcons. Mortality is high when treatment is not initiated. Many raptor species may be infected with *Leucocytozoon*, with severe clinical disease evident in the immature raptor. A complete blood count will identify these parasites.

Summary

Raptors often present to the veterinarian with multiple complex issues. Being familiar with the raptor species and their differences in behavior, nutritional requirements, and response to disease enhances the veterinarian's ability to formulate a sound diagnostic and therapeutic plan. Having a trained staff and proper hospital management of the patient increases the speed and extent of recovery.

Sources of equipment necessary for raptor medicine are

- In Flight Products by Marzo, 14321 5th Line Nass, RR #2, Rockwood, Ontario, Canada NOB 2KO (gloves and jesses).
- Cyrus Hoods, PO Box 1553, Miles City, MT 59301 (hoods).
- Hawkmasters, 2460 Turner Road, Ceres, CA 95307 (hood blocks and patterns).
- Northwoods Limited, PO Box 874, Rainier, WA 98576 (equipment and supplies).

References

[1] Joseph V. Introduction to a veterinary falconry practice. In: Proceedings of the Association of Avian Veterinarians, Tampa, 1996. Madison (WI): Omnipress; 1996. p. 255–60.
[2] Redig PT, Ackermann J. Raptors. In: Tully TN, Lawton MPC, Dorrestein GM, editors. Avian medicine. 1st edition. London: Butterworth-Heinemann; 2000. p. 180–213.
[3] Joseph V. Vomiting and regurgitation. In: Olsen GH, Orosz SE, editors. Manual of avian medicine. 1st edition. St. Louis (Missouri): Mosby; 2000. p. 70–84.
[4] Beebe FL, Webster HM. North American falconry and hunting hawks. 7th edition. Denver (CO): North American Falconry and Hunting Hawks; 1994.
[5] Joseph V. Emergency care of raptors. Vet Clin North Am Exot Anim Pract 1998;1(1):77–98.
[6] Hernandez M, Aguilar RF. Steroids and fluid therapy for treatment of shock in the critical avian patient. Seminars in Avian and Exotic Pet Medicine 1994;3:190–9.
[7] Redig PT. Management of medical emergencies in raptors. In: Bonagura JD, Kirk RW, editors. Kirk current veterinary therapy XI. Philadelphia: WB Saunders; 1992. p. 1134.
[8] Harris DJ. Care of the critically ill patient. Seminars in Avian and Exotic Pet Medicine 1994; 3:175.
[9] Joseph V. Selected medical topics for birds of prey. In: Proceedings of the Association of Avian Veterinarians. Tampa (FL): 1996. p. 261–4.

[10] Joseph V. Raptor hematology and chemistry evaluation. Vet Clin North Am Exot Anim Pract 1999;2(3):689–99.
[11] Halliwell WH. Serum chemistry profile in the health and disease of birds of prey. In: Proceedings of the International Symposium on Diseases of Birds of Prey. London: 1980. p. 111.
[12] Hernandez M. Blood chemistry in raptors. Proceedings of the First Conference of the European Committee of the Association of Avian Veterinarians. Vienna (Austria): 1991. p. 411–9.
[13] Hernandez M. Raptor clinical hematology. Proceedings of the First Conference of the European Committee of the Association of Avian Veterinarians. Vienna (Austria): 1991. p. 420–33.
[14] Lumeij JT. Avian plasma chemistry in health and disease. Proceedings of the Association of Avian Veterinarians. Nashville (TN): 1993. p. 20–6.
[15] Joseph V. Medical management of selected raptor diseases. Proceedings of the Avian and Exotic Symposium. Davis (CA): 1993. p. 67–80.

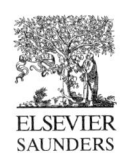

Common Procedures in the Pet Ferret

Ricardo Emanuel Castanheira de Matos, LMV,
James K. Morrisey, DVM, DABVP–Avian*

*Section of Wildlife and Exotic Medicine, Department of Clinical Sciences,
College of Veterinary Medicine, Cornell University, Ithaca, NY 14853-6401, USA*

The domestic ferret is an increasingly popular pet in North America and Europe and may easily be incorporated into the structure and workings of most small animal hospitals. Not only does treatment of ferrets provide case diversity and intellectual challenges to the veterinarian but it may increase revenue, because most ferret owners have several ferrets. The diagnostic and supportive care procedures used commonly in ferrets are similar to those used in dogs and cats. This article presents the common diagnostic and supportive care procedures used in ferrets, with special emphasis on some of the unique aspects that make these procedures easier to learn and perform.

Triage and patient assessment

Classic triage principles as they apply to dogs and cats also hold true for ferrets. Ferrets are remarkably hardy animals that can tolerate substantial illness and appear to be stable despite being critically ill. The most life-threatening problems should be treated first; these include profuse bleeding, shock, and dyspnea. Acute hemorrhage in ferrets is usually traumatic in origin; however, severe anemia may occur as a result of chronic disease or chronic low-grade blood loss, such as from a gastric ulcer. The use of transfusions and blood substitutes is discussed later in this article. Shock in ferrets is most commonly decompensatory, and the animals may have normal to slow heart rate, weak or absent pulses, severe hypothermia ($<98°F$), and profound mental depression [1]. Shock is best treated with placement of an intraosseous or intravenous catheter and the administration of colloids and crystalloids at 5 mL/kg and 10 mL/kg, respectively (these may be mixed

---

* Corresponding author.
E-mail address: jkm27@cornell.edu (J.K. Morrisey).

together), in small boluses. These boluses should continue until the blood pressure stabilizes as 90 mm Hg, at which time fluids may be given by constant rate infusion to deal with the fluid deficit and maintenance. Dyspnea in ferrets is usually related to cardiac disease, although primary pulmonary problems, such as pneumonia, may also occur. These are best distinguished using radiographs and echocardiography. Dyspneic ferrets will benefit from being placed in an oxygen cage with the oxygen set at 40% until a thorough history and diagnostic plan may be determined. Pleural fluid can accumulate with both cardiac and pulmonary disease and should be removed for diagnostic and therapeutic effects.

The physical examination in ferrets is fairly straightforward, and readers are referred to other issues for a more thorough discussion of the normal examination; only the more unique aspects are discussed here [2]. Most ferrets are tolerant of the examination procedure, although they can be difficult to hold still. It is best to perform the examination with minimal restraint to avoid urination and defecation by the ferret, although this is the easiest means of collecting such samples. If the ferret is to be restrained, it may be held by the scruff or may be stretched out for a more complete restraint, such as for cystocentesis or other procedures (Fig. 1). The examination should be thorough and systematic and should follow an organized

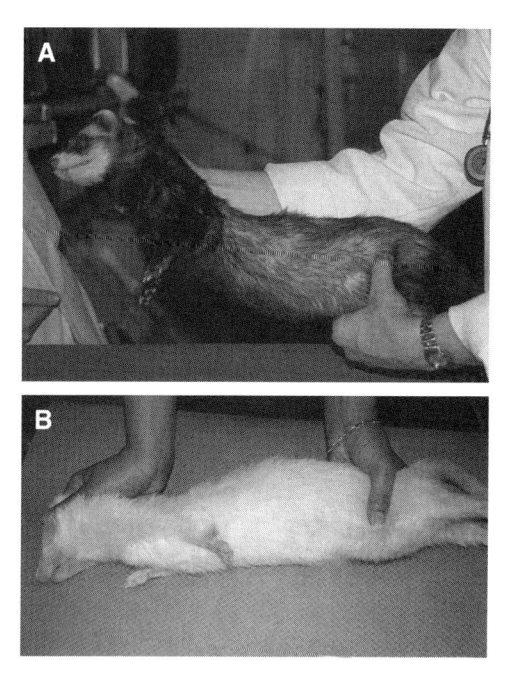

Fig. 1. Restraint for a more active ferret may be accomplished by scruffing and suspending the animal slightly (*A*) or by performing the "stretch," in which the ferret is scruffed with one hand and a circle is made cranial to the pelvis with the other (*B*).

procedure. In this way all problems are identified, even those not noticed by the owner.

Assessments of attitude and hydration status are the first steps in a thorough physical examination. A healthy ferret should be alert and actively investigating its surroundings. A ferret with its eyes closed is severely depressed and should be assessed and treated accordingly. Hydration in ferrets is assessed using skin turgor, mucous membrane examination, and eye position. Ferrets have thick skin around the neck and dorsum, and skin turgor can be harder to assess in ferrets than in other species. As part of the evaluation, it is important to determine how the skin moves over the underlying tissue. In a hydrated ferret the skin should move easily over the underlying tissue and the mucous membranes should be slick. As the level of dehydration increases, the mucosa will be sticky; with severe dehydration ($>10\%$), the eyes will become sunken into the skull. Oral examination may be performed by simply suspending the ferret by its scruff (Fig. 2) or by gently pushing down on the mandibular canine tooth while holding the cheeks firmly with the other hand. Chipped canines are common in older ferrets.

Ocular examination in ferrets is straightforward, although ferrets lack a menace response. Ferrets exhibit a dazzle response to bright light. The ears commonly have brown, waxy discharge that may be confused with

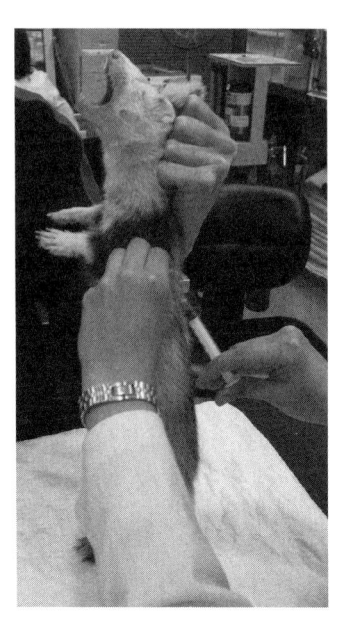

Fig. 2. Most ferrets will yawn when suspended by the scruff, which allows for visualization of the oral cavity.

mite excrement. Ferrets can have *Otodectes cyanotis*, the dog and cat ear mite, but mites tend to leave more granular material in the ears as opposed to the waxy appearance of the normal debris. Microscopic examination of the material revealing mites is definitive diagnosis for an ear mite infection. The ears may also contain two small tattooed dots placed by the commercial breeder to identify animals that have been neutered or spayed and descented.

Peripheral lymph nodes in adult ferrets, especially those that are overweight or taking prednisolone, are surrounded by large amounts of fat. This effect may make the nodes appear to be enlarged, but careful palpation will reveal soft, easily compressible fat surrounding the much firmer lymph node.

Cardiac auscultation in ferrets should be performed using a small stethoscope, such as a human neonatal unit. This reduces the noise of surrounding pulmonary tissue and allows the listener better to identify low-grade murmurs and other problems. The heart is located farther caudally than one might initially suspect and is usually three to four ribs caudal of the elbow. Many apparently healthy ferrets have a respiratory sinus arrhythmia and may occasionally drop beats. If the ferret is having any other signs of respiratory or cardiac compromise, an echocardiogram is warranted.

Abdominal palpation typically reveals a prominent to large spleen in healthy ferrets that is caused by extramedullary hematopoeisis (EMH). Careful palpation for clean edges and homogeneous consistency are helpful in differentiating EMH from lymphoma or other splenic diseases. Abdominal ultrasound and percutaneous aspiration are easily performed in ferrets and should be done if there are any inconsistencies in the palpation or if the clinician has concerns. The kidneys are easily palpable, but perirenal and sublumbar fat accumulation may occasionally be mistaken for a mass. The adrenal glands are not normally palpable but may be palpated cranially and medially to the kidneys when the glands are enlarged. The glands feel like a firm nodule within the perirenal fat in this area.

The integument should be examined for any thinning areas or alopecia. Scratch marks may be seen in ferrets with pruritus from any cause. One should check around the tail base and tail with especial care, because this area is often the first affected with adrenal disease or seasonal alopecia. Check the genitals for problems such as vulvar swelling in females associated with adrenal disease or preputial tumors in males.

Assessment of body temperature is usually postponed until the end of the examination, because it is not well tolerated and usually induces defecation and urination. This is an excellent time to collect such samples if needed. Good restraint is required to avoid damaging the rectal tissue and to obtain an accurate reading. The use of quick-read thermometers is helpful in this situation, especially those with softer, flexible tips. The normal body temperature for a ferret is 100.5°F to 102.5°F, although the range may be 100°F to 104°F (37.8°C to 40°C).

Sample collection

Blood collection

Ferrets have several accessible veins for venipuncture, including the cephalic, lateral saphenous, and jugular veins [3]. Restraint is an important aspect of ferret venipuncture. Some ferrets tolerate manual restraint well, whereas others are more fractious and may require mild sedation.

Lateral saphenous and cephalic veins may be approached as in other species, keeping in mind that ferret skin is quite tough and these veins are small and superficial. These veins are generally useful only for small quantities of blood for quick assessment tests, such as hematocrit and blood glucose. Small needles, such as 25- to 27-gauge needles and 0.5- to 1-mL syringes, are necessary for these sites. The authors find that using insulin syringes allows for repeated use of these veins, whereas a 25-gauge needle allows for a one-time use.

The jugular vein is the best choice for larger blood samples. For a classic approach to the jugular vein, the ferret is restrained like a cat at the end of the examination table with head and legs extended or is held in lateral recumbency with the forelegs and neck extended (Fig. 3). The jugular vein is held off at the thoracic inlet. This vein is frequently difficult to visualize, because it is small and superficial, and it is generally palpated as it arises from the thoracic inlet. Bending the needle will permit a more superficial venipuncture. The jugular vein may also be easily accessed as it dives under the cranial end of the sternum. This approach was previously called a cranial vena cava venipuncture, but close attention to the anatomy reveals that it is simply the thoracic portion of the jugular vein [4,5]. This is often the best approach for obtaining large volumes of blood and may be drawn in a well-restrained awake animal (Fig. 4). Distraction with sweet substances is often enough to facilitate a good blood draw, although some animals do require sedation or anesthesia. Twenty-five–gauge needles and 1- to 3-mL

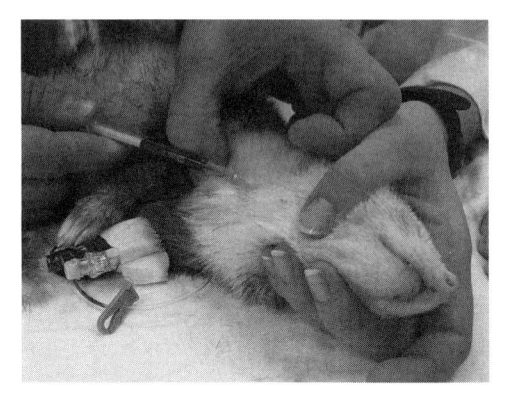

Fig. 3. Jugular venipuncture may be accomplished from a lateral or table-end positioning. The vein is difficult to visualize but may be palpated easily.

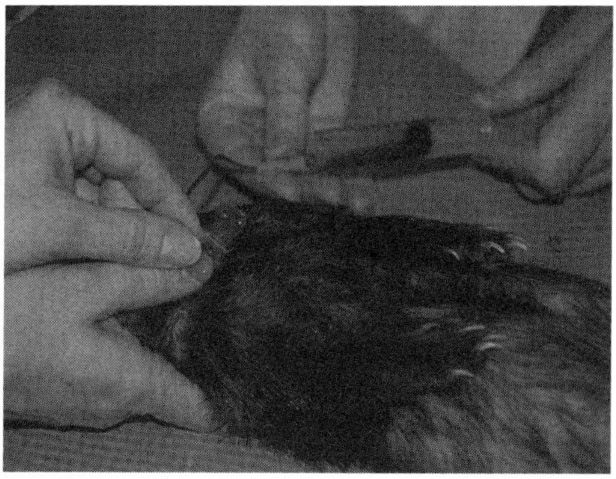

Fig. 4. The jugular vein may be easily accessed as it dives below the sternum.

syringes are used for this procedure. The animal is placed in dorsal recumbency and the forelegs held alongside the body. There is a palpable notch between the manubrium and the first rib into which the needle is advanced slowly and superficially. The needle is directed toward the opposite hip. Slight negative pressure is applied as the needle is advanced until blood begins to flow. The needle should be quickly withdrawn if the patient moves excessively, to avoid lacerating the vein.

A safety guideline for maximum blood volume to remove is 1% of body weight in grams. When the volume of blood obtained is small, use of lithium heparin collection vials rather than serum clot tubes will increase the volume of plasma retrieved.

Fecal and urine collection

When the urinary bladder is palpable, cystocentesis is the method of choice for urine collection, because this sample gives the best indication of what is occurring in the kidneys and bladder. The urinary bladder may be approached through the lateral body wall, as in a cat, with a 3-mL syringe and a 1-in, 23-gauge needle. Restraint is crucial, and distraction with a sweet substance is often successful. Obtaining the sample while the animal is scruffed is another option. Manual expression may be useful, and litter-trained ferrets' urine may be collected in a clean, litter-free box. As previously mentioned, many ferrets will urinate when restrained or when a rectal temperature is obtained. A free catch of this sample is possible when the clinician is prepared with an empty sterile vial.

Fecal samples are easily collected during examination. Ferrets will typically defecate following placement of a thermometer to determine rectal temperature. If a sample is not immediately produced, allowing the ferret a few minutes in a cage or on the floor of an examination room may be helpful.

Bone marrow aspiration

Bone marrow aspiration may be a valuable diagnostic tool and is performed in ferrets as in other small animals. Anesthesia is required. The iliac crest, proximal femur, and humerus are all appropriate sites for bone marrow collection in the ferret, although the proximal femur is most easily accessed and commonly used. The skin around the collection site must be shaved and aseptically prepared. A small skin incision is made over the site with a No. 15 scalpel blade. An 18- to 20-gauge, 1.5-in spinal needle or Jamshidi biopsy needle (Cardinal Health, McGraw Park, Illinois) may be used to collect the sample into a 6-mL syringe. The needle is inserted into the marrow cavity using a twisting motion to penetrate the bone cortex. If a bone core is present, it will prevent aspiration; in these patients the original needle may be withdrawn and a new needle of equal size may be reinserted in the same site and the marrow aspirated [6]. The marrow is aspirated using repeated suction of the syringe until 0.25 to 0.5 mL of material is present in the syringe. This material is then pushed out of the syringe onto a Petri dish containing a small amount of sterile saline, and small drops are placed on slides for examination. One should look for small spicules of bone in the bloody material in the dish to be certain a good sample was collected.

Splenic aspiration

Percutaneous splenic aspiration is a frequently used diagnostic tool in ferrets to assess the spleen for a variety of diseases. A small area of skin is shaved and aseptically prepared, and the spleen is palpated and immobilized under the prepared area in the awake ferret (Fig. 5). One should introduce

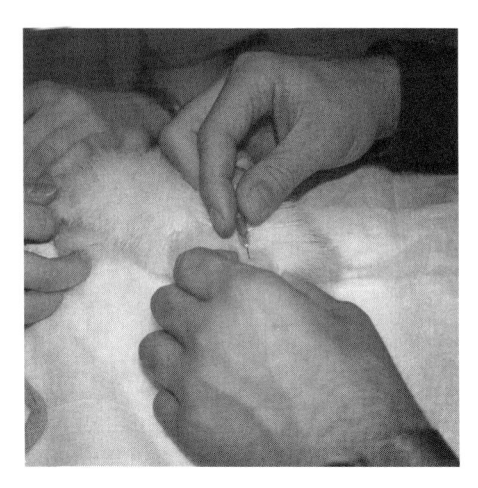

Fig. 5. The spleen is easily palpated and may be aspirated in the distracted or mildly sedated ferret. Here the spleen is held in place against the skin while a needle is inserted for sample collection.

a 22- to 25-gauge needle attached to a 3-mL syringe, aspirate, and withdraw quickly. Aspirate from two sites if possible. The aspirate will appear bloody. Place drops of this bloody material on slides and gently smear them out. The slides should display a "thicker" quality when compared with normal blood smears. Splenic aspirates are generally safe, though there may be bruising at the site. Ultrasound-guided aspirates should be performed when possible, because this allows the aspiration of focal abnormal areas and visualization of any post-aspiration bleeding. Sedation may be required for ultrasound-guided aspirates or in fractious animals.

Liver biopsy and aspiration

Ultrasound-directed liver biopsy or fine needle aspiration is performed as in the canine or feline patient. As in other small animals, it is best to acquire a coagulation panel before biopsy. Aspiration is less likely to cause serious bleeding but also supplies fewer cells that are useful for a diagnosis and cells that are more subject to trauma than a biopsy [6]. When performing a liver biopsy, the clinician should be aware of the size of the biopsy specimen acquired by the instrument in relation to the size and depth of the ferret's liver. General anesthesia is required for either procedure.

Lymph node biopsy and aspiration

Lymphadenopathy can be caused by a variety of problems, such as lymphoma, other neoplasias, and inflammation. When lymphoma is suspected by physical examination and complete blood count, popliteal nodectomy is recommended for diagnosis [7]. Lymph node aspirates may be useful but difficult to obtain in ferrets because of the large amount of fat commonly surrounding the peripheral lymph nodes. When attempting to obtain an aspirate, it is important carefully to palpate the firmer lymph node within the softer, more compressible fat that surrounds it. Once the node is palpated, one should carefully hold it so it may be aspirated with a 25-gauge needle and 3-mL syringe. After aspirating, one should stab the needle several times through the firm tissue, because this is more likely to give a true sample of the node than a pure aspirate.

To perform a lymph node biopsy, the caudal thigh is clipped and aseptically prepared. The popliteal lymph node is palpated and held against the skin. A skin incision is made over the lymph node, and the node, which is tan and firm, is bluntly dissected from the fat and removed. In many cases, there is excessive fat, and locating the lymph node can be difficult. Hemostasis is usually not a problem, and the skin is closed with sutures.

Tracheal wash

Ferrets have a small but long trachea; therefore, tracheal washes for cytology and culture must be approached through the glottis. The animal must be anesthetized and intubated with a sterile endotracheal tube (usually a 2-mm or 2.5-mm ID). A sterile 3.5-F red rubber tube or polypropylene catheter is advanced through the endotracheal tube to a premeasured point approximately halfway down the thorax. Two to three mL of 0.9% sodium chloride is injected into the catheter and immediately withdrawn, as in other tracheal wash techniques. The collected sample should be placed in a sterile tube for cytology and culture as warranted.

Skin masses

A number of skin masses occur in ferrets, such as mast cell tumors, sebaceous adenomas, cutaneous lymphoma, and other metastatic tumors. Mast cell tumors and sebaceous adenomas are benign in nature in ferrets. Several diagnostic approaches to skin masses in ferrets exist, including impression smears and fine needle aspirates, but excisional biopsies are most likely to result in a definitive diagnosis [6]. Impression smears work best for wet or exfoliative masses that are in the epidermal tissue. Simply hold the mass firmly and squeeze slightly while pressing a clean slide into the mass. Make several samples and save some slides for special stains or second opinions in case of need. Aspirates may be performed using 20- to 25-gauge needles. The larger needles may be stabbed through the mass to obtain a small core biopsy, or a syringe may be used to aspirate cells once the needle is inserted into the mass. Biopsy specimens may be taken with punch biopsies, or, ideally, the entire mass may be removed and submitted for histopathology.

Treatment techniques

Catheter placement

Placement of peripheral catheters may be performed in awake ferrets when they are weak or debilitated. More active ferrets may require sedation or general anesthesia for this procedure (see later discussion). Intravenous (IV) catheters may be placed in the cephalic, lateral saphenous, or jugular vein. The authors use the cephalic vein as first choice for IV catheter placement. Depending on the size of the ferret and the chosen vein, 22-, 24-, or 26-gauge catheters may be used.

Careful preparation of the area is essential, because the fur oil will prevent adherence of the tape used to secure the catheter in place. For placements of catheters in the limbs, shave the fur over the vessel area. Prepare the skin aseptically. The wet skin should be dried (except the skin covering the vein) to allow the tape to adhere to the skin once the catheter is in place. Because ferrets' skin is very thick, one should puncture the skin overlying or next to the vein with a 20- or 22-gauge hypodermic needle, being careful to avoid the vein. Once the catheter is taped, consider applying sterile tissue glue to the tape securing the catheter before bandaging the leg. A butterfly tape around the catheter and sutured to the skin may also be used to secure the catheter in place. Use a T connector and low-flow extension line for fluid administration. Wrap the limb in a routine way. The area distal to the catheter should be checked at least twice a day for excessive swelling or changes in coloration, and the catheter should be checked at least once every 24 hours.

For jugular catheterization, the author most often uses a 22-gauge peripheral catheter. Other types of catheters, such as a 22-gauge, 8 in through-the-needle catheter (Intracath, Becton, Dickson Vascular Access, Sandy, Utah) on a 19-gauge needle, may also be used [7]. A cut-down procedure may be necessary to access the vein [8]. Because of the bandaging necessary to secure the jugular catheter, ferrets often become depressed and do not eat when a jugular catheter is placed. The author has used this vein in debilitated ferrets when it is important to have central venous access, or in ferrets undergoing prolonged anesthesia and requiring a second vascular access port.

When repeated vascular access is required for any reason (eg, chemotherapy), a subcutaneous vascular access system (Vascular-Access-Port, Access Technologies, Sokie, Illinois) may be placed [9]. The technique used to place the catheter and port has been described and illustrated [9,10].

In ferrets that are collapsed with poor blood pressure or in young or small ferrets, placement of an IV catheter may be unsuccessful. An intraosseous (IO) catheter may be placed in the humerus, femur, or tibia [11]. The author prefers the proximal femur because it causes the least disruption to normal movement. Unless the ferret is very debilitated, local blocks, sedation, or general anesthesia is required for placement of the IO catheter. Clip the hair and aseptically prepare the area over the head of the femur. Use a 20- or 22-gauge, 1.5-in spinal needle or a 20- or 22-gauge hypodermic needle with a sterile surgical wire as a stylet to prevent occlusion of the needle with a bone fragment plug [4]. Insert the needle medial to the greater trocanter using firm pressure and gentle rotation. Once the catheter enters the marrow cavity, it should advance easily. Remove the stylet and test the patency and location of the catheter by injecting sterile saline. If the catheter is in the right location, there will be little resistance to the injection and no swelling of the soft tissues around the femur. Radiographs may be used to confirm location of the catheter. Place a butterfly tape around the needle hub and suture it to the skin [4,11]. Use an injection cap or a T connector attached to the spinal needle. Because the bone does not expand when fluid is injected through the catheter, syringe pumps should be used for fluid administration. IO catheters may be used for several days. Prophylactic use of parenteral antibiotics is recommended [4]. Once normal volemia is established and placement of an IV catheter is successful, the author discontinues the use of the IO catheter.

Because of the ferret's small size, one should use only small volumes of heparinized saline when flushing any catheter to prevent heparin overdosage [8].

Most sick ferrets will not chew on the catheters or IV lines, but the lines (and the ferrets) can become entangled in their bedding or cage furniture and must be monitored. As their condition improves, ferrets may chew the injection port of the T connector. Cover this port to prevent ingestion of the rubber material.

Fluid administration

Continuous delivery of IV or IO fluids is recommended in severely debilitated ferrets and in ferrets requiring dextrose supplementation.

Daily fluid requirements for ferrets have not been determined. Calculating fluid requirements based on rates used in cats appears to be adequate for maintenance: 60 to 70 mL/kg/d [4,12]. Additional fluid requirements (due to dehydration, ongoing losses) and fluid supplements (eg, dextrose, vitamin B, potassium) should be calculated following protocols used for small animals. Monitor the animal carefully for signs of overhydration, such as difficulty breathing, harsh lung sounds, or heart murmur [8]. Ferrets with cardiac disease or anuric renal failure are especially at risk for developing overhydration.

Colloids may be used together with crystalloids for improving fluid volume and oncotic pressure in ferrets that are hypoproteinemic or in shock [12]. Colloids such as hetastarch are given at a dose of 10 to 20 mL/kg/d. In ferrets with shock, this may be given as a bolus at 5 mL/kg over 15 minutes and repeated as needed, not exceeding a total dose of 20 mL/kg/d [12]. When colloids are given together with crystalloids, one should reduce the crystalloid fluid rate by 25% to 50%.

For accurate delivery of the volume of fluid required IV or IO, one should use a syringe pump or Buretrol device (Baxter Health Care, Deerfield, Illinois).

Blood transfusion

Consider a whole blood transfusion when the packed cell volume (PCV) is 25% or less in a ferret that exhibits clinical signs of anemia or requires surgery or in a ferret that is thrombocytopenic and exhibits ecchymosis, petechiation, or bleeding [12]. Blood groups have not been demonstrated in ferrets, and there is little risk of a transfusion reaction, even without cross-matching and after using a variety of donors [4,12,13]. The recipient ferret may be given one dose of short-acting corticosteroid IV slowly 15 minutes before transfusion to prevent reactions [8].

Estimation of the blood volume required by the recipient may be calculated thus, as for the cat [14]: Anticoagulated blood volume (mL) = body weight of recipient (kg) × 70 × [(PCV desired − PCV of recipient)/PCV of donor in anticoagulant]. For example, if one has a 0.5-kg ferret that has a PCV of 20% and one wishes to increase it to 25% and is using a 1-kg donor ferret with a PCV of 40%, the formula will look like this: Blood volume (mL) = 0.5 × 70 [(25−20)/40], so one needs 4.375 mL of blood.

Large male intact or lately neutered ferrets are preferred as blood donors because they have larger blood volumes. Collection of blood from the donor usually requires chemical restraint. Blood should be collected immediately after induction, because isofluorane anesthesia can decrease many hematology values that begin at induction and reach maximum levels at 15 minutes after induction [15]. Blood must be collected aseptically from a large vessel (jugular or "cranial vena cava"), using a butterfly catheter, directly into a syringe with anticoagulant (Table 1) [16]. The collected blood may be given immediately to the recipient ferret. The blood administration set should include a filter. The transfusion should be given within 4 hours to prevent bacterial growth, at a rate of 0.5 mL/kg for the first 20 minutes while the patient is monitored for signs of reaction [16]. For patients requiring transfusion over a greater period of time, the unit of blood should be divided and the portion to be transfused later should be refrigerated [16]. The recipient of the blood should have a PCV performed before and 1 to 2 hours after the transfusion.

Urinary catheterization

Urinary catheters may be placed in females and males. Urinary catheters are indicated in males with dysuria or stranguria secondary to urolithiasis, cystitis, and prostatic disease [12,17]. Clinical indications to place a urinary catheter in females are rare. Urinary catheters may also be used for collecting sterile urine samples and for introduction of contrast into the bladder for contrast radiographic studies [4].

The ferret should be sedated or placed under anesthesia for urinary catheterization. For the catheter, use a 3.5-F rubber feeding catheter, a 3.0-F 11-in ferret urinary catheter (Slippery Sam, Global Veterinary Products, Waukesha, Wisconsin), or a 20- or 22-gauge, 8-in jugular catheter with the stylet removed [12,17,18]. Tomcat catheters are not long or flexible enough to reach the bladder of most male ferrets [18]. A sterile stylet or metal guitar string may be used to stiffen the catheter. Placing the catheter in the freezer may also make it more resistant to bending as it is passed into the urethra.

For females, one should position the ferret in ventral recumbency with the rear quarters elevated with a rolled towel. Aseptically prepare the vulva and perivulvar area. Use a vaginal speculum or otoscope to locate the urethral opening in the floor of the urethral vestibule, approximately 1 cm

Table 1
Common anticoagulants used for blood transfusions

Anticoagulant	Anticoagulant/blood ratio	Comments
Citrate-phosphate-dextrose-adenine	1 mL/7–9 mL	Blood may be stored for 35 days
Citrate-phosphate-dextrose	1 mL/7 ML	—
Acid-citrate-dextrose	1 mL/7 mL	—
Heparin	5–10 units/1 mL	Heparin reversed; use blood within 48 hours

cranial to the clitoral fossa. Introduce a 3.5-F, red-rubber urethral catheter fitted with a wire stylet into the urethral orifice [4,12].

In males, placing a urinary catheter is difficult because of the small size of the urethral opening, the presence of a J-shaped os penis, and the acute bend of the urethra at the pelvic canal [4,12,18]. Prepare the distal end of the prepuce aseptically. If the prepuce or the tip of the penis is swollen, a small incision may be made in the prepuce to facilitate exteriorization of the penis [8,12]. Push the prepuce caudally with one hand while placing pressure on the distal end of the os penis with the other to exteriorize the penis. If needed, use a surgical magnifying loupe to help find the orifice. Localize the urethral opening on the ventral surface of the penis and pass a 24-gauge IV catheter (without the needle) to the distal end of the urethra. While flushing gently with warm saline, insert the tip of the lubricated urinary catheter in the dilated opening alongside the IV catheter. Pass the catheter carefully into the bladder, using small amounts of warm saline while introducing the catheter if needed (Fig. 6). Resistance may be found at the level of the pelvic flexure. If this occurs, lubricate the catheter again and repeat gentle flushing until it passes. Once it is in place, butterfly tape strips may be used to suture the catheter to the skin in the ventral abdomen in multiple locations. Tape the catheter to the base of the tail to reduce tension at the sutured areas and attach a closed urinary collection device (sterile standard drip set and empty sterile fluid bag). Although ferrets do not well tolerate Elizabethan collars or "body bandages," these should be used as needed to prevent removal of or trauma to the catheter and possible foreign body ingestion [4,12,17]. Antibiotics should be given when a urinary catheter is in place [8].

When a urinary catheter cannot be placed, cystocentesis followed by temporary cystotomy may be used to treat urinary obstruction resulting, for example, from adrenal disease [19].

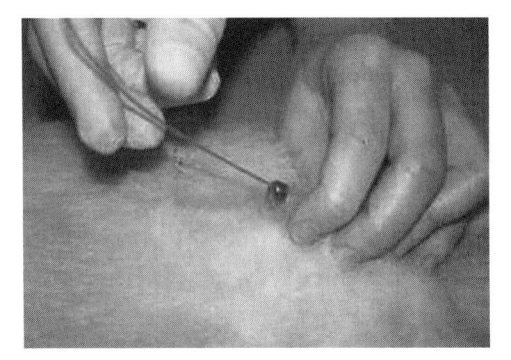

Fig. 6. Urinary catheters are more commonly needed in male ferrets that are blocked because of prostatic enlargement. Here the 3.5-F red rubber feeding tube is being slowly passed into the urethral opening.

Drug therapy

Injectable medications

Few drugs have been pharmacokinetically studied in the ferret; most drug doses are scaled down from the cat and dog [12,20].

In debilitated patients, IV and IO routes should be used for treatments. Most medications given IV may also be administered IO, except for some chemotherapy drugs. When a medication needs to be given IV and there is no indwelling catheter in place, a 25-gauge butterfly catheter may be used in the cephalic, lateral saphenous, or jugular vein.

Intramuscular injections may be given in the semitendinosus, semimembranosus, biceps femoralis, or lumbar muscles [4]. The author prefers the use of caudal thigh muscles. Care should be taken to avoid iatrogenic nerve damage. Ferrets have reduced muscle mass, which limits repeated administration of intramuscular injections.

Subcutaneous injections may be given in the dorsum and shoulder areas. The skin in these areas is thick and the subcutaneous space limited. Most ferrets react severely when a larger volume of fluid is administered subcutaneously, and adequate restraint is needed to prevent a ferret from biting its handler. When the ferret requires large doses of subcutaneous fluids daily, one should consider giving the fluids in two areas, dividing the daily volume in three or four treatments, or placing an IV catheter for continuous administration. Use small-gauge needles (23- to 27-gauge) for injections.

Oral medications

Because ferrets are difficult to pill, oral medications are best given in a liquid form. Most oral medications may be compounded to a flavored oral suspension when needed. Medicating ferrets is not difficult when the taste of the medication may be hidden in a sweet or fatty substance. Chicken baby food or liquid ferret supplements are commonly used by the author. Tablets may be crushed and mixed with Ora-Plus (Paddock Laboratories, Minneapolis, Minnesota), flavoring, and water in a 1:1:2 ratio to make them more palatable [21]. Refrigerate the medication and shake well before using. There is no guarantee of stability [21]. Avoid fish flavors, because ferrets do not like this flavor [12]. Even when flavor is favorable, the scruff hold may be necessary for giving oral medications. Medications with bitter flavors commonly used in ferrets include metronidazole, prednisolone, and bismuth subsalicylate. Ferrets may salivate excessively or paw violently at the mouth and palate following administration of these medications.

Pain management

Pain management is important in the postoperative period and for traumatic injuries. Signs of pain in the ferret include anorexia, lethargy, crying, stiff movements, inability to curl into a sleeping position, and squinting [4]. For control of major posttraumatic or postsurgical pain, opioids are often required [22]. Buprenorphine and butorphanol may be used in ferrets; heavy sedation and depression are commonly seen when the high end of the recommended dose is used. Naloxone may be used to reverse these effects as needed [4]. When pain is considered moderate or mild, nonsteroidal anti-inflammatory drugs (NSAIDs) are often sufficient. Commonly used drugs include ketoprofen, carprofen, and meloxicam [22]. The use of NSAIDs in ferrets has not been well documented, and their reaction to this type of medications is not fully known. For this reason, NSAIDs should be used with caution [12]. Like cats, ferrets are sensitive to acetaminophen toxicity [12]. Ibuprofen may also be toxic to ferrets when the dose is inappropriate [12].

Local or regional nerve block with local anesthetics may also be used, as may epidural and spinal administration of drugs [22,23]. These routes have the advantage of being more effective, allowing one to use smaller doses when compared with systemic administration and, consequently, having fewer negative side effects [23]. The technique for epidural anesthesia in ferrets has been described [23]. Most local anesthetics have a low therapeutic index, so care must be taken when calculating and preparing volumes of local anesthetic for infiltration [24].

Because there are numerous pain pathways involving a variety of different neurotransmitters, combinations of analgesics of different classes are likely to be more effective than a single agent used alone [22].

Nutritional support

Nutritional support is essential in the sick ferret to prevent hypoglycemia and hepatic lipidosis. Ferrets are carnivores with high fat and protein requirements and metabolize fat more efficiently for energy than carbohydrates [4]. Ferrets may be assist-fed meat-based soft foods marked for hospitalized dogs and cats, such as Maximum-Calorie (Iams Company, Dayton, Ohio) and Canine a/d (Hill's Pet Nutrition, Topeka, Kansas). One should give 10 to 20 mL/kg, three to four times per day [4]. Use a syringe or a tongue depressor. Once the ferret develops a taste for its favorite formula, it may eat from a bowl placed in the cage. For ferrets that refuse regular or semisolid food, one may offer high-energy paste supplements such as Nutri-Cal (Evesco Pharmaceuticals, Buena, New Jersey) or Furo-Vite (Marshall Pet Products, Wolcott, New York), chicken or beef broth, meat baby food, liquid soy-based formulas (Deliver 2.0, Mead Johnson Nutritionals, Evansville, Indiana), or mixtures of any of these [12]. These supplements are not nutritionally complete and should be used for a short period until the ferret accepts a more complete diet. Do not use any of the supplements with high carbohydrate content in ferrets with insulinoma [12].

Esophagostomy feeding tubes may be placed in ferrets for long-term management of debilitated animals or in cases of trauma or surgery to the mouth or throat tissues [4]. They may be used for feeding or long-term administration of oral medications. The technique for placement is similar to that used in felines [25]. Apply a butterfly tape to the tube, suture it in place, and add a light wrap of elastic bandaging material around the neck [4]. Feeding tubes may be left in place for as long as 6 weeks.

Gastric feeding tubes have been placed in ferrets experimentally, but the practicality of maintaining these tubes in clinical patients is still to be determined [12].

Miscellaneous procedures

Anesthesia and sedation

Inhalant anesthetics, especially isofluorane and sevoflurane, are the anesthetics of choice in ferrets, even those with chronic disease or critical injury [26]. Ideally, a ferret should be fasted for 4 to 6 hours before induction [8]. Most ferrets may be masked down easily; fractious patients may be sedated first or placed in an induction chamber. Inhalant anesthesia by mask may be used for short procedures (phlebotomy, catheter placement, bone marrow or spleen aspirates, cystocentesis) and may be used even for "longer" procedures, such as skin mass removal or castration. Ferrets undergoing intra-abdominal surgery, prolonged surgeries, or multiple short surgical procedures (eg, descenting and neutering) should be intubated and maintained using a non-rebreathing system. Intubation is easy and similar to that in a cat, using a 2- to 3.5-mm internal diameter cuffed endotracheal tube [24,27]. It is important to remember that both isofluorane and halothane anesthesia can cause changes in the complete blood count in ferrets, decreasing hematocrit, hemoglobin concentration, red blood cell count, and plasma protein levels [15]. Although sevoflurane-related changes have not been reported, a similar effect would be expected, because the changes are caused by splenic sequestration of blood.

Injectable anesthetics have been associated with several problems in ferrets, including prolonged induction and recovery, a need for premedications (eg, atropine), and, occasionally, death [26]. Hence one should avoid use of injectable agents in the debilitated ferret. The most commonly used injectable anesthetic drug is ketamine. This drug is often used in combination with diazepam, midazolam, or acepromazine to provide analgesia and muscle relaxation. These combinations may result in prolonged recovery or seizures [26]. Other injectable anesthetics, such as medetomidine and tiletamine/zolazepam, are used more commonly for short procedures. They may be combined with butorphanol, ketamine, or xylazine for a longer duration of action or deeper planes of anesthesia and muscle relaxation [26]. The authors commonly use midazolam (0.5 mg/kg) and butorphanol (0.3 mg/kg) to sedate ferrets for small procedures, such as ultrasonography, splenic aspirates, catheter placement, and so on.

Analgesics may be used during premedication for smoother induction and recovery, reduced systemic stress and stress-related diseases (eg, gastric ulcers), and a faster return to normal behavior and function [26].

During anesthesia, ECG, temperature, hemoglobin-oxygen saturation, and indirect blood pressure should be monitored closely [24]. When the anesthesia lasts longer than 20 to 30 minutes, IV or IO crystalloids with 2.5% to 5% dextrose should be given at a rate of 5 to 10 mL/kg/h [27].

Ferrets have a tendency to become hypothermic during anesthesia and recovery periods. The proper use of heat lamps, Bair Huggers (Stepic, Hixville, New York), circulating warm-water heating pads, and heated IV fluids decreased the incidence of prolonged recovery and unexpected death in postsurgical ferrets [26]. During recovery, one should monitor ferrets in heated cages closely for hyperthermia.

Imaging

Radiography in ferrets is useful in assessing intra-abdominal and intra-thoracic structures for organomegaly or other problems and in monitoring disease progression and treatment. Rigid restraint is essential to produce diagnostic films. Ferrets can be difficult to maintain under manual restraint and often need to be sedated or placed under anesthesia for radiographs. High-speed film, fine screen cassettes, and excellent machinery are important for diagnostic radiography in ferrets [6,28,29]. Cassettes are used on the tabletop with the patient positioned directly on the cassette. Standard views include dorsoventral or ventrodorsal and lateral. The whole body is typically incorporated into each view because this allows a quick and easy assessment of the entire patient [6,28].

Contrast radiography may be done in ferrets as in other mammals. Gastrointestinal disease, such as megaesophagus or obstruction and foreign body, may be delineated in an upper gastrointestinal examination. Administer 10 to 15 mL/kg of barium sulfate liquid (Novopaque 30% W/V, Picker International, Highland Heights, Ohio) orally or by stomach tube [6,28]. Mixing the barium with a human enteric supplement can increase acceptance without greatly changing the properties of the barium. Radiographs are taken at 15- to 30-minute intervals until the contrast material reaches the colon. Double contrast radiographic studies may be performed to provide superior detail of the mucosa surfaces and assess distensibility of the digestive tract [30]. When perforation is suspected, iohexol (Omnipaque, Winthrop Pharmaceuticals, New York, New York) at the same dose or diluted 1:1 with tap water should be used instead of barium for gastrointestinal radiographic contrast studies [28,31]. Esophageal structure and function may be evaluated with barium sulfate paste (Esophotrast Cream, Rhone-Poulenc Rorer Pharmaceuticals, Collegeville, Pennsylvania) [28].

Iodinated contrast agent (2 mL/kg IV) may be used for excretory urograms to evaluate for urinary tract problems such as renal, ureteral, cystic, or urethral calculi [28]. A urinary catheter may be placed to inject this material into the bladder for cystography. Expanding the urinary bladder to palpable turgidity permits detection of filling defects, diverticulae, ruptures, or aberrant bladder location [28].

Interpretation of radiographs entails an understanding of normal anatomy. Ferrets have a long thoracic cavity, and the heart is positioned more caudally than one might expect. The cardiac silhouette of a normal ferret may appear slightly elevated from the sternum on the lateral radiographs as a result of fat accumulation surrounding the ligament extending from the heart to the sternum. This finding alone should not be interpreted as pneumothorax [8]. The abdominal cavity is longer than but similarly structured to those of other companion animals. Male ferrets have a J-shaped os penis. A large fat pad may be seen around the kidneys and in the sublumbar area in obese ferrets. It is normal for ferrets to have some gas in the intestinal tract, but unusual in the stomach. The spleen is often pronounced in radiographs of even clinically normal ferrets [28].

Abdominal ultrasound and echocardiography are common imaging techniques used in the ferret. Routine restraint techniques allow for ultrasound-based imaging of most ferrets.

Performance of myelography in ferrets is similar to that described for dogs. General anesthesia is needed, and anticonvulsant drug therapy should be considered [30].

Summary

Domestic ferrets are easily incorporated into traditional small animal practices, as may be seen from the information presented in this article. A number of diagnostic and supportive procedures may be easily adapted to the pet ferret using the techniques discussed here. The authors have attempted to present these small adaptations to the reader and hope this information will benefit clinicians and their ferret patients.

References

[1] Lichtenberger M. Principles of shock and fluid therapy in special species. Seminars in Avian and Exotic Pet Medicine 2004;13(3):142–53.
[2] Ivey E, Morrisey J. Ferrets: examination and preventative medicine. Vet Clin North Am Exot Anim Pract 1999;2(20):471–94.
[3] Marini RP, Esteves MI, Fox JC. A technique for catheterization of the urinary bladder in the ferret. Lab Anim 1994;28:155–7.
[4] Brown S. Clinical techniques in domestic ferrets. Seminars in Avian and Exotic Pet Medicine 1997;6(2):75–85.
[5] Taylor B. Alternate technique for venipuncture in ferrets. Exotic DVM 2001;2(6):37–9.
[6] Antinoff N. Oncologic diagnostic sampling for the general practitioner. Exotic DVM 2001; 3(3):38–40.

[7] Brown SA. Neoplasia. In: Hillyer EV, Quesenberry KE, editors. Ferrets, rabbits, and rodents: clinical medicine and surgery. Philadelphia: WB Saunders; 1997. p. 99–114.
[8] Orcutt CJ. Emergency and critical care of ferrets. Vet Clin North Am Exot Anim Pract 1998; 1(1):99–126.
[9] Rassnick KM, Gould WJ, Flanders JA. Use of a vascular access system for administration of chemotherapeutic agents to a ferret with lymphoma. J Am Vet Med Assoc 1995;206:500–4.
[10] Orcutt C. Use of vascular access ports in exotic animals. Exotic DVM 2000;2(3):34–8.
[11] Bennet RA. Intraosseous catheters in small mammals. In: Proceedings of the North American Veterinary Conference. Orlando (FL); 1996. p. 847.
[12] Quesenberry KE, Orcutt C. Basic approach to veterinary care. In: Quesenbery KE, Carpenter JW, editors. Ferrets, rabbits and rodents: clinical medicine and surgery. 2nd edition. Philadelphia: WB Saunders; 2004. p. 13–24.
[13] Manning DD, Bell JA. Lack of detectable blood groups in the domestic ferrets: implications for transfusion. J Am Vet Med Assoc 1990;197:84–6.
[14] Bistner SI, Ford RB, Raffe MR. Blood transfusions. In: Handbook of veterinary procedures and emergency treatment. 7th edition. Philadelphia: WB Saunders; 2000. p. 579.
[15] Marini RP, Jackson LR, Esteves MI, et al. Effect of isofluorane on hematologic variables in ferrets. Am J Vet Res 1994;55:1479–83.
[16] Lichtenberger M. Transfusion medicine in exotic pets. Clin Tech Small Anim Pract 2004; 19(2):88–95.
[17] Tully T, Mitchell M, Heatley J. Urethral catheterization of male ferrets: a novel technique. Exotic DVM 2001;3(2):29–31.
[18] Orcutt C. Treatment of urogenital tract disease in ferrets. Exotic DVM 2001;3(3):31–7.
[19] Nolte DM, Carberry CA, Gannon KM, et al. Temporary tube cystostomy as a treatment for urinary obstruction secondary to adrenal disease in four ferrets. J Am Anim Hosp Assoc 2002;38:527–32.
[20] Hoefer H. Diagnostic and treatment techniques in ferrets. In: Proceedings of the North American Veterinary Conference. Orlando (FL); 2000. p. 1004–6.
[21] Rosenthal KL. New therapeutics in small mammals. In: Proceedings of the North American Veterinary Conference. Orlando (FL); 1995. p. 686–7.
[22] Flecknell PA. Analgesia of small mammals. Vet Clin North Am Exot Anim Pract 2001;4(1): 47–56.
[23] Rosenthal K. Epidural anesthesia. In: Proceedings of the North American Veterinary Conference. Orlando (FL); 1996. p. 876.
[24] Heard DJ. Anesthesia, analgesia, and sedation of small mammals. In: Quesenbery KE, Carpenter JW, editors. Ferrets, rabbits and rodents: clinical medicine and surgery. 2nd edition. Philadelphia: WB Saunders; 2004. p. 356–69.
[25] Fisher PG. Esophagostomy feeding tube placement in the ferret. Exotic DVM 2001;2(6): 23–5.
[26] Williams BH. Therapeutics in ferrets. Vet Clin North Am Exot Anim Pract 2000;3(1): 131–53.
[27] Cantwell SL. Ferret, rabbit and rodent anesthesia. Vet Clin North Am Exot Anim Pract 2000;3(1):169–91.
[28] Stefanacci JD, Hoefer HL. Radiology and ultrasound. In: Quesenbery KE, Carpenter JW, editors. Ferrets, rabbits and rodents: clinical medicine and surgery. 2nd edition. Philadelphia: WB Saunders; 2004. p. 395–413.
[29] Hoefer HL. Small mammal radiology. In: Proceedings of the North American Veterinary Conference. Orlando (FL); 1995. p. 674.
[30] Silverman S, Tell L. Radiology equipment and positioning techniques. In: Radiology of rodents, rabbits and ferrets. St. Louis (MO): Elsevier Saunders; 2005.
[31] Harrenstein L. Critical care of ferrets, rabbits and rodents. Seminars in Avian and Exotic Pet Medicine 1994;3(4):217–28.

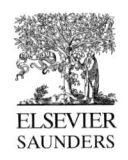

Common Procedures in Rabbits

Jennifer Graham, DVM, DABVP–Avian[a,b,*]

[a]Department of Comparative Medicine, University of Washington, Box 357190 Seattle, WA 98195, USA
[b]VCA Veterinary Specialty Center of Seattle, 20115 44th Avenue West, Lynnwood, WA 98036, USA

According to a 2002 survey of more than 54,000 individual pet owners, rabbits account for 1.7% of pets owned in the United States [1]. A recent survey completed by Griffin [2] revealed that small mammals, including rabbits, account for 44.2% of exotic species and 45.4% of revenue seen at three surveyed veterinary hospitals. It behooves the veterinarian to become familiar with basic techniques used in rabbits in a clinical setting. Clinics equipped for seeing dogs and cats may be easily adapted to accommodate rabbits [3]. This article discusses common veterinary techniques used in rabbits.

Handling and restraint

The skeleton in rabbits represents only 7% to 8% of the body weight (as opposed to 12% to 13% in cats) [3]. Because of the massive musculature on the hind limbs and the delicate nature of the skeleton, rabbits are prone to fractures of the back and hind limbs. Proper handling and housing of patients is essential to avoid injury. Rabbits are easily stressed, and care should be taken to minimize stress to the patient during handling.

Support of the hindquarters is essential when transporting rabbits to avoid injury. Rabbits used to handling may be carried with one hand under the thorax or holding the scruff and the second hand supporting the hindquarters (Fig. 1A) [4]. Stressed rabbits may be carried with the head tucked under the handler's arm to reduce stress by covering the eyes; the hindquarters should be supported at the same time (Fig. 1B). In addition, placing a rabbit in a cage with its rear facing the back of the cage while supporting

---

* Veterinary Specialty Center of Seattle, 20115 44th Avenue West, Lynnwood, WA 98036.
 E-mail address: jennifervet@yahoo.com

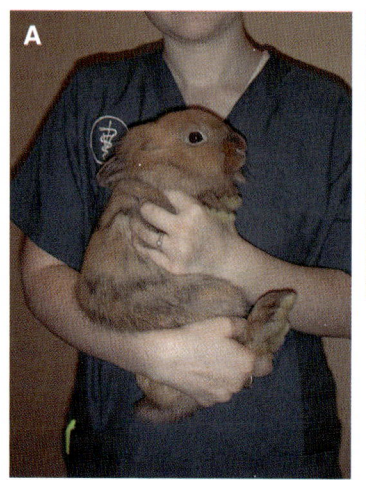

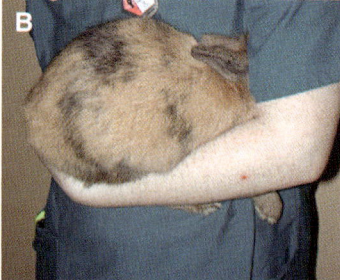

Fig. 1. (*A*) Restraint of rabbit with one hand under the thorax and second hand supporting hindquarters. (*B*) Restraint of a stressed rabbit by covering the eyes and supporting the hindquarters.

the hindquarters will help reduce the chance of injury from the rabbit's kicking [4]. When examining the rabbit or placing it in a cage, it is imperative to use a nonslip mat to avoid slipping and subsequent injury. Control of the rabbit should be maintained at all times during transport and examination to avoid injury.

When the rabbit is transferred from a carrier to a table for examination, it may be wrapped in a towel with the head covered to prevent struggling. It is important to avoid hyperthermia when using a towel to facilitate handling or examination. Alternatively, a hand may be placed over the eyes to calm the rabbit. Because rabbits are obligate nasal breathers, care should be taken to avoid obstructing the nostrils with the towel or hand. Some rabbits will become calm when placed on their backs. In this manner, the handler can sit on the floor with the rabbit in his or her lap, hindquarters toward the handler's body; examination of the incisors, belly, genitalia, and feet may be thus accomplished [4]. It is helpful to examine the rabbit in a separate room from predator species such as dogs and cats. Noises or smells from these animals may stress the sensitive rabbit.

Triage and patient assessment

Physical examination is similar to that of other species with a few exceptions. Before initiating examination, it is important to observe the rabbit at a distance. Observe the rabbit's movement in the room and document any obvious neurologic or musculoskeletal abnormalities. Note any difficulty breathing and the general stress level. If the rabbit is dyspneic, it may need to be placed in a quiet, oxygenated cage before examination. If the patient is hypothermic, thermal support should be provided until the rabbit is normothermic, taking care to avoid overheating. In rare cases, a rabbit may be too distressed to undergo an examination without sedation. It may be preferable to use a sedative, such as midazolam, to calm the rabbit as opposed to general anesthesia.

As in other species, a systemic approach is needed for the examination. It is best to take the body temperature as early into the examination as possible, because the body temperature may increase from the stress of the examination [4]. Heart and respiratory rates should also ideally be calculated before the rabbit is stressed. Care should be taken during auscultation to differentiate heart and lung sounds; lung sounds superimposed on the heartbeats may create the false impression of a heart murmur. When examining the head, one should note any ocular or nasal discharge. Otic examination should include visualization of the tympanic membrane; sedation or anesthesia may be necessary for deep otic examination in some cases. Lymph nodes are located as in other mammals; lymphadenopathy is rare in rabbits [4]. Skin and coat quality should be noted; examine the plantar surface of the feet for any signs of pododermatitis.

Thorough oral examination is a vital part of patient assessment. Palpate the ramus of the mandible and face for any signs of abscesses or tooth elongation. Although the oral cavity can be examined without anesthetizing the patient, the best examination may be made under light sedation or general anesthesia. Otoscopic cones may be used to examine the mouth of an unanesthetized patient, but approximately half the visible oral lesions are missed using this technique [5]. Nasal specula with an attached light source can give a wider field of view than the otoscopic cone (Fig. 2). Dental speculum sets are available for use in rabbits and rodents; however, approximately 25% of the visible lesions seen after death are still missed in anesthetized live patients with the use of mouth gags and cheek pouch

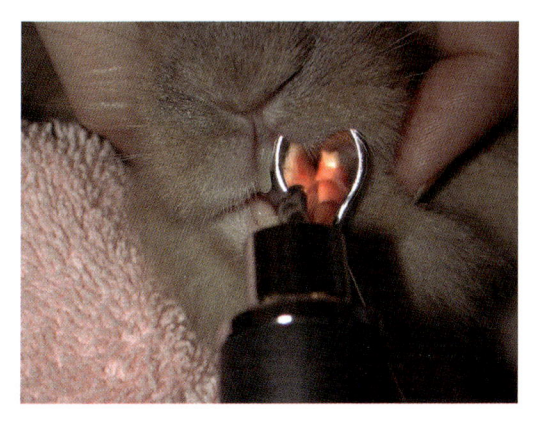

Fig. 2. Oral examination in a rabbit with a nasal speculum.

dilators (David A. Crossley, BvetMed, PhD, FAVD, DEVDC, MRCVS, personal communication, 2005). When one is using a dental speculum set, one speculum is placed over the incisors to hold the mouth open, and then a cheek pouch dilator is placed to allow visualization of the premolars and molars. The use of dental cameras or endoscopy can further aid in visualization of the oral cavity [6–8]. Good lighting, suction, and magnification can also help with the examination.

The abdomen should be carefully palpated for abnormalities; signs of discomfort may include teeth grinding and tensing of abdominal muscles. A firm or dough-like stomach, increased gas or fluid within the intestinal tract, and absence of normal intestinal sounds on auscultation may be noted in gastrointestinal disorders. Any organomegaly should be investigated.

Sample collection

Blood collection

Multiple sites may be used for venipuncture in rabbits, including the marginal ear veins, central ear artery, jugular vein, cephalic vein, and the lateral saphenous vein [3]. Use of the ear veins and artery is not ideal, because hematoma formation, bruising, or vessel thrombosis and skin sloughing may result. Alcohol may be used to part the fur and allow for visualization of the vessel. In some cases, clipping or plucking of the fur may be useful. If clippers are used, great care should be taken to avoid damaging the delicate skin of the rabbit.

The cephalic vein is a preferred site for intravenous catheter placement. When catheter placement is necessary, venipuncture of this vein should be avoided to preserve the integrity of the vessels. In addition, venipuncture of the cephalic veins may be more stressful for the patient, because the handler is working near the head of the rabbit.

An ideal site for venipuncture is the lateral saphenous vein (Fig. 3). The rabbit may be restrained in a towel with the head covered and a rear limb may be gently extended. The restrainer holds off the vein with pressure across the proximal thigh. The vessel lies across the lateral surface of the tibia just proximal to the hock. Following sample acquisition, gentle digital pressure over the venipuncture site or application of a brief pressure wrap can help prevent hematoma formation.

Jugular venipuncture should be reserved for very calm or sedated rabbits. It may be difficult to visualize the jugular vein in obese rabbits or in females with a large dewlap. This site is useful when one is collecting a larger amount of blood, such as for blood transfusion. Positioning is similar to that of a cat, with the front legs held down over the edge of the table and the head extended up. Overextension of the head should be avoided, because this can cause respiratory compromise. Alternatively, the rabbit may be

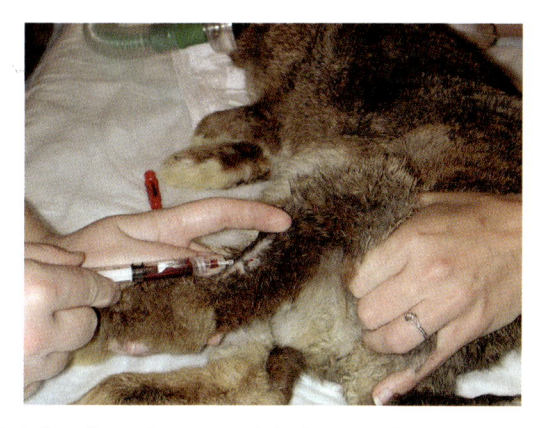

Fig. 3. Technique for venipuncture of the lateral saphenous vein in the rabbit.

wrapped in a towel and positioned in dorsal recumbency. The head and neck are extended to allow for visualization and sampling from the jugular vein.

Urine and fecal collection

A urine sample can be collected from the rabbit during examination when the bladder is gently expressed. However, care should be taken to avoid bladder rupture. Cystocentesis may decrease the chances of iatrogenic bladder rupture in some cases. Cystocentesis technique in the rabbit is similar to that in other species. In most rabbits, tranquilizers are not necessary, although sedation or anesthesia reduces the chance of struggling and damage to internal structures in stressed rabbits. The rabbit should be placed in dorsal recumbency with the handler stretching the patient by holding the hindlimbs in one hand and the scruff in the other. Alternatively, the rabbit may be wrapped in a towel and held securely with the eyes covered. The bladder is located on the ventral midline just cranial to the pelvic brim. The ventral midline area should be disinfected, and a small-diameter needle (22- to 25-gauge) attached to a sterile 6-mL syringe provides an adequate sample for complete urinalysis. Ultrasound can help with bladder visualization and detection of any bladder abnormalities (Fig. 4).

Catheterization of the urethra may be performed in sedate or anesthetized patients to collect a urine sample and allow therapeutic flushing of the bladder in cases of urinary sludging. A well-lubricated 9 French sterile catheter may be used in most rabbits [9]. The male is restrained in a sitting position to extrude the penis and allow for catheterization. The female is placed in sternal recumbency, and the urethral os is located on the floor of the vagina [9].

In most cases, fresh feces may be acquired from the rabbit's enclosure for sampling. Occasionally, a rabbit may provide a sample while the temperature is being taken. As in other species, one should examine a direct smear

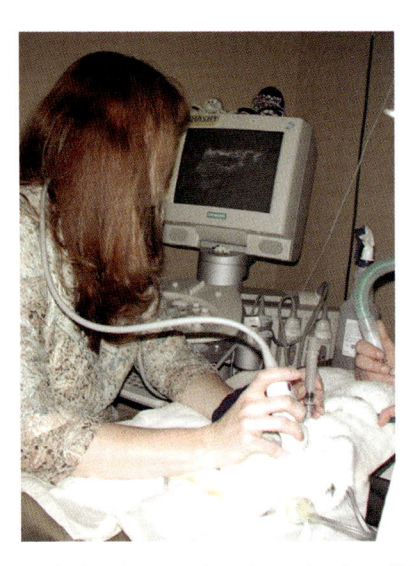

Fig. 4. Use of ultrasound to obtain urine sample and examination of bladder for abnormalities.

of fresh feces in saline microscopically for the presence of protozoal organisms, noting that several nonpathogenic protozoa may be found in the feces of rabbits [10]. Fecal flotation is used to diagnose coccidia, cryptosporidia, and helminths.

Dermatologic sampling

Some mites may be visualized under low magnification of skin brushings [11]. Acetate tape strips applied to the skin may be examined microscopically for cheyletiella, bacteria, and yeast [11]. Skin scraping is performed in the rabbit as in other mammalian species and is needed to diagnose some parasitic conditions, including sarcoptic or demodectic mange. Fungal and bacterial cultures as well as biopsies may be performed on skin lesions. In addition, darkfield microscopy is used for examination of smears for *Treponema paraluiscuniculi* [12].

Supportive care procedures

Fluid therapy

Intravenous fluids are recommended for critically ill hospitalized rabbits. A catheter can be placed in the cephalic or lateral saphenous vein. A 24- or 26-gauge catheter may be placed in smaller rabbits, whereas a 22-gauge catheter may be used in rabbits larger than 3 kg [13]. Alternatively, a butterfly catheter can be taped in place for short-term fluid therapy. Normal water consumption of rabbits is estimated to be 100 to 150 mL/kg per day [3]. Care must be taken when administering intravenous fluids to rabbits to avoid volume overload; 50 to 70 mL/kg per day can usually be tolerated intravenously. Infusion pumps help regulate fluid delivery. Direct arterial blood pressure can be measured in the rabbit by placement of an arterial catheter in the median aural artery [14]. Sloughing of the ear tip is possible with this technique. Indirect blood pressure may be monitored as in other species with a Doppler and pneumatic cuff (Fig. 5) [14]. The hair on the plantar surfaces of the feet should not be shaved in the rabbit, because this could result in pododermatitis.

A combination of crystalloids and colloids may be used to treat hypovolemic shock. If the blood pressure is below 40 mm Hg systolic, a rapid infusion of 10 to 15 mL/kg of isotonic crystalloids may be administered [14]. Hetastarch is administered at 5 mL/kg over 5 to 10 minutes [14]. Once the blood pressure is above 40 mm Hg systolic, then only maintenance fluids are given while the hypothermic patient is being warmed [14]. Once the patient's rectal temperature has reached 99°F, the blood pressure is rechecked. Hetastarch may be given at 5 mL/kg increments over 15 minutes until the blood pressure reaches 90 mm Hg systolic [14].

If peripheral vessels are collapsed from dehydration, an intraosseous catheter may be placed. Sites for intraosseous catheter placement include the proximal humerus, greater trochanter of the femur, and the tibial crest [3,15]. Fluids are given intraosseously until the patient is adequately rehydrated or an intravenous catheter is placed [3].

The subcutaneous route of fluid administration can be used on most hospitalized rabbits that have normal blood pressure and are accepting oral feedings. Rabbits can easily tolerate 120 mL/kg per day of subcutaneous fluids divided into two to three treatments daily. The loose skin on the dorsum of the rabbit is an ideal location for subcutaneous fluid administration (Fig. 6).

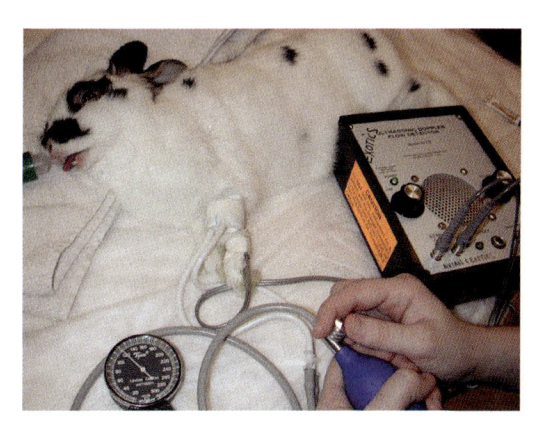

Fig. 5. Set-up for indirect blood pressure monitoring in a rabbit. Note positioning of pneumatic cuff and Doppler on the forelimb.

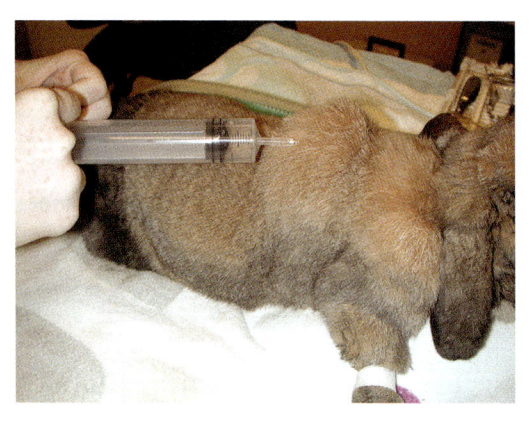

Fig. 6. Technique for administering subcutaneous fluids in a rabbit.

Medication administration

Medications may be administered by intraosseous, intravenous, intramuscular, subcutaneous, and oral routes. Intraosseous, intravenous, and subcutaneous routes are as described under fluid therapy. Intramuscular injections may be given into the large lumbar muscles on either side of the spine [3]. The rabbit should be restrained appropriately during injection to prevent injury. Care should be taken to avoid damage to the sciatic nerve when injecting into the hindlimb musculature. If the hindlimbs are used for injection, the cranial aspect of the rear leg, the quadriceps, should be used. Some medications, such as enrofloxacin, may cause pain, necrosis, or abscessation when given undiluted into the subcutaneous or muscular tissues. It is preferable to dilute such medications in fluids and administer them subcutaneously whenever possible.

When administering medications orally to rabbits, suspensions are preferable to tablets. Tablets may be compounded into flavored suspensions when needed. Owners can also crush tablets into a favorite treat or jam. For fractious rabbits, it is helpful to use a towel to wrap the rabbit in a "burrito fashion" when giving oral medications. The medication should be placed as far back as possible in the oral cavity to prevent the rabbit from spitting it out [3].

Enteral support

Anorexia as a result of illness is a common presentation in rabbits. Dental disease, gastrointestinal disease, neurologic disease, and other systemic diseases are often complicated by secondary anorexia. Because stress can worsen the condition of a compromised rabbit, veterinarians are challenged to provide adequate nutrition to the sick lagomorph in an efficient, low-stress manner. Failure to provide nutritional supplementation to an anorectic rabbit can result in hepatic lipidosis in as little as 2 to 3 days [16]. Parenteral feeding has not been completely researched in rabbits, but one study showed hepatocellular degeneration and portal tract inflammation in rabbits receiving total parenteral nutrition [17]. The changes resolved after refeeding, but portal fibrosis was permanent in four of eight rabbits. Decreases in basal bile flow and bile acid secretion (functional cholestasis) persisted following refeeding. In addition, complete colonic stasis occurred during the total parenteral nutrition period. Because maintenance of gastrointestinal motility is essential in rabbits, parenteral nutrition should probably be avoided if enteral feeding is possible until further advances are made that will help maintain gastrointestinal motility.

Different methods of enteral feeding have been evaluated in rabbits. Rabbits have specific recommended dietary requirements, including 13% to 18% dry matter dietary crude protein, 12% to 16% dietary crude fiber, 7000 IU vitamin A per kilogram of food, 40 mg vitamin E per kilogram of food, 2 mg vitamin K per kilogram of food, and 0.5% to 1% dry matter calcium [18]. Of these requirements, fiber is especially important. Because fiber is essential for the production of short-chain fatty acids and gastrointestinal motility, diets containing less than 10% crude fiber often result in enteritis [13]. Many of the commercial veterinary enteral diets are based on requirements of carnivores and are inappropriate for hindgut fermenters such as rabbits. These diets are too low in fiber, with fiber content usually less than 2% [13]. A product has become available to the veterinarian that fulfills many of the listed nutritional requirements and is an excellent diet for the convalescing herbivore. Oxbow Critical Care (Oxbow Pet Products, Murdock, Nebraska) is a timothy hay–based syringe feeding formula that is mixed with water to provide an excellent high-fiber mixture for anorectic herbivores. The product is simple to reconstitute and results in a homogeneous mixture. Although blending pellets and greens with water is an alternative to the Critical Care diet, it is more time consuming and generally results in a less homogeneous mixture. The Critical Care diet has an excellent fiber level at 21% to 25% and is highly palatable. The author and others have used the product extensively for compromised patients with positive results by syringe feeding and esophagostomy tube routes (Fig. 7). The Critical Care diet will not easily pass through a nasogastric tube owing to its high fiber content.

Syringe feeding is most often used in the anorectic rabbit but may be stressful to the patient [13]. When feeding the Critical Care formula by syringe, one may use several methods, depending on the size and demeanor of the rabbit. If the rabbit will tolerate it, it is quickest to feed directly out of a 60-mL syringe with a catheter tip. It may be easier to back-load the 60-mL syringe than to suck that material through the tip, depending on the thickness of the feeding formula. The tip is introduced into the diastema and slowly depressed. If the rabbit is smaller or resists feeding, a 1-mL syringe may be back-loaded out of the tip of the 60-mL syringe and fed to

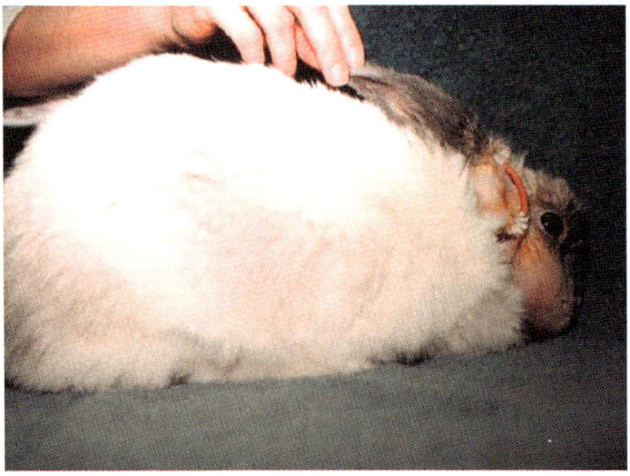

Fig. 7. Esophagostomy tube in an adult Californian rabbit following hemimandibulectomy surgery. (*Courtesy of* G. Heather Wilson, DVM, DABVP–Avian, University of Georgia, College of Veterinary Medicine, Athens, GA.)

the rabbit one syringe at a time. Although this method is time consuming, it can be an effective way to deliver the formula to some rabbits that would otherwise refuse feeding (Anna Osofsky, DVM, DABVP—Avian, personal communication, 2002). Alternatively, oral dosing syringes have a wider tip and are useful for syringe feeding.

Orogastric tubes are appropriate for single dosing but are inappropriate for chronic use [13]. For orogastric feeding, an 18 to 22 French round-tip rubber catheter should be premeasured and marked for the distance from the mouth to the last rib. A speculum should be placed to keep the mouth open. The rabbit's neck should be flexed and the tube passed through the oropharynx into the stomach. One may test placement of the tube by auscultating as air is injected through the tube into the stomach or checking for negative pressure when the tube is backed into the esophagus [13,19].

Nasogastric tubes are used in clinical settings but are not ideal, because the small diameter of the tubes precludes the use of a high-fiber diet [13]. Measurement of the tube is as described for the orogastric tube, using the tip of the nose and the last rib as landmarks. A pediatric feeding tube (3.5 to 5 French) may be used for most rabbits [13]. A topical anesthetic such as 2% lidocaine gel or several drops of proparacaine may be placed in the nasal opening several minutes before placement. The tube enters the ventral medial nasal meatus and passes ventrally and medially with the head flexed. Tube placement should be checked with a lateral radiograph or as described for orogastric tube placement. The tube can be secured with a drop of superglue on the furred area above the nose and with tape glued or sutured to the top of the head (Fig. 8) [3,13].

A study evaluating the use of pharyngostomy tubes for chronic aspirin dosing in rabbits reported complications that included accidental severing of the carotid artery or jugular vein in 3 of more than 40 rabbits, resulting

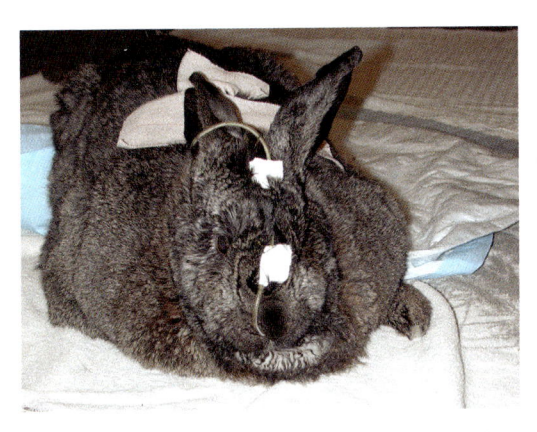

Fig. 8. Nasogastric tube in an obese adult male Flemish Giant rabbit.

in death, and insertion site abscesses in two rabbits [20]. The diameter of the pharyngostomy tubes was 1 mm; the study did not evaluate pharyngostomy feeding or histopathologic changes associated with tube placement. Percutaneously placed gastrostomy tubes have also been examined in the rabbit but had a high incidence of complications [21]. Complications associated with the gastrostomy tubes included necrosis and abscessation around the tube, tube removal by a rabbit, and gastric retention of the catheter tip following removal (the tip usually passes through the gastrointestinal tract in the dog and cat and is eliminated) [21]. A second study examining gastrostomy tube placement in rabbits reported death in one rabbit 2 days following tube placement as a result of an intra-abdominal hematoma, a second death at 7 days from no apparent cause, catheter balloon rupture in 4 of 13 rabbits, and localized fibrino-purulent peritonitis in 8 of 13 rabbits [22].

Esophagostomy tubes have been used successfully to provide nutrition in dogs and cats [23–27]. Esophagostomy tubes are preferable to pharyngostomy tubes in dogs and cats because of the high rate of complications associated with pharyngostomy tube placement, such as damage to neurovascular structures, potential for airway obstruction and aspiration pneumonia, and problems with swallowing [28,29]. In one study, a comparison of nasogastric, pharyngostomy, gastrostomy, and jejunostomy tubes showed that esophagostomy tubes were considered to be more reliable and have fewer complications [26]. A study published in 2003 showed no differences in complication rate between percutaneously placed gastrostomy tubes and esophagostomy tubes in 67 cats [30]. Potential complications that can occur with esophagostomy tubes include infection at the tube entrance site, vomiting, scratching and inadvertent removal of the tube, and kinking of the tube during placement [25–28].

Many different techniques for surgical placement of esophagostomy tubes have been described, including percutaneous intravenous needle catheter placement; intraluminally placed tube applicators or Carmalt forceps followed by esophageal perforation and tube placement; and use of a guide tube, venous catheter, and a separate tube for placement [26]. A recent report suggested that a specially designed esophageal tube applicator may have advantages over other esophageal tube placement techniques [26]. Sizes recommended for esophagostomy tubes in dogs and cats range from 10 to 30 French [23,25,26]. In some studies, 18 French feeding tubes were used in cats and were large enough to prevent displacement but did not interfere with spontaneous food consumption [24,26]. A recent pictorial in *Lab Animal Medicine* shows a step-by-step guide to placement of the esophagostomy feeding tube in the rabbit [31].

Pain control

Pain control is important for successful recovery of the compromised rabbit patient. Assessment of pain may be more difficult in rabbits than other species because they typically do not vocalize when experiencing pain. Instead, the rabbit may sit very still in the back of its cage in a crouched position while tooth grinding and be oblivious to its surroundings [32]. Pre-emptive analgesia is recommended whenever possible.

Nonsteroidal anti-inflammatory drugs (NSAIDs) are estimated to last for 12 to 24 hours in rabbits, whereas opioid drugs may only last a few hours [32,33]. Injectable formulations of NSAIDs may be preferable to oral NSAIDs when gastric motility is compromised. Pharmacokinetic parameters have been established for a variety of NSAIDs in rabbits; further study is needed to determine their long-term clinical effects. Buprenorphine is effective for 6 to 12 hours, whereas butorphanol is effective for 2 to 4 hours [32,33]. In general, abdominal or visceral pain may respond better to opioid analgesia, whereas NSAIDs may be more effective for somatic or integumentary pain [32,34]. Multimodal analgesia, combining agents from different classes, should be more effective than a single agent alone [35]. Additionally, the multimodal method allows the agents to be used at lower dosages [35]. A complete discussion of analgesia in rabbits is beyond the scope of this article; a variety of excellent references are available [13,32–38].

Miscellaneous procedures

Anesthetic delivery

A variety of ways to administer anesthetic agents to rabbits exist, including topical, injectable, inhalant, and combination protocols. Anesthesia involves many considerations, such as stability of the patient, monitoring, and anesthetic agents used. The reader should consult additional texts for complete information on anesthesia in rabbits [13,32,33,39,40].

Topical anesthesia is useful before procedures such as catheter placement. A topical preparation containing 2.5% lidocaine and 2.5% prilocaine (EMLA cream) enabled percutaneous insertion of catheters into the marginal ear vein in rabbits without causing any detectable pain or discomfort [41]. These topical preparations may take 45 to 60 minutes to take full effect.

A variety of injectable anesthetic or analgesic combinations have been used in rabbits. Injectable anesthetic protocols may include parasympatholytics, phenothiazines, benzodiazepines, alpha-2 adrenergic agonists, ketamine, propofol, tiletamine/zolazepam, and others [40]. Parenteral anesthetics are typically administered by the following routes: subcutaneous, intramuscular, intraperitoneal, intravenous, and intraosseous. Care should be taken when administering potentially irritating subcutaneous and intramuscular anesthetic preparations to rabbits, because self-mutilation could occur [40]. In addition, the veterinarian should be aware of specifics of different anesthetic drugs; for example, the use of tiletamine/zolazepam has been associated with nephrotoxicity in rabbits [42,43].

Although it is not considered a "common technique" by many practitioners, epidural anesthesia or analgesia is becoming more commonplace in small mammals. Local anesthetics, alpha-2 adrenergic agonists, and opioid agonists have been injected into the epidural space of small mammals to control pain [40,44,45]. Advantages of epidural anesthesia and analgesia include reduced to absent systemic effects compared with intramuscularly or intravenously administered drugs, quicker recovery time because of the reduced amount of gas anesthetic needed, and postsurgical pain relief [44]. Disadvantages may include inability to place an epidural catheter because of small size of the epidural and intervertebral space, potential for trauma to the spinal cord, and potential for death or serious complications when incorrectly administered [44]. Care must also be taken when calculating volumes of local anesthetic for infiltration to avoid toxicity [40].

Inhalant anesthesia is the primary component of most anesthetic regimens in small mammals [40]. Isoflurane and sevoflurane are commonly used inhalant anesthetic agents. Induction with an inhalant anesthetic is typically achieved either with an induction chamber or face mask. Premedication and supplemental injectable anesthesia are recommended for rabbits to lower the excitatory response typically seen with induction. Careful restraint to prevent injury during this period is also recommended. A variety of commercially made induction chambers and face masks are available for use in rabbits. Additionally, masks may be fashioned out of syringe cases or other materials.

For maintenance of anesthesia, endotracheal intubation is ideal to protect the upper airway and assist in ventilation. Blind and direct techniques may be used to facilitate intubation in rabbits. In either case, it is helpful if the head and neck of the rabbit are hyperextended, because this will allow for the alignment of larynx and trachea with oropharynx [40]. Care should be taken to ensure that the rabbit is adequately premedicated and relaxed to allow for atraumatic intubation. In addition, it is important to avoid overextension of the neck, which could result in damage to the spine.

For blind intubation techniques, spontaneous ventilation is required, because the breath sounds allow for appropriate tube placement [40,46]. The sedate rabbit may be placed in sternal or lateral recumbency with the head grasped in one hand to allow for its extension. The endotracheal tube is passed between the incisors and premolars and over the base of the tongue with the other hand until maximum respiratory sounds are heard. The tube is carefully and repeatedly advanced until it enters the trachea (Fig. 9). Care must be taken to avoid repeated attempts at intubation, because laryngeal edema or hemorrhage may result. Although one technique for blind intubation involves listening directly through the adapter on the endotracheal tube (ET) for respiratory noise, a stethoscope may be attached to the ET to allow for blind intubation without bending over the patient [47]. This technique involves removing the adapter from the ET and connecting a stethoscope directly to the tube; the adapter must be reattached to the ET after the rabbit is successfully intubated. As an alternative, a small piece of tubing may be used to attach the stethoscope to the adapter of the ET (Fig. 10A) (Peter Pascoe, DVM, BVSc, DACVA, DECVA, personal communication, 2000). A piece of tubing fits the adapter on the ET on one end and has a male adapter for the stethoscope on the other. The tubing that is used should ideally have a larger internal diameter than the ET. A hole should be cut into the tubing as close to the ET adapter as possible to minimize dead space (Fig. 10B). The hole should be slightly larger in diameter than the internal diameter of the ET. With this device, which may easily be made with common clinic items, there is no need to remove the adapter from the ET when using a stethoscope to assist with blind intubation.

Positioning of the rabbit for direct visualization is similar to blind intubation positioning [40]. An assistant helps position the head and can use

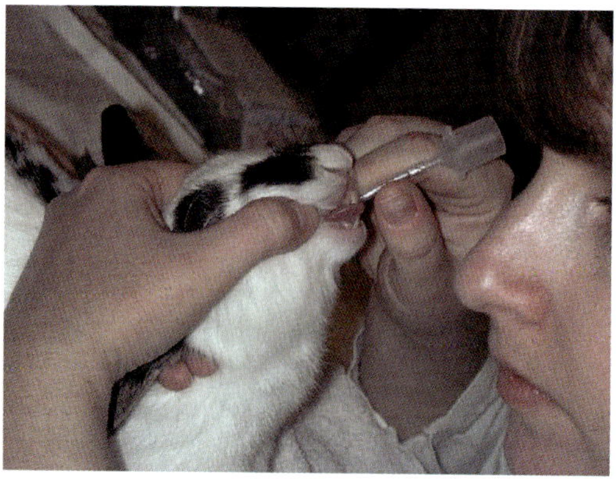

Fig. 9. Technique for blind intubation in a rabbit.

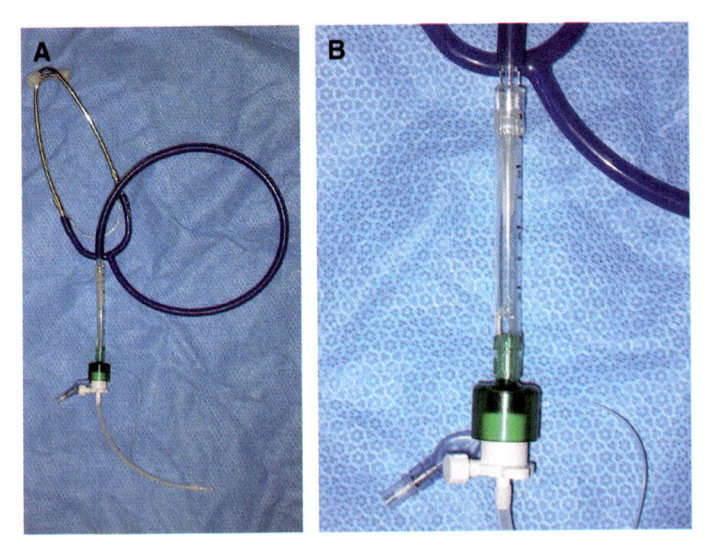

Fig. 10. (*A*) Stethoscope with adapter attached to an endotracheal tube that may be used to aid in blind intubation of a rabbit. (Courtesy of Peter Pascoe, DVM, University of California at Davis College of Veterinary Medicine.) (*B*) Close-up view of adapter in (*A*). (*Courtesy of* Peter Pascoe, DVM, BVSc, DACVA, DECVA, University of California at Davis College of Veterinary Medicine, Davis, California.)

tape or gauze strips to hold the mouth open. A laryngosope or otoendoscope may be used to visualize the glottis and facilitate intubation (Fig. 11) [40]. As an alternative, the ET may be placed over the end of a rigid endoscope so that the glottis can be visualized and the ET advanced (Fig. 12) [48,49]. Again, care must be taken to avoid laryngeal edema or hemorrhage.

Although it is still in research stages for small mammals, laryngeal mask airway (LMA) is a new method being used to deliver gas anesthetic. The LMA, designed for use in humans, is an airway device used as an alternative to a face mask or an ET [50]. In people, the LMA is inserted blindly into the hypopharynx and the cuff is inflated such that a mask surrounds the hypopharynx and provides a tight seal, allowing intermittent positive pressure ventilation (IPPV) [51]. LMA has been used in rabbits [52,53]. Although LMA provided a better airway than a face mask, its use for IPPV was associated with gastric tympany in some cases [52]. Recently, a modification of the LMA has been designed for laboratory animals [54]. Termed the airway device (AD), this device has some similarity to the LMA, but its mask portion is specifically designed for small laboratory animals. In addition, the device has an esophageal extension and, unlike the LMA, does not have a cuff associated with the mask. Although the AD is not yet commonly used, results of initial studies provide encouragement for its further development for use in small mammals [54].

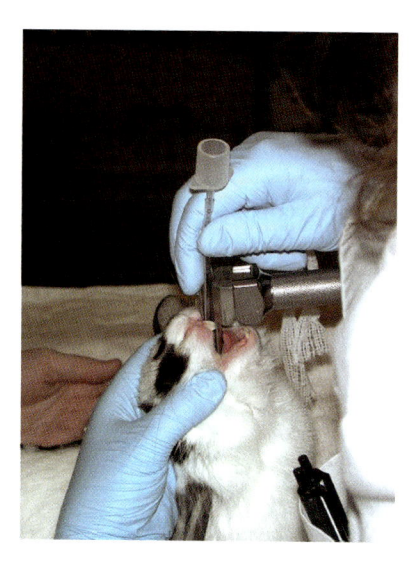

Fig. 11. Technique for direct intubation of a rabbit using a laryngoscope to aid in visualization of the glottis.

Nasolacrimal duct flush

A nasolacrimal flush is indicated to determine and restore patency of the nasolacrimal ducts when rabbits present with an ocular discharge. Common causes of nasolacrimal duct obstruction include infectious agents and dental disease. Rabbits have a single nasolacrimal duct located medial to the lid margin in the conjunctiva of the lower eyelid (Fig. 13). Most awake rabbits will allow flushing of the nasolacrimal duct after instillation of topical anesthetic drops. A lacrimal cannula or 24-gauge Teflon intravenous catheter

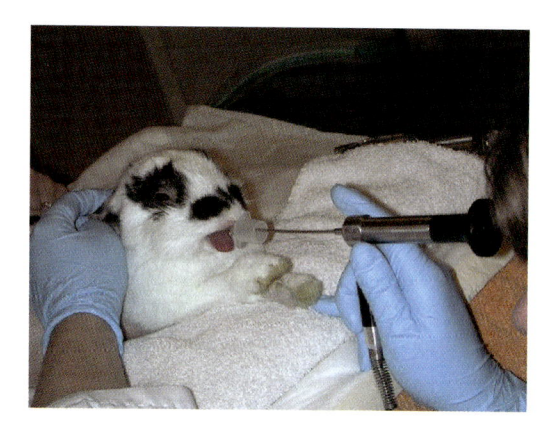

Fig. 12. Technique for direct intubation of a rabbit using an endoscope to aid in visualization of the glottis.

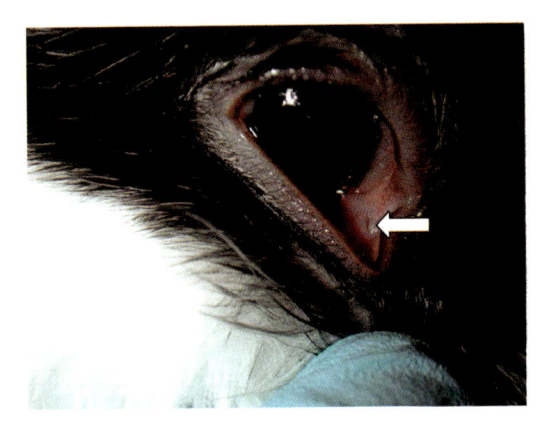

Fig. 13. Position of the nasolacrimal duct in a rabbit. The arrow shows the location of the nasolacrimal duct opening.

may be used to flush the duct (Fig. 14). When a rabbit is under anesthesia for a dental trim or other procedure, it is less stressful to flush the nasolacrimal ducts while the rabbit is still under anesthesia.

Ear cleaning

Ear cleaning may be indicated in cases of otitis. Under general anesthesia, a red rubber catheter can be passed into the ear canal, and warm saline may be used to flush the ears if a large amount of debris are present in the ear canal. Cotton-tipped applicators or an ear curette may be used carefully to "scoop" out purulent debris while using an otoscope, endoscope, or otoendoscope for visualization to minimize chances of traumatizing the ear canal (Fig. 15). Alternatively, one may flush saline into the ear with gentle massage to soften the purulent debris, followed by removal of debris with

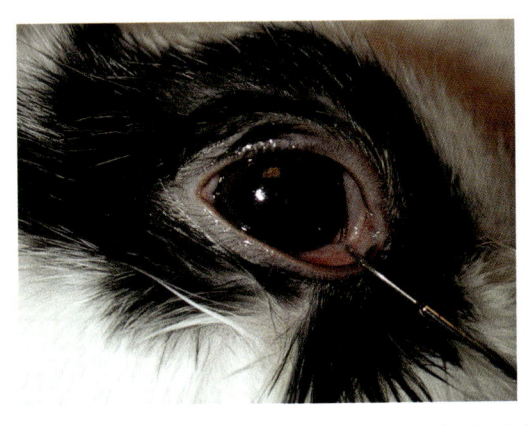

Fig. 14. Positioning of a lacrimal cannula for flushing the nasolacrimal duct in a rabbit.

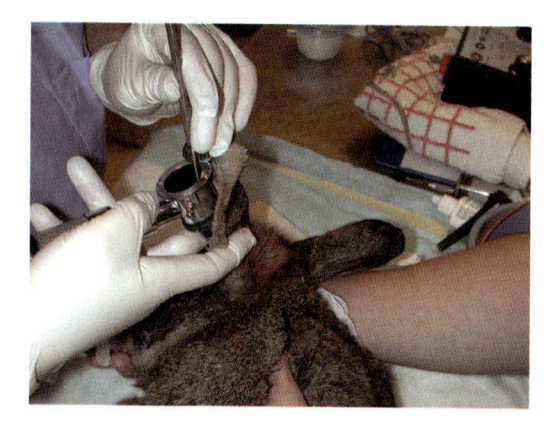

Fig. 15. Technique for using an ear curette to remove debris from the ears of a rabbit while using an otoscope to aid visualization.

a suction unit while visualizing the canal to avoid iatrogenic damage. Flushing should be avoided if the tympanic membrane is ruptured. Ear cleaning should be accompanied by appropriate medical diagnostics to determine the cause of disease. In the case of ear mites, ear cleaning is not recommended because it is painful, and treatment with ivermectin will resolve the lesions without the need for mechanical removal of crusts.

Teeth trimming

Treatment of most dental disorders involves trimming affected teeth, especially in the case of malocclusion. Traditional tooth trimming in unanesthetized rabbits has been performed with nail trimmers or wire cutters. This method is no longer recommended for several reasons: excessive force is applied to the tooth, which can damage the tooth and affect growth; the procedure is painful; the normal chisel shape of the teeth is not maintained; and longitudinal splits often occur, which may extend under the gumline and expose the pulp [55–57].

A high-speed dental drill provides the most atraumatic and accurate method of trimming teeth [55]. The pulp cavity usually extends just beyond the gingival level, and pulp exposure is unlikely when teeth are trimmed back to a level that is just below normal [55]. The chisel edge of the incisors and normal occlusal plane angulation of the premolars and molars should be maintained when trimming teeth [55]. The most effective treatment for cheek tooth overgrowth is drastic reduction of the height of all affected teeth and their counterparts, taking them out of occlusion (Fig. 16) [55].

When trimming the incisors, one may place a tongue depressor behind the incisors to protect the surrounding tissues from damage. Small spatulas may be used to protect the tongue and cheeks when performing premolar-molar trimming. A diamond bur may be useful for trimming the incisors,

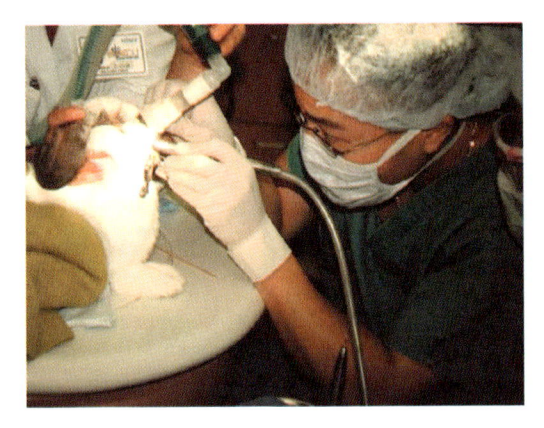

Fig. 16. Positioning of rabbit and instrumentation during a dental trim.

whereas a flat or round bur is more appropriate to use on the premolars and molars [57].

Although incisor trims may be performed with the animal awake, premolar and molar trimming should be performed under general anesthesia. Injectable anesthetics may be used alone with supplemental oxygen or in combination with inhalant anesthesia. For long or extensive procedures, such as extractions, rabbits and guinea pigs should be intubated and maintained on inhalant gas. Nasal intubation may be preferable to oral intubation because work space is less restricted. In the case of brief oral examinations and trimming, a small mask may be placed over the nose to provide inhalant anesthesia while still allowing access to the oral cavity. Careful anesthetic monitoring and support, including intravenous fluids, are vital to a positive outcome.

Depending on the rate of tooth growth and the degree of malocclusion, trimming may need to be performed as often as every 3 to 6 weeks. The client should be advised of this as soon as dental disease is diagnosed, because long-term commitments of time and money may be required.

Summary

Familiarity with common procedures specific to the rabbit allows the clinician safely to treat these unique creatures. Small mammals such as ferrets and rabbits may be more easily seen by the average veterinary practice than some of the more "exotic" species, because equipment and facility requirements are minimal. Understanding the basics of handling and restraint, triage and patient assessment, sample collection, supportive care techniques, and anesthetic delivery allows the clinician to provide appropriate care for the rabbit patient. As advances continue to be made in veterinary medicine, clients will increasingly expect and pay for quality services for their exotic pets.

Acknowledgments

The author would like to thank Dr. Tori McKlveen, DVM, MS, DACVR, Lauren Blais, LVT, and Christy Bass for assistance with asquisition of images used in this manuscript.

References

[1] Wise J, Heathcott B, Gonzalez M. Results of the AVMA survey on companion animal ownership in US pet-owning households. J Am Vet Med Assoc 2002;221(11):1572–3.
[2] Griffin C. Tracking the value of avian patients: a look inside the numbers. In: Avian practice management: dollars and sense; proceedings of the Association of Avian Veterinarians Annual Conference. Monterey (CA); 2005. p. 73–9.
[3] Mader D. Basic approach to veterinary care. In: Quesenberry K, Carpenter J, editors. Ferrets, rabbits, and rodents: clinical medicine and surgery. 2nd edition. St. Louis (MO): Saunders; 2004. p. 147–54.
[4] Antinoff N. Physical examination and preventative care of rabbits. Vet Clin North Am Exot Anim Pract 1999;2(2):405–27.
[5] Crossley D. Dental disease in rabbits and rodents. In: Bonagura J, editor. Kirk's current veterinary therapy XIII. Philadelphia: WB Saunders; 2000. p. 1133–7.
[6] Murray M. Application of rigid endoscopy in small exotic mammals. Exotic DVM 2000;2(3): 13–8.
[7] Taylor M. Endoscopy as an aid to the examination and treatment of the oropharyngeal disease of small herbivorous mammals. Seminars in Avian and Exotic Pet Medicine 1999;8: 139–41.
[8] Capello V, Gracis M. Endoscopy. In: Lennox A, editor. Rabbit and rodent dentistry handbook. Lake Worth (FL): Zoological Education Network; 2005. p. 101–7.
[9] Benson K, Paul-Murphy J. Clinical pathology of the domestic rabbit: acquisition and interpretation of samples. Vet Clin North Am Exot Anim Pract 1999;2(3):539–51.
[10] Jenkins J. Gastrointestinal diseases. In: Quesenberry K, Carpenter J, editors. Ferrets, rabbits, and rodents: clinical medicine and surgery. 2nd edition. St. Louis (MO): Saunders; 2004. p. 161–71.
[11] Harcourt-Brown F. Skin diseases. In: Textbook of rabbit medicine. Oxford (UK): Alden Press; 2002. p. 224–48.
[12] Hess L. Dermatologic diseases. In: Quesenberry K, Carpenter J, editors. Ferrets, rabbits, and rodents: clinical medicine and surgery. 2nd edition. St. Louis (MO): Saunders; 2004. p. 195–202.
[13] Paul-Murphy J, Ramer J. Urgent care of the pet rabbit. Vet Clin North Am Exot Anim Pract 1998;1(1):127–52.
[14] Lichtenberger M. Principles of shock and fluid therapy in special species. Seminars in Avian and Exotic Pet Medicine 2004;13(3):142–53.
[15] Harcourt-Brown F. The rabbit consultation and clinical techniques. In: Textbook of rabbit medicine. Oxford (UK): Alden Press; 2002. p. 52–93.
[16] Hillyer E. Pet rabbits. Vet Clin North Am Small Anim Pract 1994;24:25–64.
[17] Das J, Uzoaru I, Ansari G. Biliary lithocholate and cholestasis during and after total parenteral nutrition: an experimental study. Proc Soc Exp Biol Med 1995;210:253–9.
[18] Carpenter J, Kolmstetter C. Feeding small exotic mammals. In: Hand M, Thatcher C, Remillard R, et al, editors. Small animal clinical nutrition. Topeka (KS): Walsworth Publishing Company; 2000. p. 947–52.
[19] Reed R, Marcello J, Welzel G, et al. Gavaging a rabbit with a rubber catheter. Lab Anim 1987;16:51–2.

[20] Rogers G, Taylor C, Austin J, et al. A pharyngostomy technique for chronic oral dosing of rabbits. Lab Anim Sci 1988;38:619–20.
[21] Smith D, Olson P, Matthews K. Nutritional support for rabbits using the percutaneously placed gastrostomy tube: a preliminary study. J Am Anim Hosp Assoc 1997;33:48–54.
[22] Lindberg C, Ivancev K, Kan Z, et al. Percutaneous gastrostomy: a clinical and experimental study. Acta Radiol 1991;32:302–4.
[23] Levine P, Smallwood L, Buback J. Esophagostomy tubes as a method of nutritional management in cats: a retrospective study. J Am Anim Hosp Assoc 1997;33:405–10.
[24] Devitt C, Seim H. Clinical evaluation of tube esophagostomy in small animals. J Am Anim Hosp Assoc 1997;33:55–60.
[25] Crowe D, Devey J. Esophagostomy tubes for feeding and decompression: clinical experience in 29 small animal patients. J Am Anim Hosp Assoc 1997;33:393–403.
[26] Von Werthern C, Wess G. A new technique for insertion of esophagostomy tubes in cats. J Am Anim Hosp Assoc 2001;37:140–4.
[27] Rawlings C. Percutaneous placement of a midcervical esophagostomy tube: new technique and representative cases. J Am Anim Hosp Assoc 1993;29:526–30.
[28] Crowe D, Downs M. Pharyngostomy complications in dogs and cats and recommended technical modifications: experimental and clinical investigations. J Am Anim Hosp Assoc 1986;22:493–503.
[29] Lantz G, Cantwell H, Vleet JV, et al. Pharyngostomy tube induced esophagitis in the dog: an experimental study. J Am Anim Hosp Assoc 1983;19:207–12.
[30] Ireland L, Hohenhaus AE, Broussard J, et al. A comparison of owner management and complications in 67 cats with esophagostomy and percutaneous endoscopic gastrostomy feeding tubes. J Am Anim Hosp Assoc 2003;39:241–6.
[31] Makidon P. Esophagostomy tube placement in the anorectic rabbit. Lab Anim 2005;34(8):33–6.
[32] Harcourt-Brown F. Anesthesia and analgesia. In: Textbook of rabbit medicine. Oxford (UK): Alden Press; 2002. p. 121–64.
[33] Flecknell P. Anesthesia. In: Flecknell P, editor. Manual of rabbit medicine and surgery. British Small Animal Veterinary Association. Iowa State Press; 2000. p. 103–16.
[34] Jenkins W. Pharmacologic aspects of analgesic drugs in animals: an overview. J Am Vet Med Assoc 1987;191:1231–40.
[35] Flecknell P. Analgesia of small mammals. Vet Clin North Am Exot Anim Pract 2001;4(1):47–56.
[36] Liles J, Flecknell P. The use of nonsteroidal anti-inflammatory drugs for the relief of pain in laboratory rodents and rabbits. Lab Anim 1992;26:241–55.
[37] Flecknell P. Pain relief in laboratory animals. Lab Anim 1984;18:147–60.
[38] Flecknell P. Advances in the assessment and alleviation of pain in laboratory and domestic animals. Journal of Veterinary Anesthesia 1994;21:98.
[39] Flecknell P. Anesthesia of common laboratory species. In: Laboratory animal anesthesia. San Diego (CA): Academic Press; 1996. p. 159–223.
[40] Heard D. Anesthesia, analgesia, and sedation of small mammals. In: Quesenberry K, Carpenter J, editors. Ferrets, rabbits, and rodents: clinical medicine and surgery. 2nd edition. St. Louis (MO): Saunders; 2004. p. 356–69.
[41] Flecknell P, Liles J, Williamson H. The use of lidocaine-prilocaine local anesthetic cream for pain-free venipuncture in laboratory animals. Lab Anim 1990;24(2):142–6.
[42] Doerning B, Brammer D, Chrisp C, et al. Nephrotoxicity of tiletamine in New Zealand white rabbits. Lab Anim 1992;42(3):267–9.
[43] Brammer D, Doerning B, Chrisp C, et al. Anesthetic and nephrotoxic effects of Telazol in New Zealand white rabbits. Lab Anim 1991;41(5):432–5.
[44] Rosenthal K. Managing pain in small mammals. Presented at North American Veterinary Conference Symposium 2003: Managing pain in cats, dogs, small mammals, and birds—recognition, relief and economics. Available at: http://www.vin.com/Members/Proceedings/Proceedings.plx?CID/pain2003&PID=pro581980=VIM. Accessed September 1, 2005.

[45] Kero P, Thomasson B, Soppi A-M. Spinal anesthesia in the rabbit. Lab Anim 1981;15: 347–8.
[46] Alexander D, Clark G. A simple method of oral endotracheal intubation in rabbits (*Oryctolagus cuniculus*). Lab Anim 1980;30(5):871–3.
[47] Conlon K, Corbally M, Bading J, et al. Atraumatic endotracheal intubation in small rabbits. Lab Anim 1990;40(2):221–2.
[48] Tran H, Puc M, Tran J, et al. A method of endoscopic endotracheal intubation in rabbits. Lab Anim 2001;35(3):249–52.
[49] Worthley S, Rogue M, Helft G, et al. Rapid oral endotracheal intubation with a fibre-optic scope in rabbits: a simple and reliable technique. Lab Anim 2000;34(2):199–201.
[50] Brain A. The laryngeal mask airway—a new concept in airway management. Br J Anaesth 1983;55:801–5.
[51] Brain A, Denman W, Goudsouzian N. LMA instruction manual. San Diego (CA): LMA North America; 2000.
[52] Bateman L, Ludders J, Gleed R, et al. Comparison between facemask and laryngeal mask airway in rabbits during isoflurane anesthesia. Veterinary Anesthesia and Analgesia 2005; 32(5):280–8.
[53] Smith J, Robertson L, Auhll A, et al. Endotracheal tubes versus laryngeal mask airways in rabbit inhalation anesthesia: ease of use and waste gas emissions. Contemp Top Lab Anim Sci 2004;43(4):22–5.
[54] Imai A, Eisele P, Steffey E. A new airway device for small laboratory animals. Lab Anim 2005;39(1):111–5.
[55] Crossley D. Treatment of dental disease in rabbits and rodents. Proceedings of the 14th Annual North American Veterinary Conference. Orlando, FL, 2000. p. 995–7.
[56] Lobprise H, Wiggs R. Dental and oral diseases in lagomorphs. J Vet Dent 1991;8:11–7.
[57] Capello V, Gracis M. Dental instruments and equipment. In: Lennox A, editor. Rabbit and rodent dentistry handbook. Lake Worth: Zoological Education Network. p. 193–212.

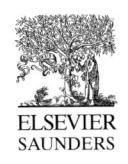

Common Rodent Procedures
Eric Klaphake, DVM, DABVP–Avian*

Avian Health Clinic, 7152 East Main Street, Reynoldsburg, OH 43068, USA

For many exotic animal practitioners, rodent clients represent a sizable portion of the clientele base. That base owns and loves pets that are often ephemeral in nature, most with life expectancies of less than 10 years, many less than 5 years. These pets often present for the first time to a veterinarian after a history of pet store–recommended therapies that did not achieve desired results or with a condition that has reached a level of significant crisis for the owner. Owners have invested several dollars to purchase the pet, a bit more for its enclosure and diet, only to be told that a veterinary visit may run them fifty dollars for just the examination, after spending five to ten dollars on pet store medications. Many clients are likewise incredulous that a patient as small as a hamster or a guinea pig should cost as much to examine as a dog or cat. However, the veterinarian often has to spend more time with these clients to educate them about proper husbandry and diet, as well as receiving additional training in unique aspects of these pets that are often not covered in any detail in veterinary schools. These are important factors to recognize before agreeing to provide veterinary care to these animals.

Always remember that clients who actually come into a veterinarian's office are already raising the standard of care for their animals, even if they decide not to pursue any further treatment or service. Some individuals cannot justify spending more money on what was supposed to be an inexpensive pet. For these individuals, as well as for a suffering animal, humane euthanasia may be considered the best option to offer in a bad situation, preferable to a flush down a toilet, release into the "wild," or a slow, painful, progressive death at home. Many practitioners find that the high incidence of euthanasia or unstoppable progression of severe disease to death in these species can be frustrating and becomes a reason why they refuse to see and treat these patients or confine themselves to simple situations, such as

---

* 5564 Sweetwater Valley Drive, New Albany, OH 43054.
   E-mail address: dreklaphake@att.net

neuters and nail trims. Each veterinarian develops a sense of which common procedures he or she feels comfortable performing on rodents. Many excellent references for practicing rodent medicine exist; Web site sources for the ones regularly used by the author are listed in Box 1. This article reviews some of the common procedures actually performed by the author in 9 years of exclusive exotic animal practice and also delves into procedures described in the literature that may elevate a practitioner's level of care.

The order Rodentia is the most numerous of all mammalian orders, with more than 2050 species and 29 families [1]. Currently rodents are organized into two suborders, Sciurognathi and Hystrichognathi, based on their mandibular structures [1]. Well-known members of the suborder Sciurognathi include squirrels (family Sciuridae), chipmunks (*Tamias* spp), marmots (*Marmota* spp), woodchucks (*Marmota monax*), prairie dogs (*Cynomys* spp), beavers (*Castor* spp), pocket gophers (family Geomyidae), desert jerboas (*Jaculus jaculus*), rats (family Muridae), mice (family Muridae), hamsters (Syrian/golden [*Mesocricetus auratus*], Siberian/dwarf [*Phodopus sungorus*]), "gerbils" (actually Mongolian jirds, *Meriones unguiculatus*, not true gerbils), voles (family Muridae), lemmings (family Muridae), muskrats (*Ondatra zibethicus*), dormice (family Myoxidae), and springhaas (*Pedetes capensis*) [2]. Well-known members of the suborder Hystrichognathi include naked mole rats (*Heterocephalus glaber*), porcupines (families Erethizontidae and Hystricidae), chinchillas (*Chinchilla lanigera*), guinea pigs (*Cavia porcellus*), Patagonian cavies/maras (*Dolichotis* spp), capybara (*Hydrochaeris hydrochaeris*), agoutis (family Dasyproctidae), degus (*Octodon* spp), and nutria (*Myocastor coypus*) [2].

The most commonly kept species include mice, rats, "gerbils," hamsters, guinea pigs, chinchillas, and prairie dogs. However, other pet species may present from time to time. The author has treated pet mara, jerboas, degus, and "rescued" squirrels. Many exotic animal practitioners will voluntarily or unexpectedly be pressed into action by an individual (often a small child) bearing injured or orphaned rodent wildlife into their clinics. From squirrels to common house mice to beaver to porcupines to woodchucks—a practitioner can never be sure what will come through his or her door. Obviously, providing veterinary services to a zoo or laboratory animal facility may also entail an ability to perform basic veterinary procedures on those rodents.

Anatomy

Although comprehensive treatment is beyond the scope of this article, it is important to be aware of some of the unique anatomic features of rodents. Most weigh between 20 g and 1 kg, with exceptions such as the beaver and the largest rodent, the capybara (30 to 50 kg) [1]. Rodents are often identified by their teeth, which are classified as heterodonts (variably shaped and classified) [1]. In fact, the word "rodent" is derived from the Latin word "to gnaw" [3]. Their incisors lack anatomic roots, instead having an open apical

Box 1. Web sites for selected rodent veterinary medicine resources

- The Association of Exotic Mammal Veterinarians
www.aemv.org
- Oxbow Pet Products
www.oxbowhay.com
- Bair Hugger Blanket
http://www.bairpaws.com/arizanthealthcare/faw_vet.shtml
- Dremel
http://www.dremel.com/

Journals
- *Veterinary Clinics of North America Exotic Pet Practice*
http://vetexotic.theclinics.com
- *Seminars in Avian and Exotic Animal Medicine*
http://www.us.elsevierhealth.com/product.jsp?isbn=1055937X
Replaced in 2006 by *Journal of Exotic Pet Medicine*
http://www.us.elsevierhealth.com/product.jsp?isbn=15575063
- *Exotic DVM Veterinary Magazine*
http://www.exoticdvm.com
- *Laboratory Animals*
http://www.rsmpress.co.uk/la.htm
- *Lab Animal*
http://www.labanimal.com/laban/index.html

Books (all published by Elsevier/WB Saunders)
- *Laboratory Medicine: Avian and Exotic Pets*
http://www.us.elsevierhealth.com/product.jsp?isbn=0721676790
- *Clinical Anatomy and Physiology of Exotic Species*
http://www.us.elsevierhealth.com/product.jsp?isbn=0702027820
- *Ferrets, Rabbits, and Rodents: Clinical Medicine and Surgery* (2nd edition)
http://www.us.elsevierhealth.com/product.jsp?isbn=0721693776
- *Exotic Animal Formulary* (3rd edition)
http://www.us.elsevierhealth.com/product.jsp?isbn=0721601804
- *Saunders Manual of Small Animal Practice* (3rd edition)
http://www.us.elsevierhealth.com/product.jsp?isbn=0721604226
- *Radiology of Rodents, Rabbits and Ferrets: An Atlas of Normal Anatomy and Positioning*
http://www.us.elsevierhealth.com/product.jsp?isbn=0721697895

pulp that results in incisors that have continuous growth and eruption [1]. The only nerve in these teeth is found at the base [2]. Only dentin is found on the buccal surface of the teeth, compared with the lingual surface's enamel [1]. This combination creates the "chisel" appearance of normal healthy rodent incisors [1]. It is important during incisor-tooth dentistry to try to recreate the chisel appearance. The two lower incisors are normally longer than the two upper incisors; this feature gives the lower incisors greater "play" or independent movement during examination and may be mistaken for a fracture below the gingiva.

A diastema is located between the incisors and the premolar/molar teeth, the latter being often referred to as "cheek teeth." Buccal velvety or furred soft tissue occupies the diastema, making visualization of the more caudal teeth challenging [2]. In some rodents, a cheek pouch lined with squamous cell epithelium may be found, with that of the hamster extending down the neck to the scapula. New owners may present these animals as having neoplasia, abscesses, enlarged lymph nodes, and so on, which are possible but unusual. Gentle pressure on these structures externally may elucidate whether seeds or other material are within; if there is any doubt, manual pressure can often express the contents through the oral cavity. In this author's experience, some rodents may have unilateral filling of a pouch. Each rodent group has its own cheek tooth grinding surface pattern, by which it is classified [2]. Guinea pigs, chinchillas, and capybaras have continuously growing molars, whereas most other rodents do not [1]. Obviously, this is important when evaluating for potential dental disease and selecting a method of treatment (Fig. 1). All rodents should have their cheek tooth arcades examined (if feasible based on the rodent's size) under general anesthesia when dental disease is suspected, in addition to skull radiographs.

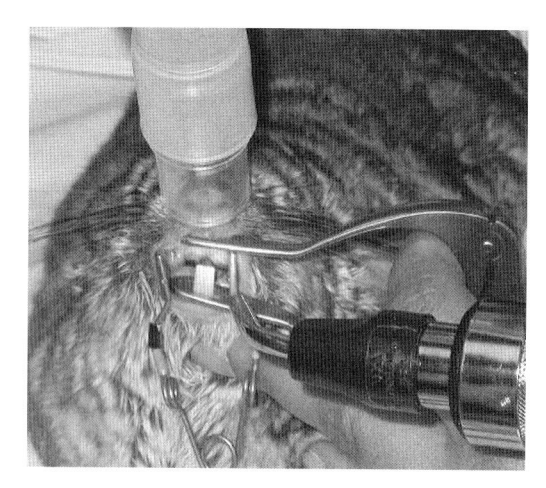

Fig. 1. Common equipment used for oral examination of a chinchilla, *Chinchilla lanigera*. Note placement of gas anesthesia tubing over chinchilla's nostrils.

However, only guinea pigs and chinchillas should require cheek tooth trimming or filing like the horse; for other rodents, dental evaluation, diagnosis, and treatment should more approximate those of a dog or cat.

The grinding motion of the teeth is also important to understand. Unlike the rabbit, rodents grind their mandibles rostrocaudally, with incisor occlusion when the mandible is positioned most rostrally and check tooth occlusion when it is positioned most caudally [1]. This pattern can lead to confusion and misdiagnosis of malocclusion on examination or in interpreting radiographs.

The gastrointestinal tract of guinea pigs and chinchillas is that of a hindgut fermenter with a large cecum where bacterial digestion of cellulose occurs [4]. This author tends to view them as miniature horses in terms of gastrointestinal disease management. The intestine of mice, rats, hamsters, and "gerbils" is of a more omnivorous variety [4]. Most rodents are cecotrophic to various degrees, with the guinea pigs and chinchillas more active in cecotrophy, particularly during pregnancy and lactation [4].

Sexing is a common request on presentation of a rodent to the veterinarian. Unfortunately, many suppliers of pet rodents misidentify the sex of the rodent, leading to inappropriate names for the animals or even aggression or fecundity issues when several are owned. When most rodents are young, no scrotum or testes are evident. Some rodents have pendulous scrotums when sexually mature or during their breeding seasons; others maintain inguinal or even intra-abdominal testes. Some rodents have a caudally directed penis that can be easily extruded with gentle pressure, such as the guinea pig or chinchilla; others, such as the beaver, have a cloaca-like opening and may require DNA sexing to confirm sex. When not extruded far enough, the female's urinary papilla in some species may resemble a penis. Many rodents also have a baculum (os penis) [2]. Often the distance between the urogenital opening and the anus is used to sex rodents, with males having a greater distance than females. However, one may easily misidentify male distance with female distance in young rodents, unless the individual is extremely experienced or has several animals of probable mixed sex to compare for the species. Sexing a single individual can be a challenging experience, and it is better to state that the sex is unknown at that time than to misidentify.

Be aware that some rodent species can be of a "hairless" variety, but be certain that the animal is not actually undergoing a pathologic alopecia, rather than one from a genetic source. This author has worked with hairless rats, mice, and guinea pigs; hairless variations of the other species may exist (Fig. 2). It is important to avoid exclusive restraint by means of the tail in some species, such as gerbils and rats, because the skin can deglove, leaving exposed muscle, tendon, and ligaments, or the entire tail may be removed by improper restraint. None of these species has sweat glands, and they lack the ability to pant, important factors to consider during stressful situations or for recommendations of ambient temperature at home. Other important species-specific anatomic variations of which to be aware are listed in Table 1.

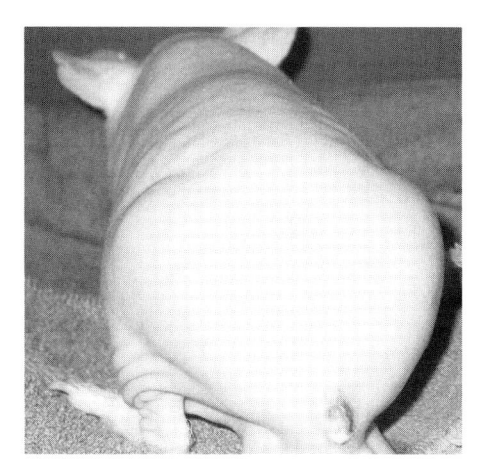

Fig. 2. Hairless variety of guinea pig, *Cavia porcellus*. Note excessive build-up of glandular debris by caudal sebaceous gland.

General triage and patient assessment

One of the first steps an exotic animal veterinarian should undertake is visual observation of the animal before stress is induced (Fig. 3). In some

Table 1
Selected anatomic features of common rodent pets

Species	Important anatomic features
Mouse	Eyes bulge with scruffing; porphyrin production; mammary glands may extend onto dorsum; yellow incisors; cecotrophic; spontaneous ovulator [8]
Rat	Eyes bulge with scruffing; porphyrin production; mammary glands may extend onto dorsum; older male rats can become brown; granular sebaceous secretions at hair base shafts; yellow incisors; cecotrophic; spontaneous ovulator [8]
Hamster	Nocturnal; eyes bulge with scruffing; porphyrin production; mammary glands may extend onto dorsum; yellow incisors; bilateral hip (flank) glands; unilateral midline ventral marking gland (only in Djungarian hamsters—*Phodopus* sp); copious vaginal discharge post-ovulation; some species can hibernate; cecotrophic; spontaneous ovulator [8]
"Gerbil" (jird)	Eyes bulge with scruffing; porphyrin production; mammary glands may extend onto dorsum; yellow incisors; unilateral midline ventral marking gland; cecotrophic; spontaneous ovulator [8]
Prairie dog	With stress or anesthesia, anal gland "flower" may protrude [15]; some species hibernate in wild; cecotrophic; complex, socially oriented reproductive cycle [2]
Guinea pig	Both sexes have nipples and mammary glands; large tympanic bullae; white incisors; cecotrophic; preputial glands; caudal sebaceous gland at tail base (especially a concern in males) [13]; commonly develop "corns" (keratinaceous growth) by 5th digits of front feet; some guinea pigs exude a milky secretion from both eyes with stress (Klaphake, personal communication); spontaneous ovulator [14]
Chinchilla	Nocturnal; yellow incisors; no toenails; plantar surface may become callused; large tympanic bullae; cecotrophic; spontaneous ovulator [14]

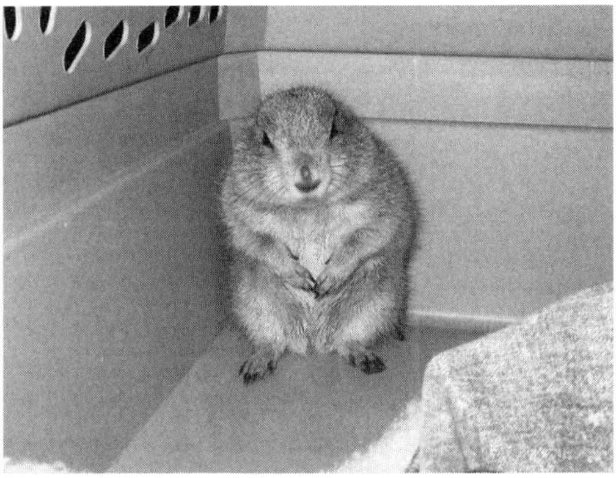

Fig. 3. Prairie dog, *Cynomys* sp, observing veterinarian from travel enclosure. Note nasal planum alopecia from chronic rubbing, common when kept in enclosure with cage bars. These rodents can be dangerous to handle without anesthesia.

cases, the client may already have begun the stressing process; in other cases the animal's condition may be too critical, and immediate action may be necessary. Observation of the animal is most safely accomplished within the container in which the animal is brought to the veterinarian's office. The animal should not be allowed onto the examination table without forethought. These animals exhibit the "flight" version of "fight or flight," having evolved as prey items, and this reaction needs to be addressed to avoid a tragic fracture or even death due to the fall from the table. Providing a small towel for the animal to gain traction on or burrow into is often helpful. Keeping the veterinarian's full attention on the animal itself is also crucial, because the animal is in an unfamiliar surrounding and may be liable to bite or bolt. Another important consideration is where the small rodent can go in the examination room if it does reach the floor. How tall is the space under doors? Are there holes along the baseboards or underneath items in the room that are small enough for the animal to fit into? Avoiding this contingency may seem like an obvious concern, but unfortunately, it is not uncommon. When flight is not an option, even the smallest of the rodents can inflict extremely painful bites to an individual, whether it is the veterinarian, technician, or owner. It is therefore highly recommended that one not allow owner restraint of the patient. When one is bitten by the rodent, it is imperative to avoid the natural response of flinging the rodent across the room or against the table, or dropping the animal and causing further problems. This suggestion may seem humorous, but it does occur. Discussing restraint method and rationale before proceeding may be useful so as to avoid the appearance to the owner of unnecessary pet brutality.

When the patient's condition is not viewed as critical by the owner or technician, a thorough history of the problem, husbandry, and diet may be gathered by the technician. In addition, getting a weight from a gram scale is crucial early in the process (Fig. 4). The author generally does not recommend taking the temperature of rodents awake, excepting guinea pigs and chinchillas; this may also be done by an experienced technician before the veterinarian enters the room. Most of these animals' temperatures may be taken using a soft, short-tipped thermometer, while covering the animal's head and extending its rear slightly over the table edge. Care must be taken to enter the anus, not the vaginourethral opening in females. Excessive struggling by the rodent, lack of lubrication, or unnecessary aggressiveness in placement of the thermometer may lead to bleeding and perforation.

An examination of most of these animals should be performed in less than a minute when the patient is critical. Again, observation before handling can provide initial information about eyes, respiration, nostrils, fur condition, and basic musculoskeletal status. At this point, one may either further evaluate any areas of concern or proceed to the palpation stage of the examination. Specific handling recommendations are described under each species-specific section. If the animal is large enough, take a quick look in the ears and perform gentle superficial swabbing of the external ear canal for potential cytology. Carefully expose the incisors by pulling the lips back either with your fingers (guinea pigs and chinchillas) or with a cotton-tipped applicator (the four smallest rodent species). Look at incisor alignment; note any debris, gingivitis, foul smells, and appearance of the mucous membranes. Some veterinarians assess the cheek teeth using an otoscope to visualize, but the author has found this stressful to the animal and a difficult method from which to gain useful information. When cheek teeth issues are suspected (eg, anorexia, selective eating, foul breath, diarrhea, drooling), then more invasive evaluation is necessary in any case. If discharge is noted around the eyes or nostrils, one should collect it with gentle swabbing material for cytology or culture. Gently palpate the maxilla and mandible externally for potential fractures, dental disease, abscesses, or

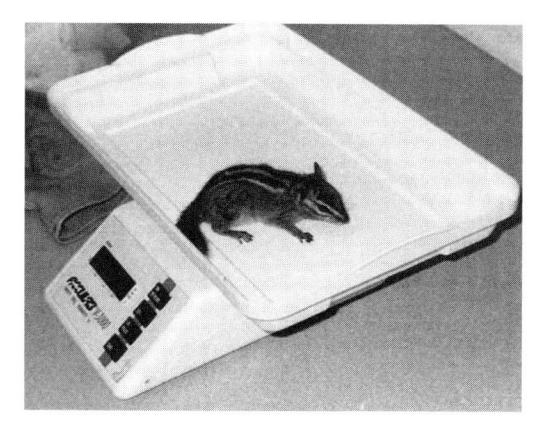

Fig. 4. Weighing wild chipmunk, *Tamias* sp, on digital scale. With many smaller rodents, technique shown here could result in animal's escaping or injuring itself.

neoplasia. For more specifics on oral or ophthalmologic examination, the author recommends other sources [5–7].

One should be aware that attempting auscultation of any of the four smallest rodents can lead to puncture of the stethoscope's diaphragm by the rodent's teeth if care is not taken. Normally rapid heart rates are often exacerbated by fear, making for a heart rate that is difficult to count and in which it is probably, for all but the most astute veterinarians, difficult to ascertain an arrhythmia or murmur except in the most severe cases. The author usually assesses whether the rate may be easily counted; if it can, then bradycardia may be a concern. Tachycardia is difficult to determine. Again because of rodents' small size, the difference between upper and lower respiratory sounds should be interpreted carefully, owing to the close proximity of the two regions and the ease with which sound transfers between them. Harsh breathing sounds have been exhibited by some guinea pigs and rats presented for routine examination with no other diagnostic evidence of respiratory disease, and, in all species, normal auscultation has been present in animals later revealed to have end-stage pneumonia or severe pulmonary neoplasia.

Palpation of the abdomen should be preceded by asking the owner whether the animal could be pregnant. When in doubt, one should assume that an animal of dubious sex, housed with another of the same species regardless of sex, or one newly acquired (<75 days ago for guinea pigs and chinchillas, <1 month for the smaller rodents) may be pregnant. A nonpregnant abdomen is generally doughy to the touch, and one has difficulty defining structures as particular organs. If something well defined, something firm that is not fecal pellets, or crepitus is noted, diagnostic evaluation is recommended.

Tactile and visual examination of the fur quality and skin should involve as much surface area of the animal as possible, including the tail. Assessing hydration of the skin is important. Beyond the normal structures described in Table 1, other "lumps and bumps" should be more thoroughly examined (Fig. 5). Generally, abscesses are painful on palpation, whereas neoplasias are not. Extremely pruritic guinea pigs have been known to enter a seizure-like state when one is palpating the areas of pruritis. In the author's experience, these animals curl their heads laterally to the site, begin twitching uncontrollably, appear to lose consciousness, and often roll onto their opposite sides. Discontinuing the stimulation usually stops the response after 10 to 15 seconds. Examine and palpate the legs and feet for toenail issues and to assess for pododermatitis (common in guinea pigs and chinchillas). Guinea pigs commonly develop keratinaceous growths on the medial surface of their front feet, which may be trimmed back as if trimming a nail (Fig. 6). Confirmation of the animal's sex and examination of the anogenital region conclude the examination.

Examinations should be rapid enough to minimize handling stress but thorough enough to gain the necessary information. Again, an explanation

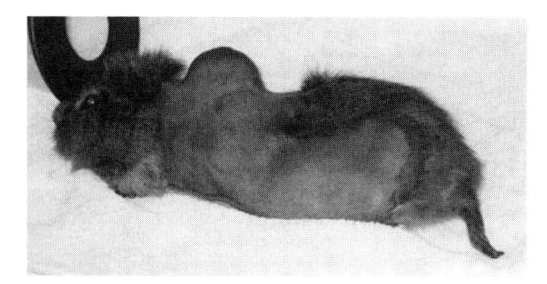

Fig. 5. Guinea pig, *Cavia porcellus*, with large dorsal mass, later determined to be an abscess. Note excessive borders shaved for procedure.

to the client before the examination may reduce client questioning of the veterinarian's experience and training with these animals.

To restrain mice, the author prefers to put on a pair of examination latex gloves before handling. The odor of mice is often difficult to remove from the restrainer's skin after examination. A small washcloth or old surgical towel may be used to scruff the mouse and minimizes the risk for being bitten when the grip allows the mouse too much latitude. Although mice may be picked up by the tail, this often causes immediate stress to the animal and the owner and may lead to degloving. Disposable plastic bag–like rat and mouse containers that cone down with the head in the smaller end may be purchased from laboratory animal suppliers to minimize the risk of biting during sample collection, but they do not allow for a thorough hands-on examination. Movement of mice is best accomplished using a container.

Hamsters and gerbils may be scruffed in a similar manner, though latex gloves do not appear to be necessary to avoid a semipermanent odor after

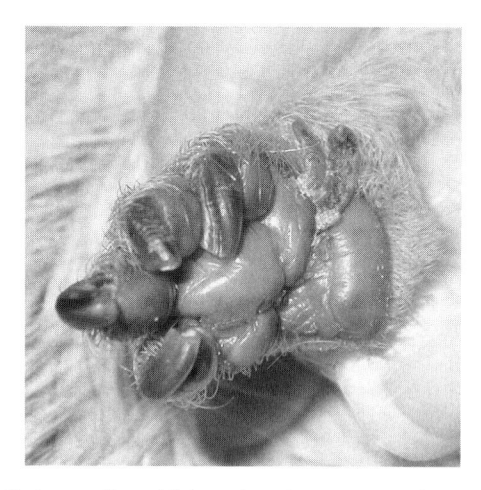

Fig. 6. Guinea pig, *Cavia porcellus*, with large keratinaceous growth on palmar surface of medial foot. Only noted by author on forefeet, usually trimmed to pad base as with toenails; nonpainful.

hand-washing. Scruffing hamsters, gerbils, and mice can cause protrusion or bulging of the eyes from the sockets, which often causes concern, especially to owners if they are observing the examination. Do not grab gerbils by the tails; this is the most common rodent the author has seen for tail slip. Hamster aggression appears to vary with handling and the species, with the Russian dwarf hamsters presenting as the most high-strung and likely to bite. Gerbils are generally easy-going, although young gerbils can be unpredictable balls of energy. Movement of gerbils and hamsters is best accomplished using a container.

Rats are difficult to scruff and, with the exception of extremely young animals, often vocalize and fight scruffing passionately. Most will allow a thorough examination with minimal restraint on a towel or other nonslick surface. Remember that an animal with painful injury and abdominal discomfort may be prone to bite when those areas are manipulated, hence the need for a good history and observation before handling. Rats may continually dribble urine, which is not considered a pathologic condition. Covering them on the table with a thin towel and restraining the head may permit a quick manipulation of the painful region. Movement of rats is best accomplished using a container or by carrying a relaxed one in one's open palms. Other suggestions for small rodents may be found in various sources [4,8–11].

Guinea pigs are the easiest to examine of the group but may still run off the table without supervision or when spooked. They rarely bite, but caution is still recommended. Initially keeping them upright on the table and allowing the head to hide under a towel can be helpful. Holding a guinea pig in a vertical position often elicits struggling. Guinea pigs tend to urinate during examinations, often copiously. Their urine is usually cloudy, and porphyrin has occasionally been noted, though not as commonly as in rabbits. Guinea pigs should be supported under the forelegs and hind end when carried.

Chinchillas may be restrained by grabbing the base of the tail and supporting the animal ventrally under the thoracic cavity with two fingers between the forelegs. Grabbing any of the fur areas will probably lead to a handful of fur, an unhappy owner, and a regrowth time of several months. Chinchillas love to run and jump, so care should be taken in allowing the animal free movement on the examination table. Chinchillas also appear prone to difficulties with fracturing hind legs in wire-sided cages, which is of concern in advising the owner and in housing the animal in hospital. They have a high propensity for leg injuries on open-wired running wheels; solid chinchilla-specific wheels are available. Although generally not aggressive, chinchillas can nip when unhappy; the author has never been painfully bitten. Chinchillas are especially sensitive to heat ($>24°C$ or $75°F$), so care should be taken to educate owners about transporting their animals to the veterinarian, particularly in the summer. Further information about guinea pigs and chinchillas may be found in [12–14].

Prairie dogs should still be considered wild animals, because they do not breed easily in true captive situations; most are currently wild caught. They are the largest of the pet rodents discussed in this article and are also the most powerful, dangerous, and problematic to restrain. To examine a prairie dog thoroughly, the author generally requires gas anesthesia to be administered. Although visual examination or minor palpation may be possible in a calm awake animal, it is not worth the risk to self, client, and animal to try to "bruticaine" these animals into a thorough conscious examination. Chambering a prairie dog down is highly recommended. Before initiating anesthesia, one should consider which diagnostics and therapeutics may need to be performed, advise the client of risks and costs, and have everything ready to go to avoid repeated episodes. Often this means that the veterinarian has to proceed under supposition of the problem and to be prepared for other possibilities as the examination, diagnostics, and therapeutics progress. Further discussion of anesthesia may be found later in the article. With stress or under anesthesia, prairie dogs may prolapse their anal glands as small protrusions that generally revert to normal form when stress or anesthesia is resolved. Prairie dogs are prone to "odontomas," which are growths that may occlude the nasal cavity in these obligate nasal breathers. A history of dyspnea should place this condition on the rule-out list, and precautions may be necessary before proceeding with anesthesia. Further information on prairie dogs may be found in other sources [15,16].

Emergency care

When an animal is evaluated as being in critical condition by the technician, veterinarian, or especially the owner, the patient should be brought into the treatment or hospitalization area immediately. Until the veterinarian is able to assess the situation, the animal should be placed into an incubator or container where oxygen may be administered in a low-stress manner (Fig. 7). Generally, flow rates do not need to exceed 1 to 2 L/min. Intubation is extremely challenging and difficult in rodents and should be attempted only as a last resort in a crashing patient. The technician should then notify the doctor and get a more thorough history, while someone experienced is monitoring the situation. When the patient is judged to be hypothermic based on an accurate rectal temperature or general handling body temperature, a previously warmed incubator set at 27°C (80°F) should house the patient during oxygen administration. In hospital, it is generally safest to house small rodents on newspaper bedding alone, with a small box serving as a hide-box, until the situation is fully evaluated. Do not offer food and water until the initial assessment is made. Often the stress of travel to the veterinarian places the small rodent in an even more precarious state, and the opportunity to be observed in a warmed, oxygenated incubator, although not standard emergency room protocol, offers the best chance for the patient to handle further evaluation and diagnostics. Many exotic animal "emergencies"

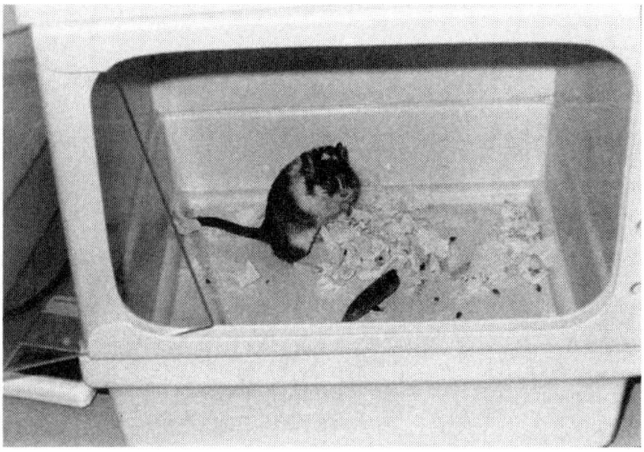

Fig. 7. "Gerbil" or jird, *Meriones unguiculatus,* in incubator for observation. Note copious quantity of feces from 1 hour in incubator for fecal sample tests.

are actually a culmination of chronic disease, in which immediate response will not change the situation and dealing with the client is of greater concern. Unfortunately, when clients are informed of the costs of emergency medical intervention, many are unable or unwilling to pay. Obtaining an early understanding of client intentions can head off unwanted and unpaid for treatments and diagnostics, to the clinic's and patient's advantage. Most true emergencies require significant financial investment, and such treatment often has a low success rate with small rodents. When an animal is bleeding, additional handling will increase blood pressure, so anesthetizing the patient often is an important first step. One should first decide which diagnostics are to be performed before administering therapeutics, to avoid treatment effects from confounding diagnostics. Many times, it is more critical to administer treatments before blood tests or radiographs may be performed.

If fluid therapy is considered necessary by the veterinarian, the most common route of administration is subcutaneous. Usually the author will use a balanced electrolyte solution containing 2.5% dextrose at an initial rate of 40 to 50 mL/kg twice daily. Based on hydration status on response to therapy, this rate may be adjusted as desired. Though fluids normally are reported to be absorbed less slowly subcutaneously in a critical animal, it has been the author's experience in rodents that absorption in a warmed environment reached the desired end result reasonably. It is not uncommon for the owner to note small scabs at the sites of injection 1 to 2 weeks post-injection, which most likely represent injection site necrosis. They rarely exceed 1 cm in diameter. The author has never seen any long-term complications from these sites, but they are important to consider when treatment of a previously pruritic and self-excoriating rodent is being evaluated. A complication of subcutaneous injections is their potential to go through two layers of skin and miss injecting the animal completely.

One should make sure to balance the stress and time needed successfully to place an intravenous or intraosseous catheter against the need for immediate fluids. The author has administered subcutaneous fluids that were completely absorbed by the time the animal was induced with anesthesia and a catheter was placed. If an intravenous or intraosseous catheter is being considered, remember that these animals are extremely efficient chewers, whether of the catheter itself or the connecting line. Rodents can chew through steel pipes and usually have minimal necks for collar placement. A patient truly requiring a catheter often has poor peripheral circulation, and placement requires general anesthesia, except in the most moribund of patients. The author has placed an intraosseous catheter in the proximal femur, using a 3.75-cm (1.5-in), 22-gauge spinal needle for guinea pigs, chinchillas, and prairie dogs. Some smaller rodents require the use of 25- or 27-gauge needles, but, because those needles lack a stylet and are of such a small diameter, occlusion commonly occurs. When the needle is bent, the catheter no longer flows, and if the animal feels better it may pull it out on its own. The author usually places a piece of white tape to form flaps laterally and sutures those flaps to the skin. In some cases, a bolus of 100 mL/kg of fluids has been administered over 15 to 20 minutes because of concerns about patency or survival of the catheter. Intravenous catheters may be placed, particularly in surgical procedures when staff is available to monitor the catheter. But kinking of the catheter, a slow rate necessitating a microfluid pump, and blown veins appear to be common complications, along with the long learning curve for those placing catheters in small structures. One should flush the catheter with a small amount of saline (heparinized only if needed) several times a day. In guinea pigs, chinchillas, and prairie dogs, the cephalic or lateral saphenous veins may have short 25- or 27-gauge catheters attempted. Jugular vein cutdowns tend to be problematic in these animals because of their short, stocky necks. Lateral tail veins are reported to be used for catheters in rats in research settings.

Intramuscular injections can be challenging to administer to rodents because of small muscle mass size, and, with the exception of injection of emergency medications such as epinephrine, these are rarely performed by the author. Anterior hind leg muscles are recommended to avoid the sciatic nerve. Intraperitoneal fluid adminstration is another option in the lower left or right abdominal quadrants [8]. Intraluminal or subcutaneous injection can occur unintentionally, and, because of the large gastrointestinal mass of rodents, positioning of the rodent does not appear to be significant [8].

In administering medications to rodents, it is important to consider several factors. Obviously, when the animal has ileus, there are significant concerns about how well the medication may be absorbed orally. Certain antibiotics in particular [17] can have an undesired impact on gastrointestinal microflora and microfauna when administered orally. What will the stress level of administering the medication be for the administrator (staff or owner) and the recipient? In most cases, oral medications are the preferred form. With some wildlife or more dangerous pet rodents (prairie dogs), hiding the medication in food or having a compounding pharmacy develop a desirable flavor is a possibility (Fig. 8). There is a reason wild rats and mice are difficult to eliminate from one's house with rodenticides, and that same concept carries over to medicating. Small volumes for the four small rodents are essential, with 0.05 mL often being the limit per dose of what may be given to the animal against its will. If larger volumes are needed, they should be given in 0.05-mL intervals with breaks in between. A syringe may be introduced into the diastema to give undesired medications for rats and mice. In the author's experience, gerbils generally are amiable about being medicated and in several cases have held the syringe to their mouths, provided the flavoring is reasonable. Hamsters also tend to be easy to medicate, because they appear to desire to attack the syringe and simply swallow as it is being plunged. Chinchillas and guinea pigs may be "burrito-wrapped" in a towel and have the syringe introduced into the diastema with intervals of 0.25 mL or more if they are swallowing.

Nutritional support comes in several different forms for these animals. Nutrition is a complicated issue for these species, one better left to an entirely separate article. Basically, it comes down to high fiber, little or no carbohydrates, low protein in adults, low calcium in adults, low calories, and no treats, although a cachectic or critical patient may require more calories, a more concentrated caloric diet, and high palatability. A first step is to offer the animal what it normally eats at home, unless there are concerns about potential toxicity issues. An anorectic animal is not an animal to switch to a more nutritionally appropriate diet. A second option is to offer items that are higher in palatability until the animal starts eating. For example, alfalfa pellets might be offered instead of timothy hay pellets. For guinea pigs and chinchillas, leafy (thin) green vegetables are often palatable and

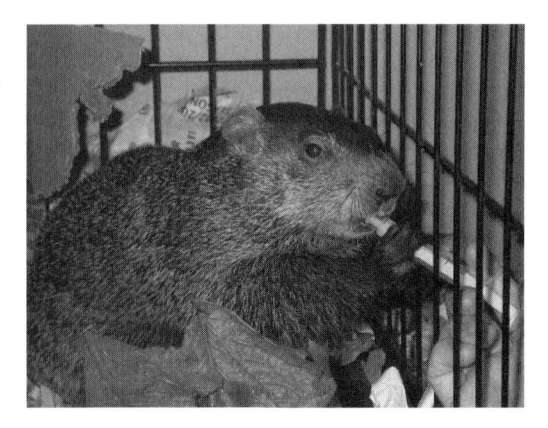

Fig. 8. Immature woodchuck, *Marmota monax,* raised in captivity, willingly taking oral antibiotics from owner owing to flavoring of medication.

provide additional moisture. Finally, supportive feedings may be necessary. The author prefers to use the Critical Care for Herbivores diet (Oxbow Enterprises, Murdock, Nebraska) (Fig. 9). It is powdered pellets that may be mixed with water and fed through a syringe (often a catheter-tipped one) to the animal. The author recommends the anise-flavored (black licorice) instead of the apple-flavored variety. Usually water is slowly added to the powder until the suspension is of a desired consistency for the patient and diluted enough to fit through a syringe. Following recommendations from the company appears to generate a paste difficult to fit into a syringe. Administration occurs using the same methods and volumes as with oral medications. Supportive feedings are labor-intensive, messy, and slow work. Patience on the part of staff or the owner is essential to avoid oral trauma or aspiration. The author finds that attempts to calculate the nutritional needs of the animal can be pointless, because the volume actually ingested by the patient rarely approaches that value. Over time, guinea pigs have been known to lap the mixture out of bowls. Nasogastric and esophageal feeding tube placement has been described, but in the author's experience and opinion, the frustration level of trying to pass a high-fiber diet into these tubes is high and the success rate of tube use in these species is low.

Pain management in these species is necessary when the veterinarian feels that the animal is experiencing discomfort. Assessing pain and management of pain may be challenging, and these are topics for another article. Remember that each animal responds differently to pain and to its management.

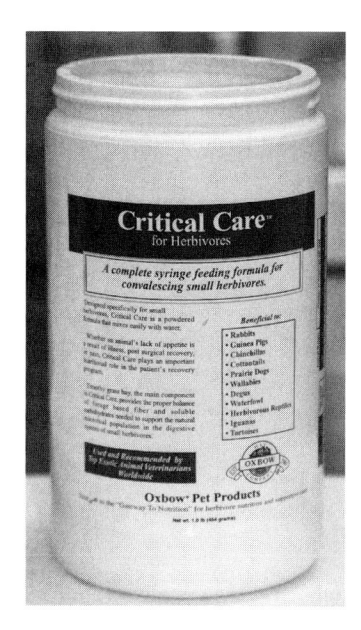

Fig. 9. Critical Care Diet for Herbivores from Oxbow Pet Products, Murdock, Nebraska.

Rodents are generally hindgut fermenters, and opioids can have an effect on the gastrointestinal system. However, opioids still tend to be a key component in attempted pain management. The author prefers buprenorphine hydrochloride administered subcutaneously, because published information suggests a longer duration of action. Dosage, frequency, and time of initial administration are dependent on the animal's health and circumstances and the ability to monitor response. Other veterinarians prefer butorphanol tartrate. Generally, the author has found no good option for oral opioid analgesia in rodents; however, an opioid-like drug, tramadol hydrochloride, may offer compounding options in the future. In certain cases of surgery, the author may "drip" several drops of 0.25% bupivacaine hydrochloride into an incision or fracture site for additional analgesia. The other category of drugs used in rodents for pain management is the nonsteroidal anti-inflammatory drugs. Injectable carprofen or flunixin meglumine may be administered, and oral meloxicam or compounded carprofen have been effective, provided one is alert for the typical side effects. Because rodents are often used as models for human or other animal drugs, other references can recommend specific regimens [17,18].

Sample collection

Generally about 1% of body weight may be removed in blood volume in an otherwise healthy animal. In a 30-g mouse, this means 0.3 mL. In a 1-kg guinea pig, this means 10 mL. Obviously, one must first decide whether the stress and challenge of blood collection are warranted to change the course of treatment based on patient status, the client's financial amenability, and the veterinarian's phlebotomy skills. In many cases, the author does not pursue phlebotomy for these reasons. General anesthesia is recommended for all the techniques described by the author. Most techniques described for hamsters, gerbils, and mice are based on laboratory animals and either require special equipment or expertise or involve terminal patients. If the reader is inclined to collect blood in these animals, the author recommends reading about the lateral saphenous vein technique described by Bihun and colleague [8], where the vein is exposed, nicked, and collected in microcapillary tubes as it wells forth. In rats, the author anesthetizes the animal, places a rubber band around the tail after warming the tail in a bowl of warm water for several minutes, and attempts to hit the superficial lateral tail veins or the ventral tail artery. The use of 1-mL syringes with 25-gauge needles is recommended. In some cases, the use of butterfly catheters or placement of the needle without an attached syringe has worked. Obviously, with the arterial phlebotomy, one should place a pressure wrap over the site.

For phlebotomy involving guinea pigs, chinchillas, or prairie dogs, the author again highly recommends the use of gas anesthesia for the benefit of everyone involved. Once the animal is anesthetized, many veterinarians will collect blood from the lateral saphenous, cephalic, or jugular veins.

The author generally performs a sternal notch phlebotomy using a short, 25-gauge butterfly catheter, carefully and gently directed at about a 20° angle to the body from the left shoulder toward the right hind leg, with the patient squared flat and as symmetrically as possible on the table and the forelegs both pulled either up or back. This is a blind stick, and it is important to remember the ramifications of phlebotomy at this site. The phlebotomist is attempting to hit one of several major veins in this region, but, in these smaller animals, one must be aware of needle length versus the location of the heart. Moreover, one cannot hold off the site, so manipulation of the needle should be as gentle as possible to minimize the risk of laceration. When the shoulder to hind leg does not provide venous access, the author has also directed the needle at the same angle but positioned directly down the midline. "Fishing" for the vein is highly discouraged. The author has used this technique for more than 6 years with minimal complications in small mammals ranging from hedgehogs and sugar gliders to guinea pigs, rabbits, and ferrets. However, other veterinarians have raised concerns about the inability to stop the bleeding when the animal has difficulties with blood clotting, when blood is collected from an artery, or when a large laceration occurs.

Urine collection in rodents can be challenging. For the larger rodents, cystocentesis may be attempted through palpation or ultrasound guidance under general anesthesia. However, most rodents will void their bladder during the stress of anesthesia or restraint, so one should always be prepared to collect the suboptimal sample from the tabletop or even to wring out a towel as a last resort. One should remember what to expect from the sample collected, in interpreting results and in deciding to submit for cultures. Collection may also be performed by housing the rodent in an appropriately sized wire-bottom cage with nonabsorbent material below, or in a solid-bottom container with nonabsorbent litter, such as may be used for domestic cats. Desert-dwelling species such as gerbils can concentrate their urine, often making each drop extremely valuable.

Fecal sample collection is rarely a problem in the healthy rodent (see Fig. 7). If a sample is needed, it is often helpful to advise clients ahead of time to bring a fresh sample with them, in case the animal does not produce one during the visit. When a sample is not provided, it may be helpful to offer the owner the option of leaving the animal for a portion of the day, though one must provide space, food, and hiding areas to make the patient comfortable. Many rodents that are healthy or boarding become constipated in a novel environment, particularly guinea pigs and chinchillas. One should also remember about cecotrophs, if softer feces are found. When a fecal culture is desired, gentle swabbing of the rectum with the appropriate-sized culturette may be performed, preferably under anesthesia to avoid contamination or perforation.

Other sampling techniques, such as skin scrapings and hair pluckings (Fig. 10), cytology, bone marrow aspirates (femur—as with an intraosseous

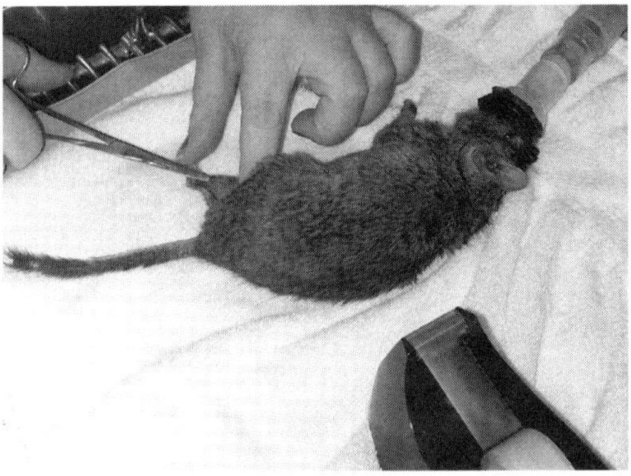

Fig. 10. Plucking hair from a degu, *Octodon* sp, with pruritis, mild alopecia, and crusting of the skin for cytology and culture. Note the transparent tape for tape preparations for microscopic examination.

catheter), skin biopsies, and superficial mass removals, are similar to those performed in other animals. Important modifications to remember are as follows. General anesthesia is highly recommended for all procedures more invasive than a skin scraping. Even with skin scrapings, one should make sure the patient may be competently restrained so that the scraping does not go too deep or too far. Remember that pruritic guinea pigs may experience seizure, as previously described. Use equipment appropriate for the size of the animal. Closure of larger wounds from biopsy procedures or surgeries may be challenging, and dehiscence due to poor planning and the patient's ingenuity can be common. In guinea pigs, chinchillas, and prairie dogs, subcuticular sutures may be easily placed and should only be avoided when patient survival is at risk, at which time the closure method the veterinarian can employ most rapidly (skin staples) should be used until the crisis is resolved. Judicious use of surgical glue may help to close edges or "pooched regions," although excessive use may cause irritation and encourage the animal to attempt immediate self-dehiscence. In smaller rodents, it is recommended to place subcutaneous sutures to reduce the size of the immediate incision. If subcuticular sutures are not possible (use small, dark-colored absorbable sutures to assess for accidental skin penetration), then numerous simple interrupted sutures may be placed to minimize dehiscence by rodent removal of several sutures. If the wound is on an extremity, bandaging may protect sutures, although excessively tight bandaging may lead to vascular compromise necrosis or self-mutilation. The author has had poor results with collaring rodents and using chemical chewing deterrents, although other veterinarians have had some success with their use. One option the author has used successfully in rodents is to grind the incisors short enough to eliminate occlusion of those teeth: use a Dremel (Robert Bosch Tool Corporation, Mount Prospect, Illinois) under anesthesia. In rats, this lasts about 1 week in the author's experience, so that either the incision site has had enough time to heal, no longer requiring suture support, or the sutures no longer bother the rodent. Concerns regarding diet provision during regrowth of the teeth should be addressed as in a rodent with fractured incisors. Analgesic therapy is also recommended with this procedure.

Miscellaneous procedures

General anesthesia is a commonly necessary procedure in working with rodents. Use of a volatile gas anesthetic, either by mask or by chamber, is the most commonly followed protocol. Most rodents do not need to be fasted long before anesthesia; often removal of food an hour before a procedure is adequate. When intubation is anticipated, injectible anesthetics are highly recommended. The author typically uses a combination of ketamine, midazolam hydrochloride, and buprenorphine. To maintain rodents on gas anesthesia, generally only a nasal mask is necessary. This method can be especially helpful for quick dental procedures; it eliminates the need for an intratracheal tube that would clutter an already small oral cavity but still permits quick reversal of anesthesia if needed. However, during a painful procedure performed with gas anesthetic alone, it has been this author's experience that many rodents need to be maintained at high levels of isoflurane, even with good mask seals.

Once the animal is anesthetized, one should aggressively swab moisture and debris from the mouth and cheek pouches using cotton-tipped applicators, particularly in guinea pigs. Make sure the eyes are immediately lubricated with artificial tears and repeat this at the end of the procedure. Intubation of rodents has been described in numerous texts. The author has only intubated guinea pigs, chinchillas, and prairie dogs successfully and generally uses endotracheal tubes 2.0 mm or 2.5 mm in diameter. Even if injectible agents were used, one should continue to provide gas anesthesia by means of the nasal mask while intubating. To intubate, a small rigid endoscope used inside the endotracheal tube has been successful, but complications leading to damage of the endoscope are possible. The scope is introduced into the glottis; then the endotracheal tube is gently slid into the trachea. The use of a defogger before attempting may be helpful.

Another intubation method involves the use of a small-bladed laryngoscope and a rubber-tipped stylet (M. Jones, personal communication, 2003). The head is extended back until it is as close to perpendicular with the table as possible, with moderate tension placed on gauze pulling the mandible from the maxilla. The tongue is gently grasped with gauze and exteriorized as much as possible without overstretching. Sometimes tongue placement to either side of the incisors improves the view. One should keep the stylet a bit longer than the endotracheal tube. When the glottis is visualized, advance the stylet into the trachea, then the endotracheal tube.

Trying to advance the tube and stylet together causes the visualization to be lost and creates a high probability of missing the trachea and instead placing in the esophagus. Cheek spreaders also improve visualization. One should make sure to measure tube length before placing, to avoid intubation of only one bronchi. A final technique described is the blind technique with variations. The author has had no success in performing this technique. To determine correct placement of the tube, one should watch for fogging of the tube or shallow movement of the anesthetic bag in parallel to the animal's respiration pattern. If edema or laryngeal trauma is noted or suspected, or more than two attempts have been made to the level of the glottis, it is recommended that one either abort the procedure and recover the animal or maintain the animal on mask anesthesia only. Overexuberance may lead to complications, including death. When intermittent positive pressure ventilation is required, the author generally provides three to six breaths per minute, applying a light pressure where the slightest resistance from the patient's lungs is noted. If the patient is intubated, do not extubate until the patient is at a proper level of anesthesia. Further information on anesthesia may be found in other sources [17,18].

Euthanasia is unfortunately a common procedure performed on these short-lived animals. Methods used in laboratory situations are rarely acceptable to clients (cervical disarticulation) or available to most private practitioners (carbon dioxide chambers). An exception for cervical disarticulation occurs when the "owner" owns those rodents for the purpose of feeding other animals, such as reptiles or raptors, and wishes to feed freshly killed rodents for the other animal's safety. In these situations, the author will teach the client to quickly and safely euthanize these animals. Proper protocols are described by the American Veterinary Medical Association. For a client-owned pet, two questions need to be answered by the client before proceeding with the euthanasia. First, will the animal have a necropsy performed, and, if so, will cardiac, hepatic, or pulmonary samples be necessary? Second, does the client wish to be present during the euthanasia? Many veterinarians will try to dissuade the client from being present, especially children, but this author feels that, provided the process and what it entails are explained to the owner, it may contribute to healing the loss of a treasured family member. The author always asks whether any female clients who desire to be present are or might be pregnant, and, if so, either advises them to leave the room or uses injectible anesthesia.

The owners are encouraged to take their time saying goodbye while materials for a successful euthanasia are collected. Once the owners are ready, the procedure is explained to them again. All necessary paperwork is signed, and billing is completed or a bill sent to the owner at the veterinarian's discretion. The owner is encouraged to be seated if feeling lightheaded. The animal is either restrained and masked or chambered with general anesthesia, using isoflurane or a similar gaseous agent. While the animal enters a deep state of anesthesia, challenges to placement of the needle and expected agonal responses are explained (open-mouthed gasping, paddling of the legs, release of urine or feces). Deep pain is accessed with toe pinches until responses are no longer occurring. At this time, the owners are asked if they are ready, and if so, are shown the syringe of euthanasia solution with its purpose explained. At this time, the needle is directed into the left thoracic cavity of the patient, using a pediatric stethoscope to guide it to the heart. If a flash of blood occurs, the syringe is slowly injected, with a final check of proper placement with approximately one fourth of the volume left. In some cases, the heart may not be easily located; depending on the veterinarian's reading of the client's emotional response to the procedure and necropsy needs, the solution may be injected into the proximity of the heart or into the lungs. Euthanasia solution is inexpensive, and, when necropsy is not the goal, greatly exceeding the recommended doses of 1 mL per 4.6 kg can be helpful to speed up the process. In some cases, the author has had to give several injections, either to speed up the process or because of lack of an appropriate response. Having some euthanasia solution on immediate reserve is recommended. The only complication seen by the author that is not routinely explained beforehand is bleeding from the nostrils or mouth. This has rarely been seen but should be expected as a possibility. Make sure the patient is dead and that all agonal responses have stopped before sending the animal home with the owner. Make sure the owner is in the proper state of mind before leaving to drive, or encourage waiting in a quiet area of the clinic until such a state is reached.

Surgical preparation of rodents also requires some considerations not relevant to larger mammals. Rodents are more quickly prone to hypothermia with their smaller size and higher metabolism. The use of a Bair Hugger blanket (Arizant Health Care, Eden Prairie, Minnesota) (Fig. 11) is highly recommended for all small mammals to minimize core temperature loss. Other forms of supplemental heat should be used cautiously to avoid the risk for thermal burns or hyperthermia. In preparing a site for surgery, one needs to strike a balance between increased anesthetic time and a properly cleaned surgical field. Most rodent hair is fine, and it requires fine clipper blades to remove in some cases. Be careful not to nick or irritate the skin or to remove nipples. The author has used small human electric clippers with success. Generally, the preparation site should be much larger than anticipated, because certain surgeries require further expansion, particularly in the removal of mammary gland masses. Remember that hair can always grow back. In some cases, removal of a layer of "fuzz" may become impossible, and excessive attempts increase the risk for anesthetic complications, particularly when the patient is unintubated or critical to begin with. Generally the author does three passes of the site with antiseptic, following each pass with a pass of minimal rubbing alcohol to rinse. Some veterinarians believe alcohol contributes excessively to hypothermia and prefer to use warmed sterile saline. The site is cleaned on each pass from the inside out, with the alcohol or saline being used to mat down edge hair if needed. The author believes that

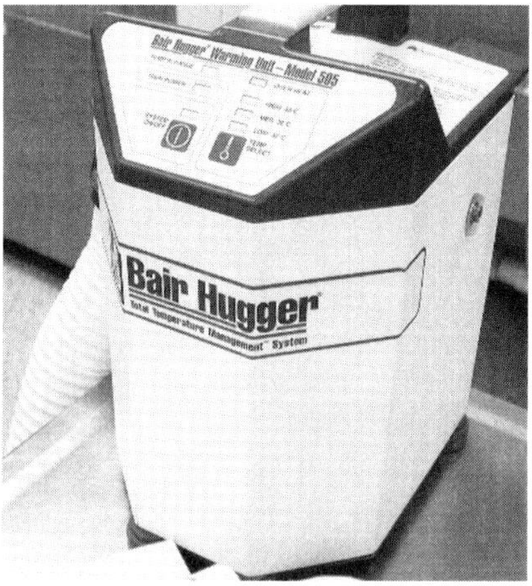

Fig. 11. Bair Blanket heating unit from Arizant Health Care, Eden Prairie, Minnesota.

his rodent patients have sometimes died because too much time was spent on preparation, leading to extended general anesthesia and hypothermia, particularly in the nonintubated animals. A golden rule to follow is that mask anesthetic times exceeding 1 hour in rodents carry a much higher risk for mortality. For animals requiring multiple surgeries, it may be worthwhile to space surgeries out over a week rather than performing them all in one anesthetic period.

The topic of particular surgical techniques is covered by other sources [19–22], but some common procedures performed by the author in these species may be noted. Often specialized surgical instruments and tools, modified from ophthalmologic surgical packs, electrocautery, and hemoclip ligation, are important for gentle tissue handling and maximum hemostasis and speed. Dentistry is another topic previously covered in other sources in detail [5,6], and the reader is advised to refer to those sources for performing these procedures or for a thorough examination of the mouth.

Radiography is best performed using general anesthesia for proper positioning. Rodents commonly can have artifactual torsion of the vertebrae due to malpositioning. One should immediately evaluate radiographs for proper technique, positioning, and labeling before discontinuing general anesthesia. All common rodents should be radiographed using a tabletop technique. The use of masking tape to position limbs and minimize fur removal is encouraged. High-detail and mammography film is likewise recommended. When dental films are desired, properly labeled oblique views are helpful. For the most sensitive evaluation of suspected otitis interna and otitis media, CT is recommended. Further information on radiology in these rodents may be found in other sources [23].

Nail trims may be performed during anesthetic recovery, between anesthetic procedures, or while the animal is awake (excepting prairie dogs). Again, chinchillas lack trimmable nails. Nails are trimmed in the same manner as those of a dog or cat, staying distal from the quick. In small mammals, it is often nail sharpness rather than length that bothers the owners. In these cases, typical trims may simply create new sharp edges. Instead, one may use a slow speed setting on the Dremel or a human nail file to dull the tips. Guinea pigs often develop "corns" on the medial surface of the forefeet (see Fig. 6). The author usually trims these back as close to the footpad as possible.

Older (or obese) male guinea pigs commonly develop a build-up of exudate around the caudal sebaceous gland, located just dorsal to the tailbase (see Fig. 2) [13]. This material is waxy and often matted in the fur. In some guinea pigs, excess build-up appears to cause an irritation and to be one of many possible causes of self-inflicted flank alopecia. Judicious plucking or shaving of the fur, followed by a warm-water soaking and removal of excess secretion, has been successful in some cases of pruritus or alopecia. Periodic repetition of such care may be necessary. Older male guinea pigs may also develop a dilatation of the rectum, with normal-to-soft feces and hair impacted within the dilatation. Often a white crème-to-brown paste, created by the anal glands, creates a potent odor that one may mistake for diarrhea. The owner can be taught to clean gently at home as needed wearing latex gloves and using lubricated cotton-tipped applicators. The cause of this condition is unknown, and, as long as hygiene is maintained, it does not appear to be life threatening. A final condition seen occasionally by the author in older male guinea pigs is impaction of the circumferentially located preputial glands. Under general anesthesia, these may be gently expressed to removed the impacted whitish exudate.

In summary, common rodent procedures are a blend of techniques and equipment developed in the world of laboratory animal medicine with cutting edge and routine procedures used in larger pet mammals, tempered by the practical concerns of patient size and the financial constraints placed by owners. Most practitioners should be able to perform basic techniques such as examination, radiology, anesthesia, phlebotomy, grooming procedures, euthanasia, and emergency care with a minimal investment in equipment beyond what most practices already provide.

References

[1] Sainsbury AW. Rodentia (Rodents). In: Fowler M, Miller E, editors. Zoo and wild animal medicine. 5th edition. Philadelphia: WB Saunders; 2003. p. 420–42.
[2] Nowak RM. Order Rodentia. In: Walker's mammals of the world, vol. 2. Baltimore (MD): John Hopkins University Press; 1999. p. 1243–714.
[3] Webster's ninth new collegiate dictionary. Springfield (MA): Merriam-Webster; 1988.
[4] O'Malley B. Introduction to small mammals. In: Clinical anatomy and physiology of exotic species. Philadelphia: Elsevier Saunders; 2005. p. 165–71.

[5] Crossley DA, Aiken S. Small mammal dentistry. In: Quesenberry KE, Carpenter JW, editors. Ferrets, rabbits, and rodents: clinical medicine and surgery. 2nd edition. Philadelphia: WB Saunders; 2003. p. 370–82.
[6] Legendre LFJ. Oral disorders of exotic rodents. Vet Clin North Am Exotic Anim Pract 2003; 6(3):601–28.
[7] van der Woerdt A. Ophthalmologic diseases in small pet mammals. In: Quesenberry KE, Carpenter JW, editors. Ferrets, rabbits, and rodents: clinical medicine and surgery. 2nd edition. Philadelphia: WB Saunders; 2003. p. 421–8.
[8] Bihun C, Bauck L. Basic anatomy, physiology, husbandry, and clinical techniques. In: Quesenberry KE, Carpenter JW, editors. Ferrets, rabbits, and rodents: clinical medicine and surgery. 2nd edition. Philadelphia: WB Saunders; 2003. p. 232–44.
[9] Brown CJ, Donnelly TM. Rodent husbandry and care. Vet Clin North Am Exotic Anim Pract 2004;7(2):201–25.
[10] O'Malley B. Rats. In: Clinical anatomy and physiology of exotic species. Philadelphia: Elsevier Saunders; 2005. p. 209–25.
[11] O'Malley B. Hamsters. In: Clinical anatomy and physiology of exotic species. Philadelphia: Elsevier Saunders; 2005. p. 228–36.
[12] Donnelly TM, Brown CJ. Guinea pig and chinchilla care and husbandry. Vet Clin North Am Exotic Anim Pract 2004;7(2):351–73.
[13] O'Malley B. Guinea pigs. In: Clinical anatomy and physiology of exotic species. Philadelphia: Elsevier Saunders; 2005. p. 197–208.
[14] Quesenberry KE, Donnelly TM, Hillyer EV. Biology, husbandry, and clinical techniques of guinea pigs and chinchillas. In: Quesenberry KE, Carpenter JW, editors. Ferrets, rabbits, and rodents: clinical medicine and surgery. 2nd edition. Philadelphia: WB Saunders; 2003. p. 232–44.
[15] Funk RS. Medical management of prairie dogs. In: Quesenberry KE, Carpenter JW, editors. Ferrets, rabbits, and rodents: clinical medicine and surgery. 2nd edition. Philadelphia: WB Saunders; 2003. p. 266–73.
[16] Pilny AA, Hess L. Prairie dog care and husbandry. Vet Clin North Am Exotic Anim Pract 2004;7(2):269–82.
[17] Carpenter JW. Exotic animal formulary. 3rd edition. Philadelphia: WB Saunders; 2005. p. 377–408.
[18] Heard DJ. Anesthesia, analgesia, and sedation of small mammals. In: Quesenberry KE, Carpenter JW, editors. Ferrets, rabbits, and rodents: clinical medicine and surgery. 2nd edition. Philadelphia: WB Saunders; 2003. p. 356–69.
[19] Bennett RA, Mullen HS. Soft tissue surgery (guinea pigs and chinchillas). In: Quesenberry KE, Carpenter JW, editors. Ferrets, rabbits, and rodents: clinical medicine and surgery. 2nd edition. Philadelphia: WB Saunders; 2003. p. 274–84.
[20] Bennett RA, Mullen HS. Soft tissue surgery (small rodents). In: Quesenberry KE, Carpenter JW, editors. Ferrets, rabbits, and rodents: clinical medicine and surgery. 2nd edition. Philadelphia: WB Saunders; 2003. p. 316–28.
[21] Helmer PJ, Lightfoot TL. Small exotic mammal orthopedics. Vet Clin North Am Exotic Anim Pract 2002;5(1):169–82.
[22] Kapatkin A. Orthopedics in small mammals. In: Quesenberry KE, Carpenter JW, editors. Ferrets, rabbits, and rodents: clinical medicine and surgery. 2nd edition. Philadelphia: WB Saunders; 2003. p. 383–91.
[23] Stefanacci JD, Hoefer H. Radiology and ultrasound. In: Quesenberry KE, Carpenter JW, editors. Ferrets, rabbits, and rodents: clinical medicine and surgery. 2nd edition. Philadelphia: WB Saunders; 2003. p. 395–6.

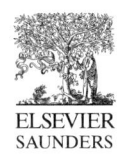

Common Procedures in Hedgehogs, Prairie Dogs, Exotic Rodents, and Companion Marsupials

Cathy A. Johnson-Delaney, DVM, DABVP–Avian Practice*

Eastside Avian and Exotic Animal Medical Center, 13603 100th NE, Kirkland, WA 98034-5212, USA

Nondomesticated species are commonly being kept as companion animals. These include the African pygmy hedgehog (*Atelerix albiventris*), the North American black-tailed prairie dog (*Cynomys ludovicianus*), and exotic rodents such as the degu (*Octodon degus*) and duprasi or fat-tailed gerbil (*Pachyuromys duprasi*). Common companion marsupials include the sugar glider (*Petaurus breviceps*), Bennett's or Tammar (Dama) wallabies (*Macropus rufogriseus rufogriseus* and *Macropus eugenii*, respectively), the Brazilian or South American gray short-tailed opossum (*Monodelphis domestica*), and the North American Virginia opossum (*Didelphis virginianum*) (Fig. 1).

Although many of these animals are now bred domestically and are fairly docile when human-raised, they are essentially wild animals and hence have strong instincts to hide illness and pain. They may also react with ferocity and quickness when handled by individuals other than their owners. It becomes a challenge to practitioners and staff to understand body language, movements, and behaviors of these animals so as to provide adequate restraint and clinical assessment, while protecting the animal, the owner, and the veterinary staff. Many of these species can inflict painful bites and deep scratches to those who are inexperienced in working with them. It is always advisable to have staff rather than the owner restrain an ill or pained animal during examination and procedures, because restraint by the owner raises liability issues when he or she is injured in the hospital. Veterinary staff should be trained in proper restraint techniques for these species, as well as being familiar with potential zoonoses [1,2].

---

* 13813 65th Avenue West, #7, Edmonds, WA 98026-3517.
 E-mail address: cajddvm@hotmail.com

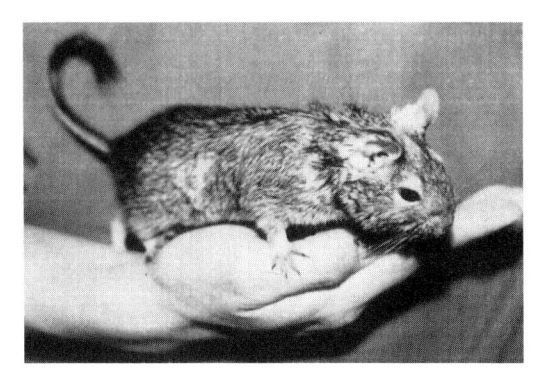

Fig. 1. Degu.

Some of the marsupial pets are more easily restrained within a cloth sack that mimics a pouch. Pet wallabies, for example, will then remain still for examination procedures, including weighing (Fig. 2). Most prairie dogs and Virginia opossums are wild-caught and potentially carry zoonotic pathogens. The other animals listed earlier are now almost exclusively domestically bred, although many are still produced from wild-caught parentage. Many breeders have not had their breeding stock adequately screened for pathogens, including parasites, so these animals may carry the pathogens described in these species in the wild. Even so, no human cases have been reported for most of the potential disease agents. Table 1 lists potential zoonoses of the animals in question [1,3,4,5].

A clinic bite, scratch, and injury protocol should be in place and should be in compliance with local, state, and federal occupational health regulations. Clinic policy should require appropriate wound care even when the

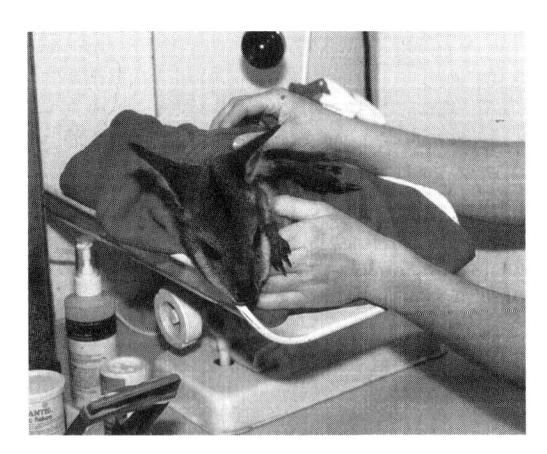

Fig. 2. Tammar wallaby being weighed in a cloth sack as the restraint device. A large pillowcase also works well if the owner does not provide a sack.

Table 1
Potential zoonoses

Species	Potential zoonotic disease	Transmission reported to humans
Bennett's Wallaby, Tammar Wallaby	*Angiostrongylus cantonensis*	None reported
	Dermatophytes: *Trichophyton spp; Microsporum spp*	None reported
Degu	None reported in domestically bred; wild may carry *Linguatula serrata, Echinococcus granulosis, Trypanosoma cruzi*	None reported
Duprasi	None reported	None reported
Hedgehog	Salmonellosis, Salmonella serotype Tilene	Yes
Prairie dog	Plague (wild-caught animals), *Yersinia pestis*	None reported
	Monkeypox (from contact with imported African rodents)	Yes
Short-tailed opossum	None reported	None reported
Sugar glider	Giardia	None reported
	Salmonellosis	None reported
Virginia opossum	*Sarcocystis spp* carriers	Horses; none reported in humans
	Salmonellosis	None reported
	Sarcoptes scabei	None reported
	Chagas disease (*Trypanosoma cruzi*)	None reported
	Dermatophytosis	Anecdotal, author's experience
	Rabies	None reported. Opossum is fairly resistant.

Data from Refs. [1,3,45].

employee believes the wound is minor; all these wounds have the potential for infection and complications. Proper equipment should always be available, disinfected, and in full working condition. This equipment includes but is not limited to various thicknesses and sizes of restraint gloves, various restraint boxes (which may double as anesthetic chambers), towels, and, in instances of animals that may jump or climb, some sort of eye or face protection. Routine wearing of safety glasses by staff may decrease the incidence of animal fluids, disinfectants, or medications getting into the eyes. Long-sleeved laboratory coats or smocks greatly decrease the incidence of scratches. Procedure gloves also provide barriers to animal body fluids, ectoparasites, infectious dermatologic pathogens, quill pricks, scratches, and even bites from smaller animals.

Practitioners should be aware of any local, state, or federal regulations that may apply to the possession of these species. They should check their state, US Department of Agriculture (www.usda.gov), county, and city Web sites for regulations concerning exotic animals [6]. Although the veterinarian is unlikely to report ownership of an illegal animal, in some jurisdictions this reporting may be required. Veterinarians also must report certain infectious diseases to local, state, or federal public health authorities should diagnosis of a reportable disease be made. Often owners can obtain prohibited exotic animals through the Internet, regardless of laws, and they may actually be unaware of restrictions. At the time the animal is presented, however, the veterinarian's responsibility is to the medical care of the animal; the legality of the particular animal may be secondary. The veterinarian should discuss regulations with the owner and document that the discussion took place. The veterinarian's role may be to influence future acquisition of exotic animals and counsel the owner on appropriate choices.

Ethically, and often legally, the veterinarian is placed in the middle when an illegal exotic animal is brought in for treatment. Regardless of whether the veterinarian judges the animal to be an appropriate or an illegal pet, the owner has sought assistance for that animal, and the veterinarian's first responsibility is to care for its health and well-being. In the author's opinion, the owner should be educated about the legality, husbandry, and dietary, behavioral, and medical needs of the animal so that the animal may have the best possible quality of life.

Recognition of pain and distress

For practitioners who are unfamiliar with the species listed earlier, recognizing the signs of pain is a priority. Many are not presented to the practitioner until they are very ill and often in severe pain and distress. There are no contraindications to administering analgesics. A rule of thumb that many laboratory animal practitioners follow is "If the given condition or procedure were performed on you, what type and level of pain relief would you want?" Although most dosages published for these species have been used anecdotally, they are often based on response to the therapy and provide a starting point. When the practitioner cannot find a published dosage for a medication, it is helpful to consider the type of physiology and metabolism for a choice of medication and dosage. Allometric scaling, though sometimes useful as a guideline, tends to require mathematical analysis that the practitioner rarely has time to perform when presented with a patient. The author has found that, in at least one published pharmacokinetic study done in marsupials, allometric scaling was extremely inaccurate [7]. In this case, it was more appropriate to consider the body weight and gastrointestinal system as equivalent to those of another, well-known animal and use that dosage.

The author generally uses this system as a guideline: For those animals that have a simple gastrointestinal tract and a diet that is insectivorous, carnivorous, or various levels of omnivorous (hedgehog, sugar glider, opossum, duprasi), use published doses for similarly sized known carnivores, such as the ferret or cat. For those animals that are herbivores with either hindgut digestion (degu, prairie dog) or foregut digestion (wallabies), follow guidelines for rabbits and guinea pigs. In the author's experience, these doses calculated by kilogram body weight have appeared therapeutic in the clinical setting. All animals should be assessed for body temperature and hydration.

Hedgehogs, sugar gliders, opossums, and prairie dogs may enter a state of torpor if ambient temperature is lower than their environmental zone and need to be warmed before extensive therapy, because metabolism has slowed. Prairie dogs and Virginia opossums appear inclined to enter torpor when they are obese and are subjected to a decreased light cycle accompanied by lower than normal home temperatures. Providing thermal assistance for these animals usually starts on the examination table. See Table 2 for guidelines for temperature requirements and thermal zones [5,8–17].

Many analgesics may also be used as preoperative medications and continued as part of the postoperative regimen. With the advent of nonsteroidal anti-inflammatory drugs such as carprofen and meloxicam, both in oral and injectable forms, administration of these is easy, economical, and effective.

Table 2
Thermal zones and body temperature

Species	Ambient range (degrees C)	Body temperature (rectal or cloacal)	Comments
Bennett's wallaby	0–33	35.0–36.0 (cloacal)	In lower temperatures, needs heated, dry shelter.
Degu	20–25	36.9–37.9	
Duprasi	20–30	36.5	Provide warm zone in cage.
Hedgehog	24–30	36.1–37.2	Provide warm zone in cage.
Prairie dog	20.5–22	35.3–39.0	Enters torpor in temperatures below 20.5°C.
Short-tailed opossum	22–37	33.0–36.0 (cloacal)	Provide warm zone in cage. May enter torpor below 22°C ambient.
Sugar glider	27–31	36.3–36.5 (cloacal)	Provide warm zone. Less than 15–16°C prolonged, may enter torpor, negative calorie balance.
Tammar wallaby	16–37	35.0–36.0 (cloacal)	In lower temperatures, provide heated, dry shelter.
Virginia opossum	Most activity: 20–35; documented activity in ambient temperatures of −2°C	35.0–36.5 (cloacal)	Wild opossums may enter torpor at lower temperatures for short time periods.

Data from Refs. [5,8–17]

Anesthetics and analgesics

Remember that these nondomesticated animals can be easily stressed during handling and examination. Stress and anesthesia can combine to produce cardiopulmonary failure. This effect may be exacerbated by pre-existing lung pathologic conditions, dehydration, or other metabolic compromise. Signs of pain include decreased appetite and thirst, increased respiratory rate, abnormal resting posture, reluctance to move, abnormal movement, and trembling or tensing on gentle palpation of an affected area. "Loud" teeth chattering or grinding while sitting in a "hunched" position is frequently seen in wallabies. Hedgehogs will tightly curl, making their condition difficult to assess. Sugar gliders may bite, vocalize, and try to flee. Prairie dogs often become extremely aggressive and reluctant to be touched. They may vocalize loudly as well. Although all these signs may also be present in dehydration, weakness, and gastrointestinal distress, the practitioner needs to include generalized pain as a likely contributor to the presentation.

One way to assess pain is to administer an analgesic. If the animal resumes a more normal attitude, the pretreatment signs were probably a result of discomfort. Table 3 lists analgesics [2,7–11,14–16,18–21].

Practical use of sedatives and analgesics in office calls

It is usually better to administer a mild sedative or light anesthesia than to fight with an animal to do diagnostics or a thorough examination. Sedatives are listed in Table 4 [2,7–11,14–16,21]. Staff should be proficient in nonstressful restraint, but for many animals, any restraint or handling by unfamiliar humans is stressful. Diagnostics obtained during severe stress are not as clinically useful and may pose a danger to the animal. When an animal's condition is too critical for it to tolerate a sedative dose of a benzodiazepine, a sedative such as medetomidine, an analgesic with sedative properties such as butorphanol, or light gas anesthesia, stressing the animal with physical restraint for a blood draw or radiographs may be inappropriate until it is stabilized. This stabilization may require fluids (subcutaneous), oxygen or nebulization therapy, heat, or just a short interval in a quiet, darkened environment to calm it. Towels, dimmed lighting, and a quiet environment can decrease stress. Work on these species should be done away from barking dogs and cats, because noise, odors, and pheromones can distress them.

Vascular access and fluid therapy

For hedgehogs, degus, duprasi, sugar gliders, and short-tailed opossums, the author uses the guideline of 50 to 100 mL/kg/d of crystalloid fluids; however, this dosage needs to be evaluated several times a day and tailored to

Table 3
Analgesics opiates

Species	Buprenorphine	Butorphanol	Meperidine	Morphine	Naloxone	Oxymorphone
Sugar glider	0.01 SC, IM q 6–8 h	0.05 SC, IM q 6–8 h	NE Dose	0.1 SC, IM q 6–8 h	NE Dose	NE Dose
Wallaby	0.01 SC, IM q 8–12 h	0.1–0.5 SC, IM, PO q 6–8 h	NE Dose	NE Dose	NE Dose	NE Dose
Short-tailed opossum	0.01 SC, IM q 6–8 h	0.1–0.5 SC, IM q 6–8 h	NE Dose	NE Dose	NE Dose	NE Dose
Virginia opossum	0.1 SC, IM q 8–12 h	0.1–0.5 SC, PO q 6–8 h	NE Dose	NE Dose	NE Dose	NE Dose
Degu	0.05 SC q 8–12 h	0.4–2.0 SC q 8–12 h	10–20 SC q 2–3 h	2–5 SC q 4 h	0.05 SC IP once	0.2–0.5 q 6–12 h
Duprasi	0.1–0.2 SC q 8 h	1–5 SC q 4 h	20 SC, IM q 2–3 h	2–5 SC q 4 h	0.05 SC IP once	0.2–0.5 q 6–12 h
Prairie dog	0.01–0.05 SC, IP q 6–12 h	0.4–2.0 SC q 8–12 h	10–20 SC q 2–3 h	2–5 SC q 4 h	0.05 SC IP once	0.2–0.5 q 6–12 h
Hedgehog	0.01 SC, IM q 6–8 h	0.05–0.4 SC, IM q 6–8 h	NE Dose	0.1 IM	0.1 SC, IM q 6–8 h	NE Dose

Nonsteroidal anti-inflammatory drugs

Species	Carprofen	Meloxicam
Sugar glider	1.0 PO, SC q 24 h	0.2 PO, SC q 24 h
Wallaby	4 SC q 24 h or 1.5 PO q 12 h	0.2 PO, SC q 24 h
Short-tailed opossum	1.0 PO, SC q 12–24 h	0.2 PO, SC q 24 h
Virginia opossum	1.0 PO, SC q 12–24 h	0.2 PO, SC q 24 h
Degu	1–4 PO, SC q 24 h	0.1–0.2 PO, SC q 24 h
Duprasi	1–4 PO, SC q 24 h	0.1–0.2 PO, SC q 24 h
Prairie Dog	1–4 PO, SC q 24 h	0.1–0.2 PO, SC q 24 h
Hedgehog	1.0 PO, SC q 12–24 h	0.2 PO, SC q 24 h

Data from Refs. [2,7–11,14–16,18–21]
Doses in mg/kg.
Abbreviations: IM, intramuscular; IP, intraperitoneal; NE Dose, no established dose; SC, subcutaneous.

Table 4
Sedatives and tranquilizers

Species	Drug (doses in mg/kg) Diazepam	Butorphanol	Medetomidine[a]
Sugar glider	0.5–2.0 IM, PO, IV	0.1–0.4 SC, IM q 6–8 h	0.05–0.1 IM with ketamine at 2–3 mg/kg IM
Wallaby	0.5–2.0 IM, PO, IV	0.1–0.4 SC, IM q 6–8 h	0.05–0.1 IM with ketamine at 2–3 mg/kg IM
Short-tailed opossum	0.5–2.0 IM, PO, IV	0.1–0.4 SC, IM q 6–8 h	0.05–0.1 IM with ketamine at 2–3 mg/kg IM
Virginia opossum	0.5–2.0 IM, PO, IV	0.1–0.4 SC, IM q 6–8 h	0.05–0.1 IM with ketamine at 2–3 mg/kg IM
Degu	1–5 IM, IP, IV	1–5 SC q 4 h	0.1 SC
Duprasi	1–5 IM, IP, IV	1–5 SC q 4 h	0.1 SC
Prairie Dog	1–5 IM, IP, IV	2 SC q 2–4 h	0.1–0.3 SC
Hedgehog	0.5–2.0 IM	0.1–0.4 SC, IM q 6–8 h	0.05–0.10 IM light sedation, 0.2 IM deeper

Variation in dosages within species depending on health status. Clinician should use lowest dosage to achieve effect. Butorphanol also has analgesic effects.

Abbreviations: IM, intramuscular; IP, intraperitoneal; IV, intravenous; SC, subcutaneous.

[a] Atipamazole for reversal: marsupials at 0.05–0.4 mg/kg IV or SC. All others: Reverse at 1 mg/kg SC, IP, IV.

Data from Refs. [2,7–11,14–16,21]

each patient and medical or surgical need. For wallabies and the Virginia opossum, the author begins with 25 mL/kg/d plus percentage dehydration as the guideline for a fluid therapy protocol. Access routes for fluid therapy are listed in Table 5 (Fig. 3) [2,5,11,14–16,21]. For subcutaneous fluid administration, the author prefers to use butterfly-style infusion catheters, because these allow for some movement of the animal without dislodging the needle or tearing the skin. Gentle pressure of the wings against the skin is sufficient to hold the needle in place and allow it to move with the animal should it move during fluid administration. The flank area skin is frequently less "tough" than skin over the shoulders and may be "looser," which allows for comfortable administration.

Intraosseous catheters may be used in sugar gliders, degus, duprasi, short-tailed opossums, and Virginia opossums and are placed in the femur using a similar procedure to that used in rabbits and rodents [22]. The procedure is outlined thus:

> Anesthetize the patient only if necessary; in very debilitated animals this will not be. Puncture of the bone is considered a painful process, so systemic analgesia is required. See Table 3 for analgesics.

Clip the hair over the hip area. When metabolic bone disease is present, extreme caution is needed to prevent fracture of the bone, so alternative intravascular routes may be more appropriate. Clean the skin in all species as in a surgical preparation.

Local skin block using lidocaine 2% may be performed, although this may not be necessary if the animal has received adequate systemic analgesia.

Make a small stab incision and place an 18- to 20-gauge needle (or smaller, depending on the size of the animal) into the bone. A short spinal needle, 22-gauge, 1-in length, is preferable to prevent bone plugs, but a regular needle may be used. Put a piece of tape (make two "wings") on the hub of the needle and suture it into place on the hip.

Administer intravenous fluids of choice, warmed to appropriate body temperature, and deliver at 5 mL/h or volume appropriate to the size of the catheter and the needs of the patient.

Choice of fluids should follow general principles used in other species, except for the marsupials. Marsupials are less tolerant of elevations in blood glucose than are placental mammals. Prolonged elevations in blood glucose may lead to development of cataracts and contribute to hepatic lipidosis and other metabolic dysfunction. As a rule, one should not use crystalloids containing dextrose in the marsupials [7].

Administration of fluids and other parenteral medications may be problematic in hedgehogs owing to the presence of the mantle. Subcutaneous administration is most reliably achieved in the furred area of skin. Access is usually easiest at the lateral junction of the furred skin and mantle, midbody. Intramuscular injections are difficult unless the hedgehog is prevented from rolling up and a hind leg may be extended; otherwise, both the quadriceps and the triceps are often tucked under the tightened mantle. It is possible to inject the gluteal or quadriceps muscles through the mantle with the hedgehog tightly curled. A hypodermic needle at least 3 in in length, such as a spinal needle, may be introduced through the mantle and directed cranially at the level of the hip. The anatomy of the curled hedgehog places muscle mass directly under the mantle, and the deepest level of the mantle is also composed of muscle. It is suggested that the practitioner become thoroughly familiar with hedgehog anatomy before trying this route. The orbicularis muscle lies deep to the dermis and epidermis and may be used for intramuscular injections. A 1.5-in to 3-in needle may be necessary to penetrate the muscle because of the length of the spines and depth of the dermis and epidermal layers [15,23].

The largest muscle mass for intramuscular injections in degus, duprasi, prairie dogs, sugar gliders, and opossums is the anterior thigh. Wallabies have large anterior thigh and proximal tail muscle masses that may be used. Most also have sufficient triceps muscle mass to accept intramuscular injections, but this holds a smaller volume than does the thigh.

Table 5
Species, injection sites and volumes, venipuncture sites

Species	SC	IM	IP	IO	Venipuncture sites; volume bolus injection
Sugar glider	Supra/intrascapular area (fluids may pool ventrally); flank ventral to patagium: 6–10 mL	Anterior thigh, triceps: 0.1–0.2 mL	Up to 5 mL in gliders over 100 g	1–2 mL bolus; slow drip at 50–100 mL/kg/24 h	Lateral coccygeal, saphenous, cranial vena cava/sternal notch, jugular; ventral tail artery; 1–2 mL
Wallaby	Supra/intrascapular area; 100–200 mL	Anterior thigh, dorsal tail muscle mass, triceps. 1–2 mL	Up to 30 mL, rarely used	Rarely used; volumes similar to intravenous	Lateral coccygeal, cephalic; ventral tail artery; 5–10 mL Catheter placement in coccygeal vein
Short-tailed opossum	Supra/intrascapular area, flank; 10–20 mL	Anterior thigh, triceps, maximum 0.1 mL	Up to 5 mL	1–2 mL bolus	Lateral coccygeal, ventral tail artery; 1–2 mL
Virginia opossum	Supra/intrascapular area, flank; 100–200 mL	Anterior thigh, triceps, 1 mL	10–20 mL	Rarely used, volumes similar to intravenous	Lateral coccygeal, ventral tail vein/artery, cephalic, saphenous, pouch vein in females, 3–5 mL
Degu	Supra/intrascapular, dorsal back, flank; 5–10 mL/site	Anterior thigh, 0.5 mL	5–8 mL	1–2 mL bolus	Saphenous, cephalic, 1–2 mL; cranial vena cava/sternal notch site for blood draw
Duprasi	Supra/intrascapular, dorsal back, flank; 3–4 mL	Anterior thigh, 0.1 mL	2–3 mL	Up to 1 mL bolus slowly	Jugular, saphenous, 0.5 maximum slowly

Prairie dog	Supra/intrascapular, dorsal back; 10–15 mL/site	Anterior thigh, 0.5 mL	5–10 mL	1–2 mL bolus	Saphenous, cephalic, 3–10 mL slow bolus; cranial vena cava/sternal notch site for blood draw
Hedgehog	Flank at junction of furred skin and spined mantle. Subcutaneous given under the mantle requires a 1.5- to 3-in needle, 5–10 mL/site.	Anterior thigh, triceps, 0.5 mL; may require sedation to reach; orbicularis up to 1 mL/site	Requires sedation for access, 5–10 mL	Requires anesthesia for tibial placement, rarely used, 0.5–1 mL slow bolus	Saphenous, jugular, 0.5–1 mL, requires sedation; cranial vena cava/sternal notch site or jugular for blood draw

Abbreviations: IM, intramuscular; IO, intraosseous; IP, intraperitoneal; SC, subcutaneous.
Data from Refs. [2,5,11,14–16,21]

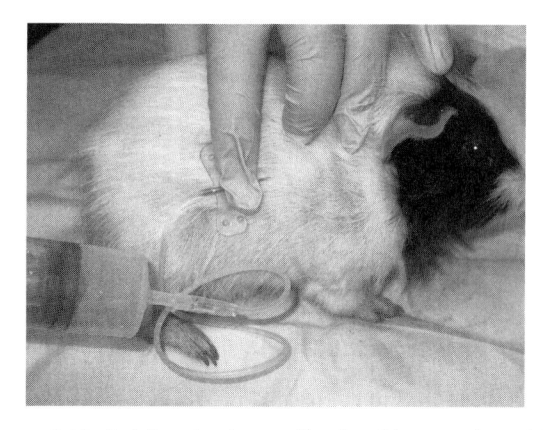

Fig. 3. Subcutaneous fluid administration in a small rodent (shown: guinea pig) using a butterfly infusion catheter. The flank skin is a site preferred by the author, because the skin is more flexible in most species, and there is ample subcutaneous space.

Subcutaneous administration of fluids in sugar gliders may result in pooling within the gliding membrane. Hence it is advisable to administer fluids and other medications ventral to the patagium rather than dorsally, as is typically done in other species. If fluids are administered dorsally over the shoulder area, the fluids may pool into the patagium.

Administration of medications and even fluids intraperitoneally is easily achieved in the smaller animals. It is problematic in female Virginia opossums, sugar gliders, and wallabies—the injection needs to avoid the pouch. This technique should not be used in animals with acute abdomens or gastrointestinal disorders or in those that may have increased abdominal pressure or may undergo abdominal surgery within a few hours. The procedure and positioning for intraperitoneal injection in degus, duprasi, and prairie dogs basically follows that used in rodents of similar size and gastrointestinal anatomy (Fig. 4) [21]. Degus may be injected following the procedure in guinea pigs. Duprasi, prairie dogs, hedgehogs, sugar gliders, and short-tailed opossums may be injected following the procedure in rats [21]. Administration by intraperitoneal injection requires adequate restraint to minimize movement. The injection should be administered just off the midline, in the lower left quadrant of the abdomen at approximately the cranial limits of a full bladder. Before the injection is made, the syringe should be aspirated to ensure that the needle has not entered the intestines or the urinary bladder [21]. For appropriate volumes for injections, see Table 5.

Appropriate volumes of blood to draw for diagnostic sampling may be calculated based on body weight. A rule of thumb used in laboratory animal medicine is the 10% rule: 10% of an animal's body weight in grams is considered to be an approximate total blood volume, although individuals and some species may actually have a higher or lower percentage. Ten percent of that figure is the maximum amount of blood that can be drawn in a 2-week

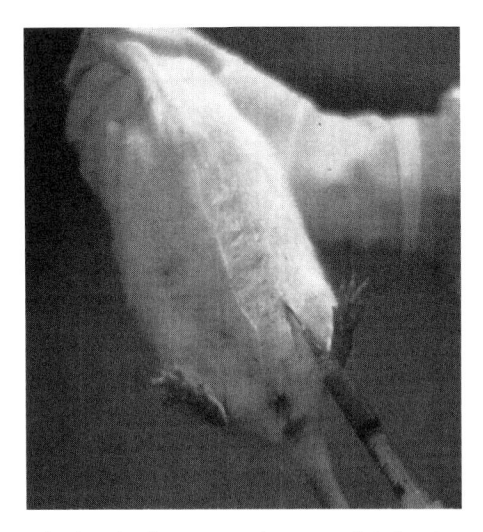

Fig. 4. Intraperitoneal injection site demonstrated on a rat of similar size to an adult prairie dog.

period in a healthy adult mammal. One should draw considerably less if the animal is ill or dehydrated. For example, a 300-g animal would have approximately 30 mL of blood, of which 3 mL total could be withdrawn in a 2-week period. The author prefers to limit volume drawn to well below the calculated maximum, particularly in ill, dehydrated, or anemic animals. If all 3 mL were withdrawn at once, replacement fluids would be necessary.

The intranasal route of administration of sedatives and analgesics has received some attention, particularly for use to achieve rapid sedation. Dosages of common sedatives in mice and rats have been published and are often slightly greater than parenteral dosages. Volume of the drug delivered can also be a limiting factor. This route deserves to be studied for sugar gliders, short-tailed opossums, hedgehogs, degus, and duprasi, because it is an easier route for drugs that are most effective by the intravenous route (Fig. 5) [24].

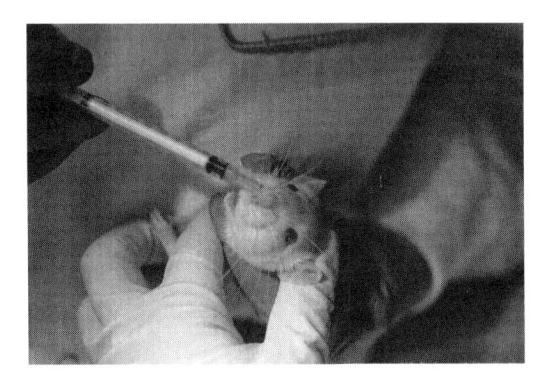

Fig. 5. Intranasal route of administration shown in a rat.

Fig. 6 shows the lateral tail vein in a short-tailed opossum. In small marsupials, the tail vein may be used as in mice: the tail is cleaned with a surgical scrub solution, dried, and the vein extended by gentle pressure proximally. The vein may be nicked with a 22-gauge needle or #11 scalpel point, and the blood is allowed to drip into a small-volume blood collection tube (Fig. 7). Hemostasis after the draw can be by direct pressure. Fig. 8 demonstrates a saphenous blood draw in an anesthetized hedgehog. Fig. 9 demonstrates the cranial vena cava/sternal notch blood draw in a hedgehog, a technique frequently used in small mammals.

Nutritional support is often needed, and gavage or assisted feeding is possible in all the discussed species. Hedgehogs, sugar gliders, and short-tailed opossums may be supported using Carnivore Care (Oxbow Pet Products, Murdock, Nebraska). Volumes for gavage are listed in Table 6. Degus, prairie dogs, and wallabies may be supported with Critical Care (Oxbow Pet Products, Murdock, Nebraska). Virginia opossums and duprasi may be supported with a 50:50 mixture of Carnivore Care and Critical Care formulas. These products can be diluted to pass easily through appropriately sized gavage tubes or syringes. Hedgehogs, sugar gliders, duprasi, and the opossums may often be stimulated to eat by the offer of gut-loaded live crickets or mealworms. Because these may not provide complete nutrition, they should be used only to get the animal eating and not as the long-term or hospital diet. The long-term or hospital diet should be a more complete diet, meeting the nutritional needs of each species. It is important that animals be hydrated and normothermic before gavage or assisted feeding is attempted. The author prefers the term "assisted" feeding to "forced" feeding when describing placement of foods in the mouth by syringe, spoon, and so forth. Many of these animals were hand-reared and respond well to the attention given them during assisted feeding.

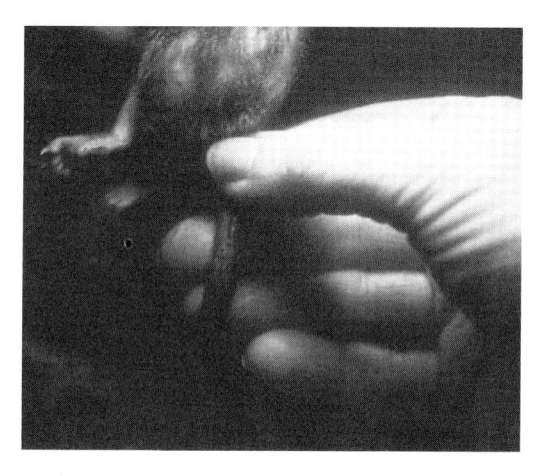

Fig. 6. Lateral tail vein in a short-tailed opossum.

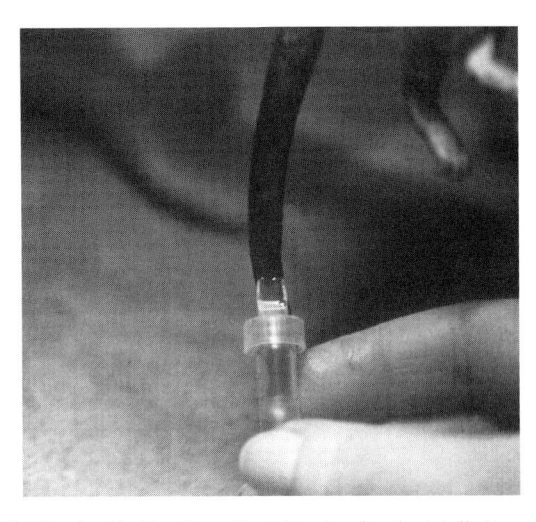

Fig. 7. Blood collection from the tail vein of a short-tailed opossum.

Oral medications may be administered in all of these species and should be formulated for the appropriate volume and flavor. The insectivore/carnivore/omnivore may like many of the flavors designed for dogs and cats, whereas the herbivore should have medications flavored as for rabbits and guinea pigs. The marsupials generally accept sweetened, fruity flavors. Administration of oral medications in hedgehogs that will not take treats from the owner or uncurl for direct placement of liquids in the mouth is a challenge. Medications can be injected into mealworms or treat foods, but volume may be an issue. Compliance by the owner may be difficult if the hedgehog is uncooperative; hence the practitioner needs to work closely with the owner to ensure that the medication is reaching the hedgehog.

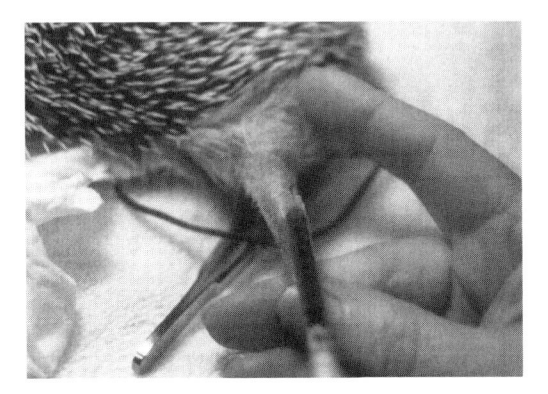

Fig. 8. Saphenous vein collection from an anesthetized hedgehog.

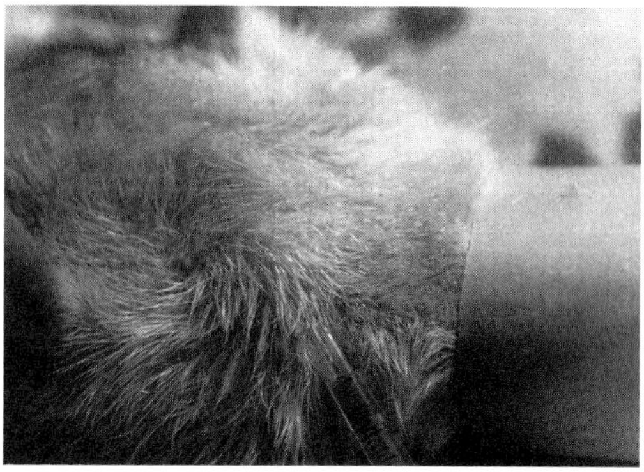

Fig. 9. "Cranial vena cava" blood draw in an anesthetized hedgehog.

Species-specific procedures

Hedgehogs

Physical examination of an uncooperative hedgehog can be a challenge. It is often necessary to administer gas anesthesia (isoflurane or sevoflurane) so that the hedgehog uncurls, rather than forcing the hedgehog to uncurl with manual restraint. Many hedgehogs have never had nail trims because the owners have been unable to do so. Overgrown and curled nails may contribute to lameness and lethargy, simply because the feet are painful and the hedgehog cannot ambulate well. Nails may be clipped easily with a small human nail clipper. Obesity is a complication to venipuncture, physical examination, and even supportive care. Hydration status may be difficult to assess in the obese hedgehog because of the mantle. Oral examination of an awake hedgehog may be facilitated by stroking the lips with a wet cotton swab. The hedgehog may bite at the swab or at least open its mouth long enough for the insertion of a small rubber spatula or bowl scraper. Cellophane tape may be used over flaky skin to obtain a sample to examine for the presence of

Table 6
Suggested gavage feeding volumes, adults

Species	Volume (mL)
Sugar glider	1–3
Wallaby	Bennetts: 30–40; Tammar: 10–30
Short-tailed opossum	0.5–1
Virginia opossum	15–20
Degu	3–5
Duprasi	0.5–1
Prairie dog	5–10
Hedgehog	May require light sedation; 2–3

All feeding volumes should be based on the estimated volume of the stomach approximately one by two to three by four full. These volumes are based on the author's experience.

mites. If quills are loose, the flaky skin attached to the quill may also be placed under the microscope. In mite-infested hedgehogs, ear canals are frequently filled with cellular debris; a cotton swab moistened with mineral oil may be used to obtain a sample for cytology and mite identification. The ears can be cleaned and treated with medications used for earmites and general ear cleaning in puppies and kittens. An ophthalmic solution containing antibiotics or corticosteroid may then be topically applied, depending on the condition of the ear canal. Parenteral nonsteroidal anti-inflammatory drugs, miticide such as ivermectin, and a return visit to check the ear canals are usually more effective than the owner's trying to continue topical ear canal treatment. Dorsal/ventral radiographs in hedgehogs are difficult to interpret because of the overlying mantle. The mantle should be elevated dorsally as far as possible for lateral radiographs. This elevation may be achieved using an Allis forcep for traction. Cotton balls may be necessary to elevate the legs to achieve a true lateral position of the trunk [2,9,15].

Degus

Degus may be restrained and examined in a similar manner to rats, with the exception of restraint by holding at the base of the tail. Degus are active and will try to climb, unlike guinea pigs. Full oral examination should be conducted under sedation; oral instruments suitable for guinea pigs work well with degus. Radiographic examination should always include views of the dentition, although dental disorders have not been reported as common problems as they are in guinea pigs and chinchillas [2,16].

Duprasi

Restraint of the duprasi patient is essentially the same as handling a large hamster or gerbil. The tail is not used to restrain the animal [2,16].

Prairie dogs

Because of the outbreak of monkeypox in the United States in 2003, the US Department of Agriculture has restricted the sale, trade, and transportation of prairie dogs. Essentially they have been removed from the pet trade, but hobby breeders are still getting some into the hands of individual pet owners. The prairie dogs already in households before the ban are approaching the geriatric age; hence an increase is being seen in odontomas and neoplastic conditions, arthritis, and renal and liver disease. Prairie dog owners have expressed concern that when their pet dies they will not be able to obtain another one. Consequently, more owners are having their prairie dogs examined and have become interested in preventive care, whereas before they did not bring the animal in for examination until they perceived a problem.

Older prairie dogs that have been housed as single animals are frequently unpredictable and excitable. They can move quickly and bite deeply with little provocation. Veterinary personnel should assume that the prairie dog will bite and should wear protective gloves and clothing as a precaution. Because dental disease with the formation of odontomas is common, radiographic examination of the head and dentition should be performed as part of the physical examination. Prairie dogs may be presented with open-mouthed breathing, which is a typical presentation of the malocclusion seen with odontoma formation. The abnormal growth of the tooth root impinges on the nasal sinus [2,10,16]. A severely dyspneic prairie dog should be provided oxygen in the examination room and may need supplemental oxygen during procedures such as radiography and blood draw. The animal may be hospitalized and placed in caging equipped with supplemental oxygen.

The author also administers an analgesic, and in some instances diazepam, to calm the severely stressed, dyspneic prairie dog. When the animal has been anorexic, it often regains appetite and shows interest in food after administration of the analgesic. Mastication of normal foods may be significantly impaired, and assisted feeding with Critical Care (Oxbow Pet Products, Murdock, Nebraska) may be necessary. Attention to hydration, gastrointestinal flora health, and pre-emptive pain and inflammation control should be initiated before surgery to remove the odontoma or odontomas. Although the prairie dog with its gastrointestinal tract motility does not appear as likely to become static and dysbiotic as the rabbit or guinea pig, choice of antimicrobials and use of gastrointestinal motility enhancers should follow guidelines for those two animals. Use of oral probiotics is often promoted; however, it is questionable whether the bacteria without protective mucus make it through the stomach as cecoliths do. Because of that factor and the retroperistaltic motility of herbivore large intestines, the author also administers probiotics by means of intrarectal insertion of a red rubber French catheter (usually number 5 or 8, depending on the size of the animal), passed approximately 1 to 2 cm into the colon. Warm, nonbacteriostatic saline is used to suspend the probiotics. One to 2 mL of suspension may easily be instilled [2,10,16].

Sugar gliders

Sugar gliders should always be provided with heat when sedated, because they may become torporous at room temperatures. The eyes should be lubricated as well, and care should be taken to prevent corneal abrasions during sedation and manipulation. Gliders are prone to bite unfamiliar handlers. The author restrains the sugar glider in a similar manner to a psittacine bird of similar weight—75 to 150 g. A towel is used, with thumb and forefinger controlling the head just below the mandibles and the rest of the hand gently surrounding the trunk. Sugar glider females have a marsupium or "pouch," which should be checked for build-up of secretions or infection. If the female has been housed with an intact male, there may be joeys present. These may be gently palpated from outside the pouch or visualized with gentle opening of the pouch. The nonpregnant pouch usually contains a small amount of sebaceous material, and the skin is soft. It should not be caked or full of congealed, waxy material or exudates, nor should it have a strong odor. A saline-moistened cotton swab may be gently inserted into the pouch in the center and moved inside the pouch for examination. If the pouch does contain exudative material, cultures may be taken for aerobic, anaerobic, and fungal/yeast assays by insertion of culturettes into the pouch. After samples have been taken, the pouch may be cleansed with a dilute chlorhexidine solution on cotton swabs. Many gliders will allow this without sedation. However, when infection or inflammation is present, pre-emptive analgesic and nonsteroidal anti-inflammatory drugs should be administered and cultures and cleansing performed under inhalant anesthesia. Sugar gliders appear to respond well clinically to the dosages and types of medications used for ferrets [2,7,8,14].

Wallabies

Most pet wallabies are easily handled; however, adults may challenge unfamiliar handlers by assuming the "boxing" position. The wallaby will lean back on its haunches and tail and reach out and try to swat with its front legs. When truly annoyed or defensive, it will lash out straight ahead with both hind feet in a single motion. This defense can inflict significant trauma, because of the force of the kick and the sharpness of the large middle toenail. When examining and working with wallabies, it is advisable to stay to the side of the animal and maintain a firm hold with one hand at the base of the tail. Many wallabies are nervous when brought to the clinic. Administration of a low dose of diazepam relaxes the animal and reduces the potential for injury, hyperthermia, and myonecrosis. Wallabies and kangaroos are prone to capture myopathy: use of diazepam is recommended before shipping or transporting these animals. Vitamin E plays a role: the author routinely administers 400 IU of oral Vitamin E to wallaby patients at the conclusion of the examination. Many appear to think it is a treat, and owners usually appreciate their pets receiving it. Cursory oral examination may be accomplished using a lighted canine vaginal speculum and a soft, narrow bowl scraper or spatula. Full oral examination requires sedation, as in rabbits. The pouch of the female wallaby should be inspected as with sugar gliders. The pouch should be free of sebaceous material and exudates. There should be no odor. Procedures for cultures and treatment of pouch infections are the same as those described earlier for sugar gliders [2,7,11,14].

Wallabies produce the same quantity of urine whether they are dehydrated or not, so urine production cannot be used to monitor hydration status. Catheterization of a macropod's bladder without a cystoscope is virtually impossible. When a clean urine sample is needed, it is possible to obtain one with ultrasound-guided cystocentesis in both males and females. Marsupials in general have unique urogenital anatomy, including a number of active secretory glands. In captivity with nonbreeding stock, it is not uncommon for glands to become impacted. These may be lanced and drained as with impacted bulbourethral or preputial glands in rats and mice. Antibiotic ointment may be instilled into the lanced gland after drainage. Parenteral nonsteroidal anti-inflammatory drugs, along with the topical/local antibiotic, are usually sufficient for resolution. The lateral tail veins provide easy access and are large enough for catheter placement [2,11,14].

Short-tailed opossums

These New World opossums do not have a pouch but carry their young on the nipples surrounded by a rudimentary flap of abdominal skin. Unlike sugar gliders, which do not have marsupial bones (pelvic ribs), short-tailed opossums have marsupial bones. Their tails are prehensile and are used to carry bedding and "treasures," as well as to aid in steadying them during climbing activities. Restraint is accomplished by holding them as one would a small rat, without using any tail restraint. They rarely bite but will snap defensively. Cloaco-rectal prolapse is a common problem in aging opossums. Reduction of the prolapse and closure of the cloaca is similar to that performed in a psittacine bird. The ventral tail vein can be accessed for blood draws [2,14].

Virginia opossums

The human-reared Virginia opossum is generally a meek animal. It may snap and bare its teeth, then roll slightly onto its back and freeze. It may also vocalize with a hissing, garbled sound resembling a wet cough. Most may be quickly controlled by draping a towel over the head and grasping the base of the tail. Restraint is then achieved by placing one hand over the back of the head, with fingers just below the ears to control the mandible. One may work with the opossum as long as the head and base of the tail are held. Many pet opossums relax as soon as their tail is restrained. The tail is prehensile, and the ventral surface is soft. In obese opossums, the ventral tail vein may be hard to palpate, but it can still be used for blood draws. In a slender opossum, the vein can be visualized and used for catheter placement. Most opossums also have front legs with accessible cephalic veins for injections and catheter placement. Dental care should mirror that of cats: brushing of the teeth and prophylactic cleaning are recommended. The author has been using the OraVet (Merial, Atlanta, Georgia) system and found it effective for maintaining dental health. The female opossum should keep her pouch free of secretions and exudates. The pouch should be checked as part of the physical examination, as with the sugar glider and wallaby [2,5,11,14].

References

[1] Johnson-Delaney CA. Safety issues in the exotic pet practice. Vet Clin North Am Exot Anim Pract 2005;8(3):515–24.

[2] Johnson-Delaney CA. Other small mammals. In: Meredith A, Redrobe S, editors. BSAVA manual of exotic pets. 4th edition. Quedgeley, Gloucester (UK): BSAVA; 2002. p. 102–15.
[3] Weigler BJ, Di Giacomo RF, Alexander S. A national survey of laboratory animal workers concerning occupational risks for zoonotic diseases. Comp Med 2005;55(2):183–91.
[4] Hankenson FC, Johnston NA, Weigler BJ, et al. Zoonoses of occupational health importance in contemporary laboratory animal research. Comp Med 2003;53(6):579–601.
[5] Williams CSF. Opossums. In: Practical guide to laboratory animals. St. Louis (MO): CV Mosby Co.; 1976. p. 142–7.
[6] Maas AK. Legal implications of the exotic pet practice. Vet Clin North Am Exot Anim Pract 2005;8(3):497–514.
[7] Johnson-Delaney CA. Therapeutics of companion marsupials. Vet Clin North Am Exot Anim Pract 2000;3(1):173–81.
[8] Pye G. Sugar gliders. In: Carpenter JW, editor. Exotic animal formulary. 3rd edition. St. Louis (MO): Elsevier Saunders; 2005. p. 343–58.
[9] Carpenter JW. Hedgehogs. In: Carpenter JW, editor. Exotic animal formulary. 3rd edition. St. Louis (MO): Elsevier Saunders; 2005. p. 359–73.
[10] Ness RD. Rodents. In: Carpenter JW, editor. Exotic animal formulary. 3rd edition. St. Louis (MO): Elsevier Saunders; 2005. p. 375–408.
[11] Holz P. Marsupialia (marsupials). In: Fowler ME, Miller RE, editors. Zoo and wild animal medicine. 5th edition. St. Louis (MO): Saunders; 2003. p. 288–303.
[12] Refinetti R. Homeostatic and circadian control of body temperature in the fat-tailed gerbil. Comp Biochem Physiol A Mol Integr Physiol 1998;119(1):295–300.
[13] Kanda LL, Fuller TK, Friedland KD. Temperature sensor evaluation of opossum winter activity. Wildl Soc Bull 2005;33(4):1–7.
[14] Johnson-Delaney CA. Marsupials. In: Johnson-Delaney CA, Harrison LR, editors. Exotic companion medicine handbook for veterinarians (supplement). Lake Worth (FL): Zoological Education Network; 1998. p. 1–52.
[15] Johnson-Delaney CA. Hedgehogs. In: Johnson-Delaney CA, Harrison LR, editors. Exotic companion medicine handbook for veterinarians. Lake Worth (FL): Zoological Education Network; 1998. p. 1–14.
[16] Johnson-Delaney CA. Special rodents. In: Johnson-Delaney CA, Harrison LR, editors. Exotic companion medicine handbook for veterinarians (supplement). Lake Worth (FL): Zoological Education Network; 1998. p. 17–38.
[17] Vanderlip S. Degus. Hauppage (NY): Barrons Educational Series; 2001.
[18] Bradley T. Recognizing pain in exotic animals. Exotic DVM 2001;3(3):21–6.
[19] Flecknell P, Waterman-Pearson A. Pain management in animals. Philadelphia: WB Saunders; 2000.
[20] Gades NM, Danneman PJ, Wixson SK, et al. The magnitude and duration of the analgesic effect of morphine, butorphanol and burpenorphine in rats and mice. Contemp Top Lab Anim Sci 2000;39(1):8–13.
[21] Hrapkiewicz K, Medina L, Holmes D. Clinical laboratory animal medicine: an introduction. 2nd edition. Ames (IA): Iowa State University Press; 1998.
[22] Mader DR. Basic approach to veterinary care. In: Quesenberry KE, Carpenter JW, editors. Ferrets, rabbits, and rodents: clinical medicine and surgery. 2nd edition. St. Louis (MO): Saunders; 2004. p. 147–54.
[23] Reeve N. Hedgehogs. London: T & AD Poyser, Ltd.; 1994.
[24] Johnson-Delaney CA, Carpenter J, Penner J, et al. Nasal administration of sedatives to mice and rats. Contemp Top Lab Anim Sci 2001;40(4):83.

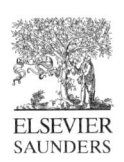

Common Procedures and Concerns with Wildlife

Debbie A. Myers, DVM

Louisiana State University, 1516 Skip Bertman Drive, Baton Rouge, LA 70801, USA

Restraint and handling procedures are stressful for wildlife. Before handling any wildlife, one should set out a clear check-list of procedures that need to be performed on the animal, as well as all equipment or medications that are needed, ready for administration or sample collection. All shore birds, waterfowl, and other water birds are handled with towels or examination gloves to protect the waterproofing of their feathers. Goggles should be worn when working with birds that have long, sharp bills (eg, herons, egrets, piscivorous birds). Long-billed birds commonly use a thrusting motion of their beaks to capture shiny fish in the water and often thrust at the face of a handler in a fighting response. Waterfowl with large necks (eg, swans, geese) should have the neck grasped with one hand and the body encircled and restrained with the other arm. As soon as the waterfowl is restrained, the legs must be grasped with one hand, placing one finger between the two legs to prevent trauma. This technique is especially important in the longer-legged waterfowl species. Geese can peck with heavily pointed bills and may strike one's body by rapidly flapping strong wings. The trachea of birds is composed of complete cartilage rings; with care, one may hold the neck without danger of suffocation. One should support a large goose by the body, controlling the neck and wings when lifted and carried (Fig. 1) [1].

Feet and claws are the most dangerous weapons of raptors, in contrast to the psittacine species where the beak is a handler's greatest concern (Fig. 2). Vultures, some large owls, and eagles will bite as a defensive behavior; however, the bite is usually not significant. All raptors should be handled with towels and leather gloves of appropriate thickness for the restrained bird's talon size. When capturing a raptor out of the cage, one should use gloves and quickly grasp the legs together with one hand, with one finger between the legs. Once the legs are restrained, the bird is brought out of the cage with

E-mail address: dmyersvet@yahoo.com

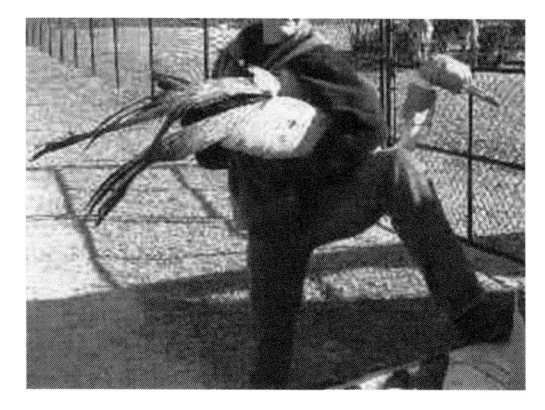

Fig. 1. Covering the head and supporting the full body aids in the restraint of large waterfowl species.

the other arm to gain control of the wings (Fig. 3). In addition, a small towel should be placed over the bird's face to reduce resistance and stress.

Small birds (eg, doves, pigeons) are generally wrapped in one hand with the head held between the thumb and the middle finger and the body held in the other hand to secure it with the wings [2].

Larger carnivores and wild small mammals often need chemical immobilization to be handled. Adult squirrels will bite, so leather gloves should be worn. One should remember that leather gloves do not prevent the penetration of rodent teeth into a hand. Grasping around the neck and holding the back legs is best; never hold a squirrel's tail, because the skin over the tail may deglove when pulled. Wild rabbits are generally not aggressive; however, around March and April breeding season–related aggression is observed. The main dangers for personnel working with rabbits are claws that can scratch and sharp incisors that can inflict deep bites. A rabbit

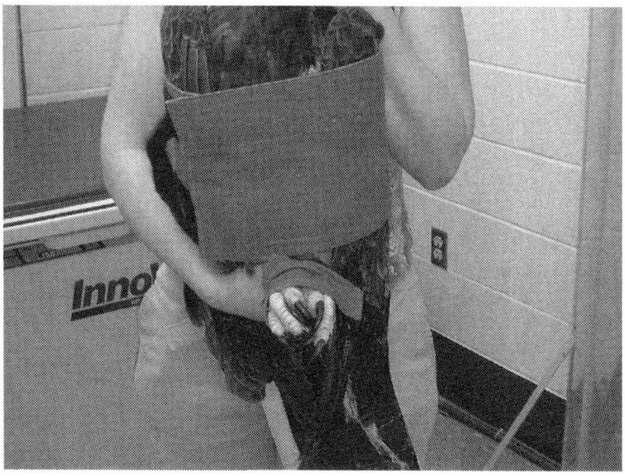

Fig. 2. Talons are the main defense mechanism of raptors. Extreme caution should be used when handling and examining raptors.

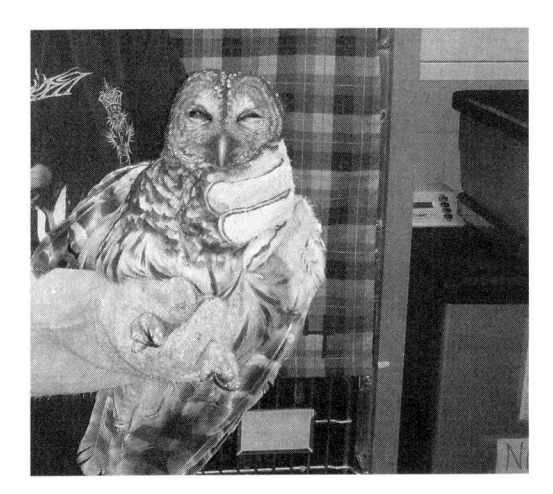

Fig. 3. Appropriate restraint for examination of a raptor. In the case of this barred owl, one finger is between the legs, the handler wears appropriate leather gloves, and the head is restrained for proper examination.

may injure itself by pushing with its powerful hind limbs, fracturing the spine or causing other spinal trauma [3]. Furthermore, stress is a looming concern with rabbits and may cause cardiac arrest [1]. For aggressive lagomorphs, scruff the neck with one hand and support the hind limbs with the other, keeping the animal close to your body. For more docile rabbits, one hand should go under the thorax, with the thumb and first two fingers encircling the front limbs while the other hand is supporting the hind limbs (Fig. 4). Always keep rabbits close to your body with the head pushed into the crook of one arm during transport. Placing the animal in a towel (similar to techniques used with difficult cats) often calms stressed rabbits [1].

Most turtles may be held by the sides of the carapace and turned slowly, as needed, to avoid torsion. Snapping turtles are best handled by grabbing the tail, but the handler should not hold the suspended animal close to his or her body while it is in midair. Snapping turtles have long, elastic necks that can extend to reach any part of the handler's body that is in close range of the head. Once the tail is grasped, run a hand over the top of the carapace and grasp the carapace just above the head.

Stress response

Stress is frequently the cause of death in hospitalized wildlife, and minimizing stress is important in the care of any animal. First, one must understand the physiology of stress. An animal is constantly stimulated by environmental changes or stressors by means of receptors for all the different senses. Somatic stressors include stimuli such as strange sounds, odors,

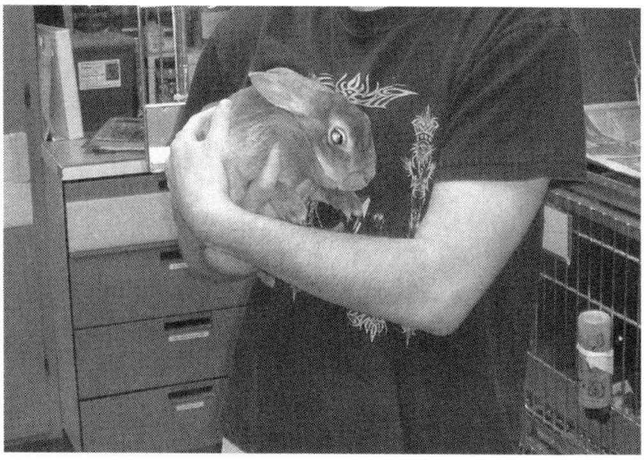

Fig. 4. Proper restraint of a docile rabbit. One finger is between the legs, and that hand supports the thorax, while the other hand controls the hind limbs.

and tastes (eg, isoflurane). Other possible stress factors include the restraint event, unexpected touches, position changes, temperature changes, and hypoxia from intense struggling. Furthermore, some drugs used for chemical restraint can cause an excitement phase and subsequent stress. These drugs can also cause fear in some wild animals, because they feel their ability to escape predators dwindling as the medication takes effect. Extreme reactions to any of these stimuli can cost the animal its life. Psychologic stressors are also involved with capture and the fight or flight reaction. When animals are consistently in a state of fright and cannot escape or defend themselves, harmful overreaction is often seen. Behavioral stressors may include changes in the animal's natural (or ecologic) rhythm, such as territorial or hierarchical upset, disruption of night and day cycles, isolation from conspecifics, and change in diet. In addition to the stresses associated with handling, there are underlying factors that may immunosuppress an animal under veterinary care, such as parasites, infectious agents, toxins, malnutrition, chemical restraint, trauma, oil exposure, and heat stress. Normally, restraint is of short duration and the animal adjusts without detriment. When any of these stresses occur for an extended period, they can overwhelm the body's ability to respond in a normal manner [1].

The sympathetic nervous system induces the fight or flight reaction by means of the adrenal medulla. The sympathetic nervous system innervates the adrenal gland; when the system is stimulated, acetylcholine is released into the adrenal medulla, causing the release of epinephrine and a small amount of norepinephrine, which then affects beta and alpha adrenergic receptors. Harmful consequences of stimulating these receptors may include ventricular fibrillation, hypoglycemia, hypothermia, and shock. The pituitary gland is also stimulated during stress by the hypothalamus and in turn releases acetylcholine. The acetylcholine causes the adrenal gland to produce cortisol, which is normally protective when released in the body. Continuous adrenal stimulation and excessive cortisol production from chronic stress may cause many harmful metabolic responses. When cortisol is released at levels significantly greater than normal, many animals display clinical signs that include muscle weakness, muscle atrophy (cortisol causes protein catabolism), enlarged abdomen (due to movement of fats and protein to the liver), weight loss, increased susceptibility to infection, impaired antibody response, vaccination failure, high blood pressure, and poor wound healing. Excessive levels of cortisol are also known to result in polyuria and polydypsia, because of the increased glomerular filtration rate and increases in blood glucose. Prolonged stress results in hypertrophy of the adrenal gland, caused by continuous stimulation by acetylcholine and excessive production of cortisol [1,4]. Some diagnostic testing values may be altered during times of chronic stress (and excess cortisol production); these include leukocyte numbers and serum chemistry values. Caution should be used when interpreting these results in stressed patients.

Eventually, the adrenal gland becomes depleted and atrophies. Handling an animal in a state of adrenal insufficiency may cause fatal shock. Lesions produced by harmful stress are often not visible on gross examination of the tissue. Many of the effects of prolonged stress are functional; they weaken tissues and organs by prolonged insults, lowering the body's resistance to disease. Decreased resistance to disease in hospitalized wildlife may result in death due to pneumonia, heavy parasitism, or bacterial infection. Stress is inevitable when wildlife are hospitalized. Even under the best conditions, the aforementioned diseases occur and may contribute to a patient's death. To minimize the detrimental effects of stress, one must provide a physical and social environment that closely resembles the animal's normal habitat. Simple changes one can make to reduce the stress on these hospitalized patients include darkening the room, minimizing speech in the animal's presence, minimizing restraint time by having all the items necessary for a procedure ready for use before handling the animal, placing a towel over the animal's eyes during restraint, and releasing the animal to a flight cage or a trained rehabilitator for release as soon as possible [1,2].

Examination

Four types of animals present to a wildlife hospital: (1) healthy animals that someone captured, perceiving a problem; (2) healthy animals that eat, defend themselves, and have no noticeable lesions but have a subclinical illness; (3) animals with no or insignificant clinical signs of disease; and (4) animals that show signs of disease [2]. Often the classification of animal presentation is made after the initial excitement of unfamiliar surroundings, people, and other animals subsides. Most animals will appear healthy and alert when they are placed in an unfamiliar environment or are injured. Many wild animals presented to wildlife hospitals are prey species, and showing any signs of illness in nature makes them more vulnerable to predation. Predators look for signs of weakness and target those animals. Therefore, these animals will act healthy until they cannot sufficiently compensate. When a wild animal presents to the clinic, the information listed in Box 1 should be obtained [2].

A health examination should be done at the time of the animal's initial presentation to the veterinary clinic. Included in the health examination is a full physical examination, along with blood work (ie, complete blood chemistry count [CBC], plasma chemistry panel) and fecal examination (ie, flotation, direct smear). The aim of wildlife veterinarians is to return a completely healthy and recovered animal to the wild as soon as possible. If an animal cannot be returned to the wild because of the extent of injury, and no other options are available, euthanasia should be performed as soon as possible to eliminate suffering. Often flight-impaired waterfowl may be released into a secure island area with a small number of animals and access to supplemental food. Likewise, some small mammals compensate well with a single malformed or amputated digit. Knowing the natural history of each wild animal encountered and its native environment can help one decide whether treatment is appropriate for ultimate release.

It is important to understand that 35% to 65% of wild avian species carry parasitic burdens [2]. Furthermore, trauma is the most common reason for a wild animal to present to a wildlife hospital. Parasitism is well tolerated by healthy wild birds, but often trauma and the stress of captivity increase the parasite burden, complicating the rehabilitation process. Hence a fecal examination and appropriate use of anthelmintics are recommended when an animal needs rehabilitation time before release.

Once the animal has been moved to a quiet place, examination should take place. The form reproduced in Table 1 provides a systematic approach to the physical examination; this consistent approach decreases the likelihood that any part of the examination will be overlooked. First, start with the "hands-off" assessment and examine any feces that may be on

---

Box 1. Information to be obtained at the time of admission of wildlife

- Name of rescuer
- Address of rescuer
- Telephone number of rescuer
- Exact location of rescue
- Circumstances of rescue
- Date and time of rescue
- Nature of any traumatic incident witnessed
- Nature of fluid, food, or treatment administered
- Signature of rescuer releasing wildlife to your care, dated

the bottom of the animal's transport box or carrier. Checking the respiratory rate at that time is preferred, because heart and respiratory rate will increase once the animal is restrained for full examination. Notice if the animal is aware of its surroundings, has a good coat or feather quality, and has a normal posture or perching ability. Partially closed eyes, hunchbacked appearance, fluffed-feather appearance, labored breathing, open-mouth breathing, or a tail bob in birds are all signs that indicate poor health and should be noted. Once the observational examination is finished, a slightly dark room and secure handling will help with the "hands-on" physical examination. Auscultation at the inception of the examination facilitates a more accurate cardiac assessment; in small patients a pediatric stethoscope is recommended for this procedure.

Examine each wild animal fully. If an animal becomes overly stressed during the examinations, simply place it back in its cage to relax and re-examine it at a later time. When examining birds, start with the head; examine the beak and the cere and note whether the area is healthy, shiny, symmetric, and has normal occlusion. Likewise, in mammals and reptiles, check for jaw alignment, symmetry, and fractures. In birds, the eyes, sinuses, and rhinarium are interconnected; therefore, an infection involving one area could influence the other structures. Also in birds, the periorbital area should be checked for swellings that can indicate sinusitis. In birds, reptiles, and mammals, the eyes should be clean, moist, and shiny with no epiphora or other abnormalities. Slight digital pressure should be applied to both globes to assess for any masses or fluid accumulation behind the eye.

Mammals should have a pupillary light response; birds and reptiles have an inconsistent response. The pupillary light response may be difficult to assess in all animals with a very dark iris color. The following technique may help: Reduce the ambient light level to low. Stand 3 ft away from the patient with its head facing you. Look through the direct ophthalmoscope at the patient's face to see the tapetal reflection. Now test the papillary light response. Constriction of the pupil should be easily seen as the shrinking of the area of tapetal reflection. Fluorescein stain may be used to detect corneal ulceration in any animal. Clinical signs of ocular problems include discharge, matted hair or feathers in the periocular area, conjunctivitis, and swelling. The cornea, anterior chamber, iris, lens, and retina should be inspected with direct and indirect ophthalmoscopy.

After the ocular examination, the nares or nasal area should be inspected. The nares should be clean, round, and open (and, in birds, have a shiny, centrally placed operculum). When there is any question of patency, a glass slide should be held over the nares or nasal passages to see if fogging occurs and air flow is present. Look for signs of occlusion, discharge, or rhinoliths and normal symmetry of the nasal openings. A small nasal opening in birds is often the result of scarring from a previous or chronic infection.

The aural area infrequently has problems; however, neoplasia or infection, in the form of a granuloma, may occur. A pen light and otoscope is

Table 1
Physical examination check sheet

Date					
Wildlife examination sheet					
Species					
Age					
Weight					
Feeding:	Amount:	Frequency		Remaining amount	
General	Specific	Normal	Abnormal		Notes
Auscultation	Cardiovascular				Heart rate:
	Respiratory				Resp rate:
Beak/Cere/Jaw/Mouth					
Oral cavity	Mucous membranes				
	Choanae				
	Glottis				
	Teeth/Occlusion				
Esophagus/Trachea					
Crop if present					
Abdominal palpation	Cranial				
	Caudal				
	Lymph nodes				
Hydration status				$<5\%$, $5\%-10\%$, $>10\%$	
Body condition					
Ears					
Nares/Nose					
Eyes					
Neurologic examination	Awareness				
	Extremity movement				
	Posture				
	Palpation				
Legs	Range of motion				

Wings
    Talons/Nails
    Plantar surface/Pads
    Scales
    Patagium
    Range of motion
    Position
    Palpation

Uropygial gland
Vent/Rectum
Feather/Coat quality
    Contour
    Flight
    Coat

External parasites _____

Diagnostics

Fecal exam:
CBC: Total WBCs _____ Heterophils _____ Lymphs _____ Monos _____ Eos _____
Packed cell volume/total protein: _____
Blood parasites: _____
Chemistry panel (if submitted) list Abnormalities: _____
Radiographs: _____

Treatment plan

	Yes	No	Type	Dose/Frequency
Antihelminthics				
Steroids				
Antibiotics				
Fluids				
Heat source				
Critical care diet				
Other medications				

List abnormal physical exam findings/differential diagnoses:

used to illuminate the inner ear. The aural area in most birds is located ventrocaudal to the lateral canthus of the eye. Blowing air on feathers against the direction of feather growth often helps to find the aural opening in birds. An owl's ears are set at different levels on each side of its head. They may be found under the feathers as two large, clean orifices, one level with the eyes and the other a little lower. The unique asymmetry of their ears enables them to locate prey even in full darkness. The aural area of reptiles is located just caudoventral to the eye and is covered by either an enlarged cutaneous scale or a transparent-to-translucent tympanum. Snakes lack an external ear. In reptiles, aural abscesses may be found.

When inspecting the oral cavity in all species, examine the tongue and membrane color. In reptiles the mucous membranes can vary in color from gray to pale pink. The glottis is located on the floor of the oral cavity in snakes. In lizards and chelonians, the glottis is located at the base of the tongue. In birds, membrane color is better assessed at the cloacal opening (especially in species with a dark tongue color). The choanae, choanal papillae, oral membrane, and glottis should be assessed in avian patients. Any areas that are discolored, appear necrotic, or have discharge or plaques should be sampled (swabbed or scraped) for microscopic evaluation.

In mammals and reptiles, examine the neck and palpate the esophagus; determine whether a cough may be elicited on tracheal palpation. In birds the crop should be palpated. Crop flushes may be collected, when indicated, to screen for fungal, bacterial, or parasitic organisms. Once the head and neck area has been assessed, the overall coat, skin, or feather quality should be evaluated. General palpation (for any masses or swellings) should be performed, noting any lesions. Each long bone, joint, and soft tissue area should be examined for normal range of movement. The plantar surface and pads of each foot should also be examined. In birds, one should evaluate the scales covering the extremities. In reptiles, look for discolored skin and retained sheds.

The body condition of the animal on a scale of one (thin) to five (obese) should be noted. Loss of body condition is an indication of an animal's general condition and possible disease chronicity. In mammals, palpating the spine and abdomen will help obtain a body condition score. In birds, body condition is assessed on either side of the keel over the pectoral muscles, and in reptiles it is assessed at the base of the tail. Weighing patients daily is ideal, but for wild animals the process can be extremely stressful. Therefore, weigh animals daily only when the situation is warranted. For instance, daily weigh-ins are required in conditions of anorexia, regurgitation, or while the animal is under anesthesia for another procedure.

Abdominal palpation in unfamiliar species can be daunting, but the procedure is essentially the same as that performed in cats and dogs. Examine the abdomen to assess the internal organs, any masses, enlarged lymph nodes, and other significant features. In reptiles, eggs and impactions may be discerned on palpation. Coelomic palpation in birds is often not as fruitful as abdominal palpation in other species, but each avian patient should be examined for obesity, coelomic distension, masses, organ enlargement, and eggs. The uropygial gland, located dorsally and cranial to the insertion of the central tail feather, should also be examined in birds. This gland secretes oil used in preening for feather conditioning. The gland should be symmetric and smooth and should produce a small volume of oily secretion from its medial aspect when expressed. Examination of the cloaca of an avian patient should include an inspection of the plumage around the cloaca for soiling and eversion of the inner cloacal mucosa to reveal any abnormalities. In reptiles, the cloaca should be examined in a similar manner. In mammals, examine the rectum for good sphincter tone and perineal staining. In larger animals, perform rectal palpation to detect masses or swellings. All animals should be weighed to the nearest gram before the conclusion of the examination [1–3,5–8].

Venipuncture is helpful in assessing a patient's disease status. One should always remember, especially in smaller animals, to take no more than 1% of body weight for blood collection. For example, in a 100-g bird, 1 mL is the maximum amount that may be safely collected. In smaller animals that do not have a medical need for hydration therapy, fluids may be administered subcutaneously to replenish blood volume lost during collection. Most "in-house" plasma chemistry analyzers can run a complete plasma chemistry with less than 1 mL of blood. With just a few drops of blood, a blood smear may be made and a hematocrit and total protein evaluated. The white blood cell count can be estimated with a Unopette 5877 (Becton Dickinson Vacutainer Systems, Franklin Lake, New Jersey), and a white blood cell differential may be obtained from a blood smear. By combining that information with a pack cell volume and total protein and a fecal examination, both flotation and direct, one may inexpensively gather the means to assess the patient when developing an appropriate treatment protocol. In birds, cloacal and choanal swabs may also be collected and Gram stained. Aspirates of masses and lesions may be evaluated microscopically. Radiology, especially in wildlife, yields the best results when the patient is under general anesthesia with an endotracheal tube in place. Keep a log of the species, age (juvenile, adult), and weight of each wild animal that has had a radiographic examination. Additional information to keep in the record includes radiographic techniques used, assessment of radiographic quality, and region examined. This information will provide a readily accessible reference table of the best techniques to use for future wildlife cases [2].

Neonates

Behavior of animals is primarily controlled by reflex actions. These actions are modified during development by external stimuli. In an animal's native habitat, stimuli related to social behavior are provided by the parents, especially the mother; in captivity, the stimuli may be modified to a greater or lesser extent by the handler. In avian species, the normal imprinting process bonds the baby birds to the parent. Newly hatched chicks (and young mammals) show no fear of new objects or events. As young animals develop ocular and auditory senses, their fear responses also develop. As fear responses develop, the ability to become imprinted decreases. The period of imprinting varies (from 18 days to 16 weeks) depending on the species and situation. When baby animals are reared without true (conspecific) parental contact, they will most likely imprint to their keeper or keepers. Many animals in this situation fail to recognize other animals of the same species as mates and develop other undesirable behaviors. Adverse imprinting may be minimized by limiting human contact with wild animals staying in the clinic, by covering cages, and by using puppets as surrogate parents so animals do not constantly visualize humans [2].

Many diseases are seen in young animals presented to a wildlife clinic.

Splay leg is caused by a lack of support for a well-nourished growing chick. The bird attempts to stand, but its leg muscles are not strong enough, or the surface is too slick to provide secure footing, causing the legs to splay out. Splay leg can lead to a permanent deformity. The chick should be placed in a suitably sized, high-sided bowl with padding. If the bird is part of a group of chicks, the temperature may be decreased to encourage huddling and support. Hobble bandages may also be used above the hock region to prevent developmental leg abnormalities during rehabilitation [2,9].

Hypoglycemia is another problem encountered when rearing young wildlife. Young animals have higher glucose requirements than do most adults of their species. This increased requirement is a result of the high level of energy needed for maintaining metabolic function, growth, and normal blood glucose levels.

Neonates use all nutrients faster because of accelerated growth rates. Maintaining blood glucose levels is important in young, growing animals. One should know how often to feed the young, based on their age and species requirements, to foster optimum growth and recovery. Clinical signs of hypoglycemia begin to appear when levels drop below 60 g/dL in mammals and avian species. Animals suffering from hypoglycemia will frequently show neurologic signs, such as ataxia or seizures leading to a loss of consciousness. For rapid response in mammals and birds, apply Karo syrup (Bestfoods, Englewood Cliffs, New Jersey) to the gums or oral mucosa, then give fluids with dextrose via gavage tube, either subcutaneously, intraosseously, or intravenously (IV). Begin an IV drip of lactated Ringer's solution and dextrose, or continue subcutaneous fluids with dextrose at this time. Recheck the blood glucose levels 2 hours after the start of the therapy and modify the amount of dextrose in the fluids according to the changing glucose levels [2,9]. In many wildlife, the subcutaneous route is the only feasible way to give fluids. In the author's opinion, one or two doses of a 5% dextrose solution subcutaneously are acceptable. After those first doses of fluids, the concentration should be tapered to 2.5% dextrose for any longer therapy. Dextrose given subcutaneously can be irritating and painful and should be used only when medically necessary.

Neonates are also susceptible to hypothermia. A high mortality is associated with hypothermia when injured animals are presented to a wildlife hospital. Hypothermia occurs when heat loss exceeds heat production. Situations that cause hypothermia include exposure to harsh weather conditions, anesthesia or sedation, overaggressive treatment for hyperthermia, severe sepsis, hypoglycemia, head trauma, debilitation, and shock. Clinical signs of hypothermia include pale mucous membranes, cold appendages, low rectal temperature, and cardiac arrthymias. Core body temperature is maintained by homeostatic balance of heat loss and heat retention, controlled in the hypothalamus. In response to cold, both heat retention and production are initiated to maintain normal temperature. To retain heat, neonates will often huddle together. Peripherally, mammals initiate the reflexes of piloerection (which traps a layer of warm air against the skin) and vasoconstriction. Increased metabolism and shivering also help generate heat. When the mechanisms mentioned fail to maintain core body temperature, hypothermia will occur. Therapy depends on the cause and level of hypothermia, with mild, moderate, and severe categories identified. The following are guidelines for rewarming patients:

- Mild hypothermia (patients with a 5°F to 6°F decrease): Passive rewarming may be effected with blankets, towels, and environmental control. Normothermia is restored by means of intrinsic heat by shivering. If an animal's temperature drops by 5°F to 6°F, the quickest way to warm it is to place it in a warm water bath at a temperature of approximately 100°F and gently massage it. Remove the animal after 5 minutes and dry with a heated dryer.
- Moderate hypothermia: Active surface rewarming may be effected using circulating hot water blankets, hot water bottles (conductive heat), heated, water-filled gloves, Bair Hugger (convective heat; Arizant, Inc., Prairie, Minnesota), heat lamps (radiant heat), or warm IV fluids. Animals that have severe hypothermia of more than 6°F will not return to normal after warming and should not be rapidly warmed; instead, gradual increases in body temperature using an incubator, warming bags, or warmed fluids are preferred. Active surface rewarming can cause vasodilatation, hypotension, and hypovolemic shock through decreases in circulatory blood volume. To prevent hypovolemic shock associated with warming a cold patient, one should apply heat only to the thorax, leaving the extremities cool while allowing the body's core temperature to rise. Once the body is able to meet metabolic demands, the extremities may be perfused and warmed.
- Severe hypothermia: Active core rewarming may be effected with warm IV fluids, warm air via mask or endotracheal tube, warm peritoneal lavage, or warm water enemas.

Because of dehydration, fluid therapy should be considered after warming at 35 to 40 mL/kg/d, in addition to normal fluid replacement. Use saline fluids over lactated Ringer's solution, because of a compromised liver's inability to metabolize lactate. Supplemental dextrose may also be needed, because the suckling response is diminished as newborns chill. Furthermore, hypothermic birds may become hypoglycemic in an attempt to maintain body temperature. All rewarming measures should be halted when the patient reaches approximately 96°F to prevent hyperthermia [2,4,9,10].

Septicemia may be defined as a microbial infection involving the entire body. Septicemia is common in young animals because of immunosuppression and the conditions that may lead to immunosuppression (eg, overcrowding, unsanitary enclosures, contaminated environment or feed, malnourishment). Ineffective antibiotic therapy and improperly treated infections (or wounds) may also lead to septicemia. Stress can lead to sepsis by means of gastrointestinal ulceration that allows bacteria vascular access.

Endotoxin, a lipopolysaccharide found on cell membrane surfaces of all gram-negative bacteria, is composed of three components: the lipid, the core, and the O-specific side chain. Endotoxin binds to receptors on macrophages, monocytes, and vascular endothelium, causing the secretion of several cytokines from mononuclear cells. Tumor necrosis factor (TNF) and interleukin 1 (IL-1) are two of these cytokines, which have direct and indirect effects on all organ systems by means of initiation and amplification of others. TNF and IL-1 can change the core body temperature set-point, inducing fever or hypothermia, decrease vascular resistance, increase vascular permeability, depress cardiac and inotropic function, affect bone marrow (eg, increase white blood cell count), initiate the release of myocardial depressant factor, and adversely affect enzymes involved in energy use by tissues. These primary cytokines also initiate secondary cytokines that lead to derangements in cardiac hemodynamics, systemic oxygen delivery, and pulmonary gas exchange. Animals with septicemia may potentially be febrile or hypothermic and may exhibit signs of weakness, lethargy, inappetence, dyspnea, pallor, diarrhea, and swollen joints. Weight loss occurs because of a TNF (cachetin) that causes adipocytes to break down fat globules and release fatty acids as part of the acute-phase reaction. Lethargy stems from IL-1, IL-6, and TNF triggered by injured endothelium, macrophages, and fibroblasts at the inflammatory site. Anorexia or loss of appetite is initiated by the effects of TNF. Myalgia or muscle pain is due to TNF-induced myoglobin breakdown. Fever results from neutrophils' and other inflammatory cells' releasing cytokines (such as IL-1 and other pyrogens). These cytokines initiate metabolic responses that result in increased body temperature, respiration, and heart rate. Body heat loss may be mitigated by cutaneous vasoconstriction, heat production, and shivering. Diagnosis of septicemia is made by clinical signs, a CBC, and a low (less than 60 g/dL) blood glucose level. This lowered glucose during septicemia has not been studied in reptiles, so the response may be variable. Every effort should be made to determine the cause of the infection and to correct underlying problems.

Mammals have passive immunity passed to them by means of colostrum in their mother's milk. In many cases an orphan will have received colostrum and will not need any more. In birds, passive immunity is transmitted to the embryo in the egg. Artificial incubation and rearing may result in young and immunocompetent chicks' having a slightly different immune protection from neonates that are parent-reared in their natural habitat. Exposure to infectious agents usually takes one of several routes: through the eggshell (birds and reptiles), via the umbilicus (mammals), and orally with food (often before the new gastrointestinal system is immunocompotent or before normal intestinal flora are established). Pathogenic bacteria are usually gram negative. Supplemental heat, fluid administration, and appropriate antibiotic therapy may often save a patient diagnosed with acute septicemia. A 5- to 7-day course of broad-spectrum antibiotics, such as enrofloxacin combined with metronidazole and a beta-lactam antibiotic (eg, ampicillin), is the recommended treatment for a diagnosed case of septicemia. (IV administration is often most effective, but in neonates IV access is difficult. Intramuscular administration would be the second choice, followed by oral and subcutaneous.) Probiotics may be given to young animals considered at risk for septicemia [2,4,9,10].

Aspiration pneumonia is a common reason for fatality in orphaned animals. Aspiration often occurs as a result of poor feeding techniques. Using sterile water for the first feeding will often prevent aspiration (by allowing the caretaker to become accustomed to nursing technique using a solution that is easy to administer). Nursing young animals takes patience, because forcing too much food rapidly can cause aspiration of the formula into the respiratory system. Gram-negative bacteria are the primary pathogens associated with aspiration pneumonia. Clinical signs may include labored breathing, potentially open-mouthed breathing, and an audible respiratory "click" (heard when the affected patient is breathing). Injectable amoxicillin or amikacin and supportive care can be helpful; however, long-term therapy should be based on culture and sensitivity obtained by means of a transtracheal wash. Furthermore, once pneumonia is present, animals are more prone to subsequent aspiration because of the incompatibility of suckling and dyspnea. Therefore, maintaining energy requirements for growing orphans can be difficult. Fluids administered with dextrose IV or subcutaneously, along with maintenance of good thermal control and frequent small feedings, can aid in recovery. Nebulization and careful coupage (gently but forcefully tapping on the sides of the thorax) to help break up debris in the lungs are warranted in some cases. To reduce aspiration in birds, one should always treat orally or feed immediately before setting the bird back in its enclosure (after all other treatments). This precaution decreases the likelihood of aspiration's occurring as the bird struggles. In birds, the glottis (tracheal opening) may be visualized, and this should be done when tube feeding to ensure that the tube goes past the glottis [2,4,9,10].

Self-induced preputial suckling in young or by conspecifics is also a common behavioral vice. The urge to suckle in mammals is strong, and neonates not raised with their mothers may mistake preputial structures for nipples and suckle them. If this behavior is not stopped, it can lead to inflammation, irritation, and possibly infection of the prepuce [9].

The preputial area should be cleaned with dilute chlorhexidine solution as needed. Topical agents such as an antimicrobial cream (Silvadene Crème, Boots Pharmaceuticals, Lincolnshire, Illinois) and Preparation H (Whitehall-Robins Health care, Madison, New Jersey) or Desitin (Pfizer, Maris Plains, New Jersey) may be applied topically to the area two to four times a day. Affected animals need to be closely observed during treatment, because it is common for other individuals to lick off the medication; however, housing young neonates alone solely for medication purposes is stressful and usually unwarranted. In most mammalian species, urination needs to be stimulated by gently but rapidly brushing a damp piece of paper towel (or cotton ball) over the genital region. If this procedure is not performed, urine may be retained. The penile tissue can become reddened and inflamed with penile suckling as well as urine retention. Stimulating of urination needs to be done before and after each feeding. The mother normally stimulates young, but orphans need assistance [9].

Hand-rearing orphaned birds and mammals is a common task for any clinician treating wildlife. However, one needs to establish whether the animal presented to the clinic is an actual orphan that needs veterinary assistance. Often young birds leave the nest before they are ready to fly. By placing the young in various concealed locations, parents lower the risk that all the young will be victims of a predator. Therefore, young birds in this situation need to be left for the parents to rear. If the animal is injured, if it is in danger from local cats, other predators, proximity to traffic, or other environmental hazards, or if the parents have been killed, then intervention may be warranted. Potential orphans (not in immediate danger) may be watched for a time, allowing the parent birds to return and feed their offspring. Avian parents generally should return within 1 to 2 hours. Remember that the parents do a better job of raising their young than veterinarians do; only take an orphan from the wild when there is no other option and the animal is in a life-threatening situation. However, sometimes intervention is necessary. To nurse young mammals, a small dropper, syringe, or baby bottle may be used, depending on the size of the animal. Hold the animal slightly upward or position its neck tilted upward to prevent aspiration (Fig. 5) [2,3]. Most avian and reptile patients need to be tube fed as part of their nursing care.

Often the first few feedings of orphans are slow, and one must let a drop or two into the mouth as they learn to nurse. Once the animal starts to take the formula, it will be more receptive to hospital feeding. Generally four

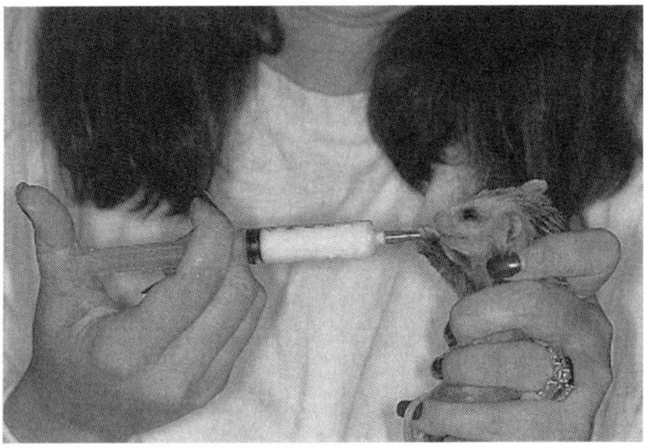

Fig. 5. Supplemental feeding of young opossums. Note the position for appropriate presentation of the bottle.

feedings are necessary: early morning, lunchtime, late afternoon, and late in the evening. Rabbits, however, only need two feedings a day. The face and fur should be wiped clean after each feeding. To house smaller mammals and birds, a small, clean plastic storage container with holes punched through may be used, with some newspaper and a towel placed on the bottom. The container may then be placed half on the heating pad and half off, so the animal can move away from the heat if it is too warm.

It is important to recognize that improper imprinting can occur during the hand-rearing of orphans. If possible, one should place at least two orphans of the same species together, not talk to orphans (especially after weaning), not handle animals at times other than during feeding and toileting, and not let children handle these young animals. Weaning occurs at different intervals for different species; adding whole foods that are in the adult diet of that species before weaning may stimulate the orphan to try these foods, increasing the likelihood of weaning in an appropriate time-span. Some animals may be resistant to weaning and may prefer formula to the more solid foods. In this case, formula thickness can be reduced by increasing the percentage of water in the mixture. Water is generally less palatable and may result in a faster switch to whole (and juvenile or adult) foods. It is vital that any wild animal considered for release first be completely weaned and maintaining its body weight. The location of release should be appropriate (and as safe as possible) for each species [9].

Wounds

Trauma-induced skin wounds are commonly treated in animals of all types and ages.

The main purpose of wound management is to clean a wound for closure and prevent further secondary infection [3]. Closing an unclean wound is unproductive, because skin may not heal correctly with the cumulative debris of dead leukocytes, cellular material, and bacteria; in many cases, closing a "dirty" wound leads to abscess formation. The two primary classes of wound healing are first- and second-intention (or granulation) healing. First intention is the type of healing that occurs when uninfected tissues are brought into apposition. Occasionally wildlife casualties fall into this category. Many wildlife wounds have considerable soft tissue damage, with wound edges that are impossible to bring into apposition. These wounds will heal from the inside outward by the granulation process [11]. During first-intention healing, the blood clot is formed in 24 hours, and mitotic basal epithelial cells are seen, along with neutrophils, at the wound margin. By day three, macrophages are the dominant cell type found in the healing wound; granulation tissue with collagen is present, and epithelial cell migration covers the wound. By day five, granulation tissue fills the incision site, angiogenesis peaks, and the epithelium is at normal thickness with surface keratinization. By the second week, fibroplasia is maximal and leads to wound contraction. Delayed primary closure may be an option in some instances; in this case, the skin edges can close over the course of a few days or longer. The edges are brought closer and closer together with horizontal mattress sutures (tightening sutures daily or every other day) until the wound may be closed entirely. During this delayed contractility, the wound should be cleaned and topical medications applied [3,11].

During the granulation (or second-intention healing) process, the body controls healing in four stages: inflammation, granulation, re-epithelization, and maturation [3]. Inflammation is more intense during granulation than in first-intention healing, because of the greater extent to which fibrin and necrotic tissue are present, the greater amounts of granulation tissue, and the larger extent of necessary wound contraction. During the inflammatory phase (which occurs immediately after the insult), an increase in blood flow and fluid release from interstitial fluid and increased capillary permeability to the damaged areas results in increased hemorrhage. This accelerated blood flow delivers fluids to the injury that are high in protein and leukocytes. The wound exhibits redness, heat, swelling, and pain. Redness is caused by hyperemia resulting from vasodilatation and increased blood flow to the inflamed area. A corresponding increase in blood vessel permeability allows for the concentration of antimicrobials (administered by staff) and leukocytes in the wound area. In major inflammatory reactions, this diversion of blood to the wound area may lead to an additional decrease in circulating blood volume, resulting in shock and an increased state of debilitation. Heat is due to the combined effects of systemic increase in body temperature (fever) and increased blood flow. Swelling results from accumulation of fluid (ie, edema) and other exudates due to increased vascular permeability. Pain results from stimulation of nerve endings by cytokines and other inflammatory mediators. During the initial bleeding, blood flow will flush debris out of the wound. Subsequent inflammation and release of chemical compounds from responding cells eventually closes off damaged blood vessels, allowing a clot to form [3,11].

At this point, neutrophils and macrophages begin to phagocytize bacteria, foreign matter, and necrotic tissue in a debridement phase. The resulting exudate of dead leukocytes (with ingested debris and bacteria) is commonly found in the wounds of wild animals. The exudates described here are essential to the healing process, because white blood cells destroy infective material and bacteria in mammals; unlike in birds and reptiles, the exudate is a liquid that can flow away from the wound. In late stages of wound inflammation, reconstructive processes are initiated that repair skin damage. Angiogenesis, fibroplasia, and epithelial regeneration flourish in a protein- and growth factor–rich tissue matrix that may be established early in the inflammation process. Leukocytes persist and continue to clean up debris associated with wound healing. During the granulation phase, there is proteolytic degradation of the basement membrane of the parent blood vessel and endothelial cell migration toward angiogenic stimuli (ie, vascular endothelial growth factor and fibroblast growth factor); endothelial proliferation and mitosis occur behind the leading edge of migrating cells. Next, maturation and remodeling of the new blood vessels occur, as well as migration and mitosis of fibroblasts with collagen production. These vessel endothelial growth factor–stimulated blood vessels are leaky, resulting in soft and edematous granulation tissue. To enhance healing, growth factors and cytokines are released.

Once the wound is devoid of infected tissue and exudates (usually after 3 to 4 days of treatment), fibroblasts migrate into the wound and form the matrix that will fill the wound. Capillaries then proceed into the matrix and provide an extensive blood supply for healing. Fibroblasts start to contract and pull wound edges together. This granulation tissue and associated blood supply appear bright pink and are resistant to infection. However, because this phase of the granulation tissue is so vascular, it bleeds profusely when damaged; lavage rather than debridement is the treatment of choice during this time. The formation of new capillaries is stimulated by angiogenesis factor, which stimulates endothelial cells to replicate and invade healing inflammatory tissue. Fibrosis is the production and deposition of collagen by fibroblasts. Existing fibrocytes are the source of fibroblasts in healing wounds.

Granulation tissue is essentially a mass composed of capillaries and fibroblasts, often with infiltration of inflammatory cells. This tissue is a foundation over which re-epithelization may occur as the basis of wound closure. Basal cells of the surviving epithelium at the periphery of the wound slide across the bare, fibrin-covered wound surface to facilitate the healing process. Migrant epithelial cells have blunt pseudopods that project by means of amoeboid movement into fibrin stands. Epithelial cells also cover gaps in epidermis by growing up to form skin appendages like hair follicles if they are still intact. Mucosal surfaces regenerate rapidly; therefore, a wound anywhere can be covered with epithelium. However, granulation tissue is usually required for prompt epithelization.

In uncomplicated skin wounds that are small and linear, the wound will completely bridge in 5 to 7 days. In the subsequent 2 to 3 weeks, the wound is repaired, and fibrosis increases as the scar tissue becomes organized. By 4 weeks, collagenization and fibrosis are largely completed. Myofibroblasts and elastic fibers appear and are responsible for wound contraction. Once the first layer of epithelium is in place, more cells are added, gradually thickening the layer during the maturation phase. This process often takes weeks to complete. At this stage, it is beneficial to protect the healing wound area with a semiocclusive dressing. During this time, capillaries supplying the granulation tissue recede. Eventually, the new epithelium develops into a scar that is not as strong or flexible as the original skin layers.

Wound repair is suppressed when contamination (eg, bacteria, debris, oil) is present, blood supply is inadequate, systemic hormonal deficits exist (eg, diabetes, Cushing's), nutrition is inadequate (especially protein or Vitamin C deficiency), the patient is older, or there is excessive movement or restraint failure at the wound site [3,10,11].

Skin wounds in birds heal differently from similar wounds in mammalian patients. Initially, birds bleed and bruise and the wound becomes contaminated, but avian blood clots much faster than mammalian blood; the higher body temperature of birds makes them more resistant to infection [12]. Because of this greater resistance, wounds are cleaned and sometimes sutured quickly; avian species will produce granulation tissue rapidly underneath debris. White blood cells and bacteria produce exudates that are solid to semisolid in birds, reptiles, and some small mammals like guinea pigs. As wounds granulate, dry necrosis (a mixture of dead tissue and debris that forms into a solid mass) occurs; this may usually be removed with tissue forceps. Every 2 to 3 days the dry necrotic exudate should be debrided, until re-epithelization reduces the quantity of exudates and fills the wound cavity. Eventually, granulation tissue will seal off the wound area, and no further cleaning will be required [3,13].

Wound treatment

All patients that present with a wound injury should be treated for shock and dehydration before any effort is made to address wound treatment. For birds, the maintenance fluid requirement is 100 mL/kg/d. For mammals, the requirement is 60 mL/kg/d; for reptiles, it is 30 mL/kg/d. When calculating fluids, one should add the maintenance requirement to the percentage of dehydration (deficit replacement fluid volume [mL] = percentage dehydration × body weight [kg] × 1000 × 0.8) and to the ongoing losses (2 × estimated volume lost), if present. These fluids may then be given over 24 to 48 hours. Usually, these fluids may be administered subcutaneously and split into four separate fluid administrations (total volume of fluid to replace ÷ 4 = each fluid treatment). Once the patient is stabilized, any fracture may be temporarily treated to ease the patient's discomfort and prevent further injury. At this time, pain medication should also be administered. For lacerating wounds, cleansing of the contaminated area should be considered once the patient is stable and less stressed and has been given pain medication. Chronic malodorous or infected wounds that have been on the animal for some time are not as important as patient stabilization. Bacteria can spread into the bloodstream from a wound, resulting in a septicemia over a 24-hour period. Care must be taken to prevent this development when possible. The basic approach to wound care is to

- Remove any bandaging put in place before hospital admission
- Control any bleeding or seeping
- Obtain culture and submit for culture and sensitivity; also obtain Gram stain
- Clipwound or pluck feathers around wound area to decrease contamination
- Clean around the wound with antiseptics and lavage the area, removing debris. The wound should be lavaged with sterile saline, using an 18-gauge needle to dislodge debris and bacteria, and debrided as necessary. A lavage of 50% dextrose (allowed to maintain contact with the wound for 30 seconds) should be followed by a sterile saline flush. Application of topical silver sulfadiazine cream (Silvadene Crème, Boots Pharmaceuticals, Lincolnshire, Illinois) is recommended, and covering the wound with a nonadherent dressing (Tegaderm, 3M, St. Paul, Minnesota; Adaptix, Johnson & Johnson, Arlington, Texas) is advisable before placing a bandage. This may be more necessary in situations where the animal is licking the wound.
- Broad-spectrum antibiotic therapy should continue until culture and sensitivity results are available [3,13]. At this time, specific antibiotics regimens may be initiated.

Bone healing

A few aspects of avian bone healing require examination. The avian skeleton is compact and strong and has an increased content of calcium and phosphorous compared with mammalian bone. Mammalian bones are too cumbersome to lift in the air; birds therefore have adapted their skeletal structure by decreasing the number of bones they have, fusing some together and decreasing the weight of the entire skeletal system by including air spaces in many bones. Because these bones are so light, they may easily shatter as a result of their high tensile strength. The female's bones are denser during the breeding season, because the cavities are filled with new bone. This "new bone" is the extra calcium that is needed for eggshell production and is stored in the medullary cavity of long bones. This extra calcification, when noted radiographically, may be mistaken for a pathologic process. Birds have a tibotarsus bone instead of a separate tibia and fibula. They have a single bone, the tarsometatarsus, replacing the tarsal bones and metatarsus. At the carpal joint, they only have one radial bone and an alula bone, instead of the two rows of bones that form the carpus of mammals. Birds also have fused vertebrae, a prominent fused sternum, and a pelvis that is open laterally to facilitate egg laying. Unlike mammals, avian species vary in the number of cervical vertebrae. Pneumatized bone in avian species replaces the thick medullary bone marrow present in the center of mammalian bone, producing a light trabecular structure. Because bone is pneumatized by air sacs, they are effectively extensions of the respiratory system. Diverticula of the air sacs extend through the pneumatic foramen into the medullary cavity of neighboring bones, filling a considerable part of the foramen with air. The clavicular air sacs aerate the humerus; hence a compound fracture of the humerus can introduce infection to the air sacs and lungs. In every bird, the sternum, humerus, and skull are always pneumatized to decrease the overall weight. However, depending on the species and sometimes on the individual, some or all of the following bones may be pneumatized: cervical vertebrae, thoracic vertebrae, synsacrum, ribs, scapula, coracoid, femur, and pelvis. Most notably, all raptors have a pneumatized femur. An important consideration for pneumatized bone is that it should be covered before irrigation to prevent aspiration, air sacculitis, and pneumonia [2,3,8,12,14–16].

Fracture healing in mammalian, reptilian, and avian bones is essentially the same, based on extraosseous blood supply and callus formation. However, avian bone healing is very rapid, and a significant amount of scar tissue and bony callus forms quickly, possibly even before a wild bird would be presented for treatment. After a fracture, fibrous tissue rapidly begins stabilizing the fracture. Shortly thereafter, cancellous bone is laid down in the callus until, after several weeks, a bony union is in place and the bird can use the limb again. Owing to its speed, healing may be less than perfect when the fracture is not aligned properly and stabilized, jeopardizing the use of the limb and return to the wild [2,3,8,12,14–16].

Avian wound treatment faces several unique challenges in addition to pneumatic bones. Purulent material in birds is solid and does not flow away from the wound; drainage of this material does not occur in birds as it does in mammals. When long bones suffer an infection, the cortical bone may become distorted by the growth of the inspissated material in the medullary cavity. In many cases, flushing an inspissated abscess pushes the pathogenic organism (infection source) farther into the cavity—especially in the femur.

The antibiotic of choice for bone and joint infections is clindamycin. Surgical removal of the cellular debris and weekly radiograph rechecks to re-evaluate the case are also recommended. When osteomyelitis is unresponsive to clindamycin and the wound therapy outlined here, the wound should be cultured for *Mycobacterium avium*. Birds that have a leg injury usually perch on their good leg, which causes greater pressure on the plantar aspect of the foot of the unaffected leg. This pattern may result in the development of pressure sores and infection commonly known as bumblefoot. To prevent this complication, perches made of Astroturf (Textile Management Associates, Inc., Dalton, Georgia) or other padding may be used. Use of a ball bandage may help to prevent this progressive disease, which starts as a mild localizing hyperemia and can advance to osteomyelitis.

Bird fractures are usually grossly displaced, owing to the pull of the muscle masses on the long bones. Even in such cases, the callus forms within a few days, linking the fragments together. Once in place, this fibrous tissue is hard to remove to get a better reduction. The build-up of this fibrous tissue callus may be exceptional and may entrap vital soft tissue mechanisms like tendons. Ankylosis may be forgotten until it is too late. This "joint fusing" is most likely to occur when a fracture near the joint results in excessive fibrous tissue build-up on or around that joint, significantly decreasing its range of motion. This may not be a preventable occurrence. However, it appears that simple disuse of the joint can also cause it to ankylose; if the shoulder, elbow, or carpal joints are affected, the bird will not be able to fly normally in the future. Therefore, any long-term immobilization of a wing fracture, exceeding 5 days, should not involve the joints distal or proximal to the fracture (as is standard practice in mammals). When immobilization over the joint is necessary, physical therapy and stretching should be performed every 3 to 5 days. In contrast, pelvic fractures (in birds and mammals) are supported by sufficient muscle mass to heal with no external support [2,3,8,12,14–16].

Summary

Wildlife patients have special needs compared with pet patients in regard to handling and restraint, the importance of the stress response, physical examination, and neonatal concerns. Because many wildlife patients present with wounds and fractures, a good understanding of the pathophysiology of these processes is also important. The primary goal of all wildlife rehabilitation procedures is the ultimate release of the animal back into its natural environment.

References

[1] Fowler M. Restraint and handling of wild and domestic animals. 2nd edition. Ames (IA): Iowa State University Press; 1995.
[2] Beyon P, Forbes N, Harcourt-Brown N. BSAVA Manual of raptors, pigeons, and waterfowl. Ames (IA): Iowa State University Press; 1996.

[3] Stocker L. Practical wildlife care. Ames (IA): Blackwell Publishing; 2000.
[4] Nelson R, Guillermo C. Small animal internal medicine. 2nd edition. St. Louis (MO): Elsevier Mosby; 1998.
[5] Orcutt C. Physical examination and preventive medicine. Vet Clin North Am Exot Anim Pract 1999;2(2):333–404.
[6] Moore A, Joosten S. Principles of wildlife rehabilitation: the essential guide for novice and experienced rehabilitators. St. Cloud (MN): National Wildlife Rehabilitators Association; 1997.
[7] Girling S. Veterinary nursing care of exotic pets. Ames (IA): Blackwell Publishing; 2003.
[8] Dyce KM, Sack WO, Wensing CJG. Textbook of veterinary anatomy. 2nd edition. Philadelphia: WB Saunders; 1996.
[9] Gage L. Hand-rearing wild and domestic mammals. Ames (IA): Blackwell Publishing; 2002.
[10] Murtaugh R. Quick look series in veterinary medicine. Critical care. Jackson (WY): Teton NewMedia; 2002.
[11] Cheville N. Pathobiology. Dubuque (IA): Kendall/Hunt Publishing Co.; 2002.
[12] Tully T. Basic avian bone growth and healing. Vet Clin North Am Exot Anim Pract 2002; 5(1):24–9.
[13] Ritzman T. Wound healing in psittacine species. Vet Clin North Am Exot Anim Pract 2004; 7:87–104.
[14] Atlman R. Disorders of the skeletal system. Diseases of caged and aviary birds. p. 382–91.
[15] Remedios A. Bone and bone healing. Vet Clin North Am Small Anim Pract 1999;29(5): 1029–44.
[16] Dunning D. Basic mammalian bone anatomy and healing. Vet Clin North Am Exot Anim Pract 2002;5(1):115–27.

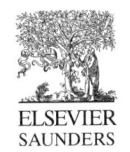

Index

Note: Page numbers of article titles are in **boldface** type.

A

Abdominal examination, of ferrets, 350, 364
  of rabbits, 370
  of rodents, 397
  of wildlife, 446–447

Abdominocentesis, in psittacines, 291

Abscesses, aural, in turtles, 263–266
  examination of, in ferrets, 355
  in rodents, 397–398

Adrenal gland, stress response role of, in wildlife, 440–441

Air sacs, cannulation/intubation of,
  in birds of prey, 340
  in psittacines, 297–298
  in avian species, pneumatized bone from, 458–459
  infections of, in birds of prey, 342

Airway intubation. See *Endotracheal intubation.*

Alanine aminotransferase, in birds of prey, 337

Alkaline phosphatase, in birds of prey, 337

Alopecia, in rodents, 393–394, 412

Amphibians, common procedures in, **237–267**
  dysecdysis and, 261–262
  educational material for, 240
  herpetologic herpetoculture review for, 237–238
  history taking for, 238–240
  imaging as, 253–254
  physical examination as, 240–242
  restraint and handling techniques for, 242–243
  sample collection as, 247, 250–252
  therapeutic techniques as, 254–255

Analgesia, for examination, of nondomesticated species, 420–421, 427, 432
  of rodents, 404–405, 408
  for pain control. See *Pain management.*

Anamnesis, in amphibian examination, 238–239
  in reptile examination, 238–239

Anemia, in birds of prey, 340, 343

Anesthesia, for examination, of birds of prey, 330
  of fish, 225
  of invertebrates, 207–209
  of nondomesticated species, 420–421
  of rodents, 400
  of turtles, 247
  for miscellaneous procedures, in avian species, 310–314
  in ferrets, 362–363
  in rabbits, 378–382
  in reptiles, 264
  in rodents, 405, 408–411
  in venomous reptiles, 281
  for respiratory emergencies, in birds of prey, 340
  monitoring parameters for, in avian species, 312–315
  in ferrets, 363
  in invertebrates, 209

Anesthetic solutions, for fish, 225

Anorexia, in avian species, 308–309
  in nondomesticated species, 432
  in rabbits, 374–375

Antibiotics, for bone and joint infections, in wild birds, 458–459
  for respiratory infections, in birds of prey, 341
  for skin wounds, in turtles, 265–266
  in wildlife, 457

Anticoagulants, for blood transfusions, in ferrets, 358

Antifungals, for respiratory infections, in birds of prey, 341

Antivenoms, for viperid reptile bites, 271

Arterial catheters, placement of, in rabbits, 373

Aspartate aminotransferase, in birds of prey, 337

Aspiration, of foreign body, in birds of prey, 339, 342

Aspiration pneumonia, in birds of prey, 334
    in neonatal wildlife, 451–452

Aspiration procedures, in ferrets, bone marrow, 353
    liver, 354
    lymph node, 354
    spleen, 353
    in fish, coelomic cavity, 230–231
    in wildlife, 447

Attitude assessment, for ferrets, 349

Aural abscesses, in turtles, 263–266

Auscultation examination, of amphibians, 241
    of ferrets, 350
    of rabbits, 369
    of reptiles, 241
    of rodents, 397
    of wildlife, 443

Avian influenza subtype H5N1, 307–318

Avian species, common procedures in, **303–319**
    anesthesia as, 310–314
    bone healing and, 457–459
    handling and restraint techniques for, 303–305
    influenza diseases and, 317–318
    medication administration as, 307–309, 314–316
    nutritional support as, 308–309, 316–317
    patient assessment as, 304–305
    preventive medicine as, 316–317
    sample collection as, 305–307
    supportive care as, 307–310
    treatment techniques as, 307–310
    vaccinations as, 317

B

Bacterial infections, in birds of prey, respiratory emergencies with, 339–341

Bagging/bagging systems, for venomous reptiles, 274–276

Bair Blanket heating unit, for rodents, 411

Ball-tipped metal gavage needles, for avian species, 308–310

Basal metabolic rate (BMR), of psittacines, 295

Baths, medicated, for amphibians, 255, 261–262
    for reptiles, 257–258, 261–262

Beak examination, of birds of prey, 328–329

Beak trimming, for psittacines, 301

Bile acid, in birds of prey, 338

Biopsy procedures, for ferrets, liver, 354
    lymph node, 354
    for fish, gill, 230–231
    for psittacines, crop, 289–290
    for rodents, 407

Birds, wild, common procedures in, 437–460
    bone healing and, 457–459
    health examination as, 441–447
    neonatal, 447–453
    prey species, **321–345**. See also *Falcons;Raptors*.
    restraint and handling techniques for, 437–439
    wound care as, 453–457

Birds of prey, educational, common procedures in, **321–345**
    caging for, 325
    diagnostic procedures as, 329–332
    equipment for, 323–325, 330
    nutritional support as, 335–336
    physical examination as, 327–329
    respiratory emergencies as, 339–342
    restraint and handling techniques for, 323–325
    supportive care as, 330, 332–335
    technical support for, 325–327
    terminology for, 321–323
    toxin exposures and, 342–343
    traumatic injuries as, 341–342

Bites, by amphibians, 243
    by nondomesticated species, 416–417, 431
    by reptiles, 244

by rodents, 395
by venomous reptiles, after
    decapitation, 283
    emergency protocol for, 273
    examination planning and, 274
    severity versus outcome of,
        272–273
    signs and symptoms of,
        270–272
Blood collection, procedure for, in
    amphibians, 247
    in avian species, 305–307
    in birds of prey, 330–331
    in ferrets, 402
    in fish, 228
    in nondomesticated species,
        426–430
    in psittacines, 288–289
    in rabbits, 370–371
    in reptiles, 248–250
    in rodents, 405–406
    in wildlife, 447
Blood glucose level, in birds of prey, 338
    decreased, 343
    in neonatal wildlife, physiology of,
        449–450
        septicemia impact on, 450–451
    in reptiles, elevated, 251
Blood pressure monitoring, in avian species,
    313, 315
    in rabbits, 373
Blood transfusions, for birds of prey, 343
    for ferrets, 357–358
Blood urea nitrogen, in birds of prey, 339
Body temperature, monitoring during
    surgery, in avian species, 312, 314
        in ferrets, 363
        in rodents, 410–411
    procedure for taking, in avian species,
        305
        in ferrets, 350
        in nondomesticated species, 419
        in rabbits, 369
        in rodents, 396, 400
Body weight, procedure for obtaining, in
    amphibians, 241, 243
    in birds of prey, 324–325, 335
    in nondomesticated species, 416
    in reptiles, 241, 258
    in rodents, 395–396
    in wildlife, 446
Bone fractures, in birds of prey, 342
    in wildlife, 458–459
Bone healing, in avian species, 457–458
    fracture treatment based on,
        458–459
Bone infections, in wild birds, antibiotics
    for, 458–459
Bone marrow aspiration, in ferrets, 353
Bumblefoot, 459

C

Caging, for examinations, of birds of prey,
    325
    of rabbits, 367–368
    for hospitalization, of avian species,
        310
Calcium level, in birds of prey, 338
    decreased, 343
Caloric requirements, of birds of prey,
    335–336
    of psittacines, 295
    of reptiles, 258, 260
    supportive feedings for. See *Nutritional
        support.*
Capture techniques, for avian species,
    303–305
    for psittacines, 287–288
    for wildlife, 438
Capybaras, oral examination of, 392
Cardiac arrest, in birds of prey, 342
Cardiac catheterization, of snakes, 255
Cardiocentesis, in snakes, 248, 255
Cardiogenic shock, in birds of prey, 332
Cardiovascular assessment, of amphibians,
    241
    of ferrets, 350
    of rabbits, 369
    of reptiles, 241
    of rodents, 397
    of wildlife, 443
Carnivore Care diet, 428
Carnivores, reptiles as, 252
    nutritional support for, 259–260
    wild, common procedures in, 437–460
        health examination as, 252,
            441–447
        neonatal, 447–453
        nutritional support as,
            335–336
        restraint and handling
            techniques for,
            437–439
        wound care as, 453–457

Casting, of birds of prey, 329–331

Catheter placement, urinary, in ferrets, 358–359
　vascular procedures for, in amphibians, 255–256
　　in birds of prey, 333–334
　　in nondomesticated species, 420, 422
　　in psittacines, 293–295
　　in rabbits, 373
　　in reptiles, 255–257
　　in rodents, 402

Cere examination, of birds of prey, 328

Cheek pouch, in rabbits, 369–370
　in rodents, 392, 396

Cheek teeth, in rodents, 392–393

Chelonians. See *Turtles/tortoises*.

Chemical restraint. See *Anesthesia*.

Chemistry tests, for birds of prey, indications for, 332, 339
　interpretation of, 337–339

Chicks, for birds of prey diet, 336

Chinchilla, examination guidelines for, 399
　gastrointestinal tract of, 393
　oral examination of, 392–393
　temperature taking of, 396

"Chinese finger-trap" technique, for pharyngostomy tube suturing, 259–260

Choanal sample collection, in psittacines, 290

Cholesterol level, in birds of prey, 338

Clinical history, in amphibian examination, 238–239
　in fish examination, 226–227
　in reptile examination, 238–239
　in rodent examination, 395–396, 400

Cloaca examination, of wildlife, 446–447

Cloaca-rectal prolapse, in opossums, 434

Cloth restraint, for avian species, 303–304
　for birds of prey, 324–325
　for nondomesticated species, 416

Clove oil, for fish chemical restraint, 225

Coelomic examination, of amphibians, 241
　of reptiles, 241
　of wildlife, 446

Coelomocentesis, in fish, 230–231
　in psittacines, 291

Colubridae reptiles, common procedures in, 270, 281–282
　safe handling techniques for, 274–281
　treatment techniques for, 281–284

Complete blood count (CBC), in birds of prey, 340

Computed tomography (CT), diagnostic, in amphibians, 254
　in reptiles, 254

Cones, anesthetic, for avian species, 311–313

Constriction, by snakes, prevention of, 246

Contrast radiography, for ferrets, 363
　for invertebrates, 213–214
　iodinated, for ferrets, 363–364

Cortisol, in stress response, of wildlife, 440–441

Costs, of rodent care, 389, 401

Creatinine kinase (CK), in birds of prey, 337

Critical Care diet, for nondomesticated species, 428
　for psittacines, 295
　for rabbits, 375

Critical Care for Herbivores diet, 404

Crocodilians, blood collection in, 249–250
　restraint and handling techniques for, 245
　urogenital examination of, 242

Crop, assessment of, in wildlife, 446
　cytology of, in psittacines, 289–290
　infusion into, for psittacines, 295–296

Cultures/culturing, indications for, in amphibians, 243
　in avian species examination, 307
　in reptiles, 251–252, 263
　in rodent examination, 396
　in wildlife examination, 447
　of wildlife wounds, 457, 459
　procedures for, in amphibians, 243, 247
　in invertebrates, 213
　in reptiles, 251–252
　in sugar gliders, 432–433

Cystocentesis, for urine collection, in reptiles, 251

Cytokines, septicemia and, in neonatal wildlife, 450

Cytology, sample collection for. See also *Biopsy procedures*.
in fish, 229–231
in psittacines, 289–290
in reptiles, 252

D

Debridement phase, of wound healing, 455–456

Degus, common procedures in, fluid therapy/injections as, 420, 422–424, 426
medication administration as, 424–427, 429
species-specific, 431

Dehydration, fluid therapy for, in birds of prey, 332–335, 340
in ferrets, 349
in fish, 226, 232
in invertebrates, 210–211
in nondomesticated species, 422, 433
in psittacines, 291–292
in rabbits, 372–373
in reptiles, 257–258
in rodents, 401
in wildlife, 447, 450
wound stabilization and, 456–457

Dentistry, common procedures for, in nondomesticated species, 430, 432–434
in rabbits, 369–370, 384–385
in rodents, 392, 396–397, 411

Dermatology procedures. See *Skin entries*.

Diabetes mellitus, in reptiles, 251

Diagnostic procedures, for birds of prey, 329–332
interpretation of, 337–339
for reptiles, 251, 262–263
for wildlife, 441, 447
imaging as. See *Imaging*.

Diastema, in rodents, 392

Diet. See *Nutritional entries*.

Doppler flow probe, for anesthesia monitoring, in avian species, 312, 314
in ferrets, 363
for cardiovascular assessment, in amphibians, 241
in reptiles, 241

Duodenostomy feeding tube, for psittacines, 296

Duprasi, common procedures in, fluid therapy/injections as, 420, 422–424, 426
medication administration as, 424–427, 429
nutritional support as, 428
species-specific, 431

Dysecdysis, in amphibians, 261–262
in invertebrates, 216–217
in reptiles, 261–262

Dyspnea, in ferrets, 348
in prairie dogs, 432
in psittacines, 298–299

E

Eagle meat, for birds of prey, 336

Ear cleaning, for rabbits, 383–384

Ear examination, of amphibians, 241
of birds of prey, 328, 341
of rabbits, 369
of reptiles, 241
of wildlife, 443, 446

Ecdysis, in reptiles, 261

Echocardiography, for ferrets, 364

Educational material, for reptile and amphibian care, 240

Elapidae reptiles, common procedures in, 271–272
safe handling techniques for, 274–281
treatment techniques for, 281–284

Elastic fibers, in wound healing process, 456

Electrocution, in birds of prey, 342

Electrolyte imbalance, in reptiles, 259
treatment of, 258, 260

Electrolyte solutions, for reptiles, 258

Emergency care, for rodents, 400–405
for venomous reptile bites, 273
respiratory, for birds of prey, 339–342

Endoscope, for airway intubation, of rabbits, 381–382

Endoscopy, diagnostic, for invertebrates, 213–214
in amphibians, 254
in reptiles, 254

Endotoxin, septicemia related to, in neonatal wildlife, 450–451

Endotracheal intubation, of avian species, 311–312
of rabbits, 379–380
blind versus direct, 380–382
of rodents, 408–409

Energy requirements, of birds of prey, 335–336
of psittacines, 295
of reptiles, 258, 260
supportive feedings for. See *Nutritional support.*

Enteral nutrition, for avian species, 308–309, 316–317
for ferrets, 361–362
for fish, 232
for psittacines, 295–296
for rabbits, 374–378
for rodents, 403–404

Envenomation, after decapitation, 283
emergency protocol for, 273
examination planning and, 274
severity versus outcome of, 272–273
signs and symptoms of, 270–272

Environmental assessment, for amphibians, 238–240
shedding problems and, 261–262
for reptiles, 238–240
shedding problems and, 261–262

Epidural anesthesia, in rabbits, 379

Epinephrine, in stress response, of wildlife, 440–441

Esophagostomy tubes, for ferrets, 361–362
for psittacines, 296
for rabbits, 377
surgical placement of, 377–378

Eustachian tube lavage, for aural abscess, in turtles, 264

Euthanasia, of invertebrates, 219–220
of rodents, 400, 409–410

Exoskeleton trauma, diagnosis of, in chelonians, 253
repair procedures for, in invertebrates, 215–217

Exotic rodents, common procedures in, **415–435**
anesthetics and analgesics for, 420–422
bite wound care as, 416–417
fluid therapy/injections as, 420, 422–426
handling and restraint techniques for, 415–416
medication administration as, 424–427, 429
nutritional support as, 428
pain and distress recognition and, 418–419
potential zoonoses from, 416–417

Extramedullary hematopoiesis (EMH), in ferrets, 350

Extremity examination, of birds of prey, 329

Eye caps, retained, of snakes, 262

Eye examination, of birds of prey, 328
of ferrets, 349–350
of reptiles, 263–264
of wildlife, 443

F

Falcons, common procedures in, **321–345**
caging for, 325
diagnostic procedures as, 329–332
equipment for, 323–325, 330
nutritional support as, 335–336
physical examination as, 327–329
respiratory emergencies as, 339–342
restraint and handling techniques for, 323–325
supportive care as, 330, 332–335
technical support for, 325–327
terminology for, 321–323
toxin exposures and, 342–343
traumatic injuries as, 341–342

Fasting, preanesthetic, for avian species, 311

Feather examination, of birds of prey, 328
of wildlife, 453–456

Feather trimming, flight, for psittacines, 299–300

Fecal collection/examination, in amphibians, 239, 250–251
in birds of prey, 329
in ferrets, 352
in fish, 228–229
in invertebrates, 213
in psittacines, 289
in rabbits, 371–372
in reptiles, 239, 250–251
in rodents, 406
in wildlife, 447

Federal regulations, on nondomesticated species, as companions, 417–418

Feeding tubes. See *Gastric feeding tubes.*

Feet/foot care, for rodents, 412

Feet/foot examination, of birds of prey, 327–329, 343

Ferrets, common procedures in, **347–365**
    handling and restraint techniques for, 348, 363
    imaging as, 363–364
    medication administration as, 360
    miscellaneous, 362–364
    patient assessment as, 348–350
    sample collection as, 351–355
    supportive care as, 360–362
    treatment techniques as, 355–359
    triage as, 347–348

Fibroblasts, in wound healing process, 455

Fight or flight response, in reptiles, 243
    in rodents, 395
    in wildlife, 439–441

Fin trauma, in fish, 229–230

Fish, common procedures in, **223–235**
    equipment suggested for, 224
    imaging as, 231–232
    medication administration as, 232–234
    safe handling for, 223–225
    sample collection as, 226–231
    supportive care as, 226, 232–234
    trauma-related, 229–230
    triage as, 223–224
    water quality testing and, 223, 226
    for birds of prey diet, 336

Flight reduction, for psittacines, 299–300

Fluid therapy, for birds of prey, 332–335
    for ferrets, 357
    for fish, 232
    for invertebrates, 210–211
    for nondomesticated species, 420, 422–426
    for psittacines, 291–295
    for rabbits, 372–373
    for reptiles, 257–258
    for rodents, 401
    for wildlife, 447
        neonatal indications for, 448–449, 453

Fluoroquinolones, FDA approval of, for avian species, 315–316

Food Animal Residue Avoidance Databank (FARAD), 315–316

Force-feeding, of avian species, 308–309
    of nondomesticated species, 428, 430
    of reptiles, 258

Forcep restraint, for examination, of invertebrates, 208

Foreign body inhalation, in birds of prey, respiratory emergencies with, 339, 342

Fractures, bone, in birds of prey, 342
    in wildlife, 458–459

Frostbite, in birds of prey, 343

Fungal infections, in birds of prey, 332
    respiratory emergencies with, 339, 341

Fur examination, of rodents, 397–398, 412

G

Gas anesthesia, for avian species, 311
    for birds of prey, 330
    for ferrets, 362
    for invertebrates, 207–209
    for rabbits, 381
    for rodents, 408

Gastric feeding tubes, for avian species, 308–309
    for ferrets, 362
    for fish, 232
    for psittacines, 296
    for rabbits, 376–377
    for reptiles, 258–260

Gastrointestinal tract, anatomy of, of rodents, 393
    of rabbits, 370
        intubation for nutrition, 376–378

Gavage feedings. See *Gastric feeding tubes;Nutritional support.*

Gerbils, examination guidelines for, 398–399

Gila monster, common procedures in, 270
    safe handling techniques for, 274–281
    treatment techniques for, 281–284

Gills, in fish, biopsy of, 230–231
    respiration function of, 230

Glandular disorders, in older guinea pigs, 412

Gloves, for capture, of psittacines, 287
    of wildlife, 438
    for examinations, of amphibians, 242–243
    of birds of prey, 323, 325–327
    of fish, 224–225

Gloves (continued)
    of invertebrates, 206
    of rodents, 398, 412

Glucose level. See Blood glucose level.

Granulation, in wound healing process, 454–456

Grooming procedures, for psittacines, 299–301

Guinea pigs, abscesses in, 397–398
    examination guidelines for, 399
    gastrointestinal tract of, 393
    older, common conditions of, 412
    oral examination of, 392–393
    temperature taking of, 396

H

Hair, anatomy of, in rodents, 393–394
    examination of, in rabbits, 369
        in rodents, 397, 412

Hair removal, for surgical procedures, in rodents, 410

Hair sample collection, of rodents, 406–407

Hamsters, examination guidelines for, 398–399

Hand feeding, of avian species, 308–310
    of neonatal wildlife, 452–453
    of nondomesticated species, 428, 430

Hand-rearing, of orphaned wildlife, 452

Handling containers, for venomous reptiles, 276

Handling techniques, for examination, of amphibians, 242–243
    of avian species, 303–305
    of birds of prey, 323–325
        by technical staff, 326–327
    of ferrets, 348, 363
    of fish, 223–225
    of invertebrates, 206–208, 213
    of nondomesticated species, 415–416
    of rabbits, 367–368
    of reptiles, 242–247
    of rodents, 395–396, 398–399
    of venomous reptiles, 274–281
    of wildlife, 437–439
        stress response to, 439–441

Handouts, general, for reptile and amphibian care, 240

Head trauma, in birds of prey, 342

Health examination. See also Physical examination.
    of wildlife, 441–447
        checklist for, 444–445

Heart rate/rhythm, assessment of, in amphibians, 241
    in ferrets, 350
    in rabbits, 369
    in reptiles, 241
    in rodents, 397
    in wildlife, 443

Heart sounds, assessment of, in ferrets, 350
    in rabbits, 369

Heating equipment, for surgical procedures, in rodents, 410–411

Hedgehogs, common procedures in, **415–435**
    anesthetics and analgesics for, 420–422
    bite wound care as, 416–417
    fluid therapy/injections as, 420, 422–423, 425–426
    handling and restraint techniques for, 415–416
    medication administration as, 424–427, 429
    nutritional support as, 428
    pain and distress recognition and, 418–419, 421
    patient assessment as, 430–431
    potential zoonoses from, 416–417
    species-specific, 430–431

Helodermatidae reptiles, common procedures in, 270, 272
    safe handling techniques for, 274–281
    treatment techniques for, 281–284

Hematology tests, for birds of prey, indications for, 329, 339
    interpretation of, 339–340

Hemolymph, collection of, in invertebrates, 212
    loss of, in invertebrates, 216

Heparin, for blood transfusions, in ferrets, 358

Heparin flushes, for catheters, in ferrets, 356

Herbivores diet, Critical Care for, 404

Herbivorous reptiles, nutritional support for, 259–260
    urinalysis of, 252

Herpetologic herpetoculture, in reptiles and amphibians, 237–238

History taking, for amphibian examination, 238–239
  for fish examination, 226–227
  for reptile examination, 238–239
  for rodent examination, 395–396, 400
  for wildlife examination, 442–443

Hoods, for birds of prey, 323–325, 330

Hospitalization, of avian species, 310
  of birds of prey, 326–327
  of venomous reptiles, 281

Husbandry, as preventive medicine, for amphibians, 238, 261–262
    for avian species, 317
    for reptiles, 238, 261–262
  assessment of, for amphibians, 238–240
    for reptiles, 238–240

Hydration status, assessment of, in amphibians, 241
    in birds of prey, 332–335, 340
    in ferrets, 349
    in invertebrates, 209–211
    in nondomesticated species, 419, 430, 432
    in rabbits, 372–373
    in reptiles, 241
    in rodents, 401

Hyperglycemia, in reptiles, 251

Hyperthermia, prevention during examination, of rabbits, 368

Hypocalcemia, in birds of prey, 343

Hypoglycemia, in birds of prey, 343
  in neonatal wildlife, 448–449
    hypothermia-related, 449–450

Hypokalemia, in reptiles, 259–260

Hypophosphatemia, in reptiles, 259–260

Hypothermia, for examination, of invertebrates, 207
  in neonatal wildlife, physiology of, 449
    rewarming protocols for, 449–450
  prevention during examination, of rabbits, 369
  of reptiles, 258
  prevention during surgical procedures, in ferrets, 363
    in rodents, 410–411

Hypovolemic shock, in birds of prey, 332–333, 335
  in psittacines, 291–292
  in rabbits, 373

I

Iguanas, restraint and handling techniques for, 243–245

Imaging, diagnostic, in amphibians, 253–254
  in birds of prey, 332, 343
  in ferrets, 363–364
  in fish, 9–10
  in invertebrates, 213–214
  in reptiles, 253–254
  in rodents, 400, 411

Immobilization techniques, for bone fractures, in birds, 459
  for examination and treatment. See *Restraint techniques*.

Immune system, of reptiles and amphibians, herpetologic herpetoculture basis for, 237–238

Immunity, passive, in neonatal wildlife, 451

Immunizations, for avian species, 317

Imprinting, in neonatal wildlife, 448, 453

Incisors, in rabbits, examination of, 369–370
    trimming of, 384–385
  in rodents, 390, 393
    examination of, 396
    suture chewing and, 407–408

Incubators, for hospitalization, of avian species, 310
  in emergency care, of rodents, 400–401

Infectious disease, in birds of prey, 332
  of blood, 343–344
  respiratory emergencies with, 339–342
  in neonatal wildlife, aspiration pneumonia and, 451–452
    septicemia related to, 450–451
  in nondomesticated species, 418
    pouch-related, 432–433
  in reptiles, 262–263
  integument-related, in ferrets, 350
  in fish, 229
  in invertebrates, 215, 218–220
  in wildlife, 442
  wildlife trauma-related, of bones, 458–459
    of skin, 453–454, 457

Inflammation, in wound healing process, 454–455

Inhalant anesthesia, for ferrets, 362
  for invertebrates, 209
  for rabbits, 379

Injectable anesthesia, for ferrets, 362
    for invertebrates, 208–209
    for rabbits, 379
Injectable therapeutics, for amphibians, 254–255
    for avian species, 307–308
    for birds of prey, 333
    for ferrets, 360
    for fish, 233
    for invertebrates, 210–211
    for nondomesticated species, 422–426
    for psittacines, 296–297
    for rabbits, 374
    for reptiles, 254–255
    for rodents, 402–403
Injection sites, for nondomesticated species, 423–425
    necrosis of, in rodents, 401
Injuries. See *Trauma assessment.*
Integument examination. See *Skin examination.*
Intracoelomic injections, in reptiles, 254
Intranasal route, for medications, in nondomesticated species, 427
Intraosseous catheters, placement of, in avian species, 307–308
    in birds of prey, 333
    in ferrets, 356
    in nondomesticated species, 422–423
        fluid administration guidelines, 424–425
    in psittacines, 293–295
    in rabbits, 373
    in reptiles, 255–257
    in rodents, 402
Intraperitoneal injections, in nondomesticated species, 426–427
Intravenous catheters, placement of, in amphibians, 255–256
    in avian species, 307–308
    in birds of prey, 333–334
    in ferrets, 355–356
    in psittacines, 293–294
    in rabbits, 372
    in reptiles, 21, 255–257
    in rodents, 402
Intubation, air sac, of birds of prey, 340
    of psittacines, 297–298
    airway. See *Endotracheal intubation.*
    gastrointestinal. See *Gastric feeding tubes.*

Invertebrates, common procedures in, **205–221**
    euthanasia as, 219–220
    exoskeleton repair as, 215–217
    fluid therapy/injections as, 209–211
    handling and restraint techniques for, 206–208
    imaging as, 213–214
    integumental disorders and, 215–219
    medication administration as, 210–211
    resources on, 205–206, 220
    sample collection as, 211–213
Iron storage disease (ISD), in avian species, 316–317

J

Jesses, for birds of prey, 323–325
Joint infections, in wild birds, antibiotics for, 458–459

K

Kidney disease, in reptiles, 251

L

Laboratory tests, for birds of prey, 329–330, 332
    interpretation of, 337–339
    for reptiles, 251, 262–263
    for wildlife, 441, 447
Lactate dehydrogenase (LDH), in birds of prey, 337
Laparoscopy, for invertebrates, 213–214
Laryngeal mask airway (LMA), for gas anesthesia, in rodents, 408
Laryngoscope, for airway intubation, of rabbits, 381–382
    of rodents, 408
Lead exposures, in birds of prey, 342–343
Leashes, for birds of prey, 323–325
Liver aspiration, in ferrets, 354
Liver biopsy, in ferrets, 354
Lizards, common procedures in, blood collection as, 248–249
    cardiovascular assessment as, 241
    intraosseous catheter placement as, 255–257

INDEX

intravenous catheter placement as, 255
restraint and handling techniques for, 243–245
urogenital examination as, 242

Local anesthesia, for ferrets, 362
for rabbits, 379

Lonestar retractor, for surgical procedures, in avian species, 313, 315–316

Lung sounds, assessment of, in rabbits, 369
in rodents, 397

Lungs, sample collection from, in reptiles, 252

Lymph node aspiration, in ferrets, 354

Lymph node biopsy, in ferrets, 354

Lymph nodes, examination of, in ferrets, 350

M

Magnetic resonance imaging (MRI), for amphibians, 254
for reptiles, 254

Maintenance energy requirement (MER), of psittacines, 295

Malocclusion, in rabbits, 385
in rodents, 393, 407

Mammals, wild, common procedures in, 437–460
bone healing and, 457–459
health examination as, 441–447
neonatal, 447–453
restraint and handling techniques for, 437–439
wound care as, 453–457

Manual restraint, of avian species, 303–305
of birds of prey, 326–327
of reptiles, 243–247

Marsupials, companion, common procedures in, **415–435**
anesthetics and analgesics for, 420–422
bite wound care as, 416–417
fluid therapy/injections as, 420, 422–426
handling and restraint techniques for, 415–416
medication administration as, 424–427, 429
nutritional support as, 428
pain and distress recognition and, 418–419
potential zoonoses from, 416–417

Masks, for gas anesthesia, in avian species, 311, 313
in birds of prey, 330
in ferrets, 362
in rabbits, 381
in rodents, 408

Masses. See *Soft tissue masses.*

Maturation, in wound healing process, 454, 456

Medication administration, in amphibians, 254–255
in avian species, 307–309, 314–316
in ferrets, 360
in fish, 232–234
in invertebrates, 210–211
in nondomesticated species, 424–427, 429
in psittacines, 296–297
in rabbits, 374
in reptiles, 254–255
in rodents, 402–403

Mercury exposures, in birds of prey, 342–343

Mice, examination guidelines for, 398

Mites, in ferrets, 350
in hedgehogs, 431
in invertebrates, 218–220

Mollusks, hemolymph loss in, 216

Molting disorders, in invertebrates, 216–217

Monkeypox, in prairie dogs, 431

Mute examination, of birds of prey, 329

Myelography, for ferrets, 364

Myofibroblasts, in wound healing process, 456

Myopathy, in wallabies, 433

N

Nail trimming, for hedgehogs, 430
for psittacines, 300–301
for reptiles, 244
for rodents, 412

Nasal examination, of amphibians, 241
of reptiles, 241, 263–264
of wildlife, 443

Nasal flush, in psittacines, 290

Nasogastric tubes, for rabbits, 376–377

Nasolacrimal duct flush, for rabbits, 382–383

Nebulized therapeutics, for birds of prey, 341
　for psittacines, 297

Necropsy, of venomous reptiles, 283

Neurologic examination, of amphibians, 241
　of reptiles, 241

Neurotoxins, of venomous reptiles. See *Envenomation*.

Nondomesticated species, common procedures in, **415–435**
　　bite wound care as, 416–417
　　fluid therapy/injections as, 420, 422–426
　　handling and restraint techniques for, 415–416
　　medication administration as, 424–427, 429
　　nutritional support as, 428
　　pain and distress recognition and, 418–419
　　potential zoonoses from, 416–417
　　sample collection, 426–430
　　species-specific, 430–434
　　vascular access as, 420, 422–426

Nonsteroidal anti-inflammatory drugs (NSAIDs), for ferrets, 361
　for nondomesticated species, 419, 421
　for rabbits, 378

Nutritional assessment, for amphibians, 238–240
　for reptiles, 238–240

Nutritional support, feeding tubes for. See *Gastric feeding tubes*.
　for avian species, 308–309, 316–317
　　product suggestions for, 309
　for birds of prey, 335–336
　for ferrets, 361–362
　for fish, 232
　for neonatal wildlife, 452–453
　for nondomesticated species, 428
　　gavage feeding volumes, 430
　for psittacines, 295–296
　for rabbits, 374–378
　for reptiles, 258–260
　for rodents, 403–404

O

Obesity, in avian species, 316
　in hedgehogs, 430

Ocular examination, of birds of prey, 328
　of ferrets, 349–350
　of reptiles, 263–264
　of wildlife, 443

Odontomas, in prairie dogs, 432

Off-label drug use, for avian species, 314–315

Omnivorous reptiles, nutritional support for, 259–260

Ophthalmic drops/ointment, for amphibians, 255
　for turtles, 265–266

Ophthalmologic examination, of rodents, 396–397

Opiates/opioids, for pain control, in nondomesticated species, 419–421
　in rodents, 405

Opossums, common procedures in, anesthetics and analgesics for, 420–422
　　fluid therapy/injections as, 420, 422–424, 426
　　medication administration as, 424–427, 429
　　nutritional support as, 428, 453
　　pain and distress recognition and, 419, 421
　　species-specific, 434

Oral care. See *Dentistry*.

Oral examination, of amphibians, 241, 243
　of birds of prey, 329
　of ferrets, 349
　of nondomesticated species, 430, 432–434
　of rabbits, 369–370
　of reptiles, 241, 244, 246
　　during abscess surgery, 265
　of rodents, 392, 396–397
　of wildlife, 446

Oral fluid replacement, in birds of prey, 333, 335–336
　in psittacines, 292
　in reptiles, 257

Orogastric tubes, for rabbits, 376

Osmotic balance, in fish environment, 226
　in reptiles, 259

Osteomyelitis, in wild birds, antibiotics for, 458–459

Otic procedures. See *Ear entries.*

Outpatient treatment, of venomous reptiles, 281

Oxygen therapy, for birds of prey, 340–341
  for psittacines, 298–299

P

Packed cell volume (PCV), in birds of prey, 340
  in reptiles, 257

Pain assessment, in nondomesticated species, 418–420
  with euthanasia, of rodents, 410

Pain management, for ferrets, 360–361
  for fish, 233–234
  for nondomesticated species, 419–421, 432
  for psittacines, 299
  for rabbits, 378
  for rodents, 404–405

Palpation examination, of wildlife, 446
  abdominal, 446–447

Paramyxovirus-1 vaccine, for avian species, 317

Paramyxovirus infection, in venomous reptiles, 282–283

Parasite infestations, in birds of prey, of blood, 343–344
    respiratory emergencies with, 339, 342
  in ferrets, 350
  in fish, 229
  in hedgehogs, 431
  in invertebrates, 218–220
  in reptiles, 252
  in wildlife, 442

Parenteral nutrition, for rabbits, 375

Passerine meat, for birds of prey, 336

Passive immunity, in neonatal wildlife, 451

Patient assessment, of amphibians, 240–242
  of avian species, 304–305
  of birds of prey, 327–329
  of ferrets, 348–350
  of hedgehogs, 430–431
  of psittacines, 288
  of rabbits, 368–370
  of reptiles, 240–242
  of rodents, 395–400
  of venomous reptiles, 274
  of wildlife, 441–447
    checklist for, 444–445

Penile suckling, in neonatal wildlife, 452

Per os (PO) fluid administration. See *Oral fluid replacement.*

Perches, for birds of prey, 323–324, 326
  size of, 325

Peritonitis, sample collection for, in psittacines, 291

Personal protection equipment, for examinations, of amphibians, 242–243
  of birds of prey, 273–275, 323
  of invertebrates, 206
  of nondomesticated species, 417, 432
  of rodents, 398, 412
  of venomous reptiles, 272
  of wildlife, 437–438

Pesticide exposures, in birds of prey, 342–343

Pharyngostomy tubes, for rabbits, 376–377
  for reptiles, 258–260

Phlebotomy procedure. See *Blood collection; Venipuncture.*

Phosphorus level, in birds of prey, 338

Physical examination, of amphibians, 240–242
  of avian species, 304–305
  of birds of prey, 327–329
  of ferrets, 348–350
  of hedgehogs, 430–431
  of psittacines, 288
  of rabbits, 368–370
  of reptiles, 240–242
  of rodents, 395–400
  of venomous reptiles, 274
  of wildlife, 441–447
    checklist for, 444–445

Pigeon meat, for birds of prey, 336

Pit vipers, common procedures in, 270–271
  safe handling techniques for, 274–281
  treatment techniques for, 281–284

Pituitary gland, stress response role of, in wildlife, 440–441

Plasma protein, total, in birds of prey, 339–340
  urinary, in reptiles, 251–252

Plastic food wrap, for examination, of invertebrates, 207–208

Plastic tubes, for examination, of invertebrates, 207

Pneumatized bone, in avian species, 458
    bone healing and, 458–459
Pneumonia, aspiration, in birds of prey, 334
    in neonatal wildlife, 451–452
Posture, assessment of, in birds of prey, 328
Pouch, cheek, in rabbits, 369–370
    in rodents, 392, 396
    of nondomesticated species, infections of, 432–433
        medication administration and, 426
Poultry, for birds of prey diet, 336
Poxvirus vaccine, for avian species, 317
Prairie dogs, common procedures in, **415–435**
    anesthetics and analgesics for, 420–422
    bite wound care as, 416–417
    examination guidelines for, 400
    fluid therapy/injections as, 420, 422–423, 425–426
    hair characteristics and, 395
    handling and restraint techniques for, 415–416
    medication administration as, 424–427, 429
    nutritional support as, 428
    pain and distress recognition and, 418–419, 421
    potential zoonoses from, 416–417
    species-specific, 431–432
Preferred optimal temperature zone (POTZ), for amphibians, 240
    for nondomesticated species, 419
    for reptiles, 240, 258
Preputial suckling, in neonatal wildlife, 452
Preventive medicine, for avian species, 316–317
    husbandry as, for amphibians, 238, 261–262
    for avian species, 317
    for reptiles, 238, 261–262
Probiotics, oral, for neonatal wildlife, 451
    for prairie dogs, 432
Procedures, common. See also *specific species.*
    in amphibians, **237–267**
    in avian species, **303–319**
    in birds of prey, **321–345**
    in exotic rodents, **415–435**
    in falcons, **321–345**
    in ferrets, **347–365**
    in fish, **223–235**

in hedgehogs, **415–435**
in invertebrates, **205–221**
in marsupials, **415–435**
in nondomesticated species, **415–435**
in prairie dogs, **415–435**
in psittacines, **287–302**
in rabbits, **367–388**
in raptors, **321–345**
in reptiles, **237–267**
in rodents, **389–413**
in venomous reptiles, **269–285**
in wildlife, **437–460**
Psittacines, common procedures in, **287–302**
    capture and restraint techniques for, 287–288
    grooming as, 299–301
    medication administration as, 296–297
    physical examination as, 288
    sample collection as, 288–291
    supportive care as, 295–299
    therapeutic delivery as, 291–295
Pulmonary edema, in birds of prey, 342

Q

Quail meat, for birds of prey, 336

R

Rabbits, common procedures in, **367–388**
    handling and restraint techniques for, 367–368
    medication administration as, 374
    miscellaneous, 378–385
    patient assessment as, 368–370
    restraint and handling techniques for, 439–440
    sample collection as, 370–372
    supportive care as, 372–378, 453
    triage as, 368–370
    for birds of prey diet, 336
Radiography, procedures for, in amphibians, 253
    in birds of prey, 332, 343
    in ferrets, 363–364
    in fish, 231–232
    in invertebrates, 213–214
    in reptiles, 253
    in rodents, 400, 411
    in wildlife, 447, 458–459
Raptors, common procedures in, **321–345**
    caging for, 325
    diagnostic procedures as, 329–332

equipment for, 323–325, 330
nutritional support as, 335–336
physical examination as, 327–329
respiratory emergencies as, 339–342
restraint and handling techniques for, 323–325, 437–439
supportive care as, 330, 332–335
technical support for, 325–327
terminology for, 321–323
toxin exposures and, 342–343
traumatic injuries as, 341–342

Rats, examination guidelines for, 399

Re-epithelization, in wound healing process, 454–456

Recommended dietary requirements, for rabbits, 375

Rectal disorders, in older guinea pigs, 412

Red blood cell count, in birds of prey, 340
in reptile urinalysis, 252

Red rubber feeding tube, Sovereign, for reptiles, 258–259

"Refeeding syndromes," in reptiles, 259–260

Reflex actions, of neonatal wildlife, 447–448

Renal function, in reptiles, 251

Reporting requirements, on infectious disease, 418

Reptiles, common procedures in, **237–267**
aural abscesses and, 263–266
dysecdysis and, 261–262
educational material for, 240
herpetologic herpetoculture review for, 237–238
history taking for, 238–240
imaging as, 253–254
nutritional support as, 258–260
physical examination as, 240–242
restraint and handling techniques for, 242–247
salmonellosis and, 262–263
sample collection as, 248–252
therapeutic techniques as, 254–260
venomous, **269–285**. See also *Venomous reptiles.*

Respiratory emergencies, in birds of prey, 339–342

Respiratory rate, assessment of, in amphibians, 241
in birds of prey, 328
in ferrets, 350
in rabbits, 369
in reptiles, 241
in rodents, 397
in wildlife, 443

Restraint techniques, for emergency care, of rodents, 400–401
for examination, of amphibians, 242–243
of avian species, 303–305
of birds of prey, 323–325
by technical staff, 326–327
of ferrets, 348, 363
of fish, 225
of invertebrates, 206–208, 213
of nondomesticated species, 415–416
of psittacines, 287–288
of rabbits, 367–368
of reptiles, 242–247
of rodents, 395–396, 398–399
of venomous reptiles, 274–281
of wildlife, 437–439
stress response to, 439–441

Restraint tubes, for venomous reptiles, 279–280

Rewarming protocols, for neonatal wildlife, 449–450

Rodents, common procedures in, **389–413**
anatomy review, 390, 392
selected features, 394
costs of, 389, 401
emergency care as, 400–405
euthanasia as, 400, 409–410
exotic, **415–435**. See also *Exotic rodents.*
handling and restraint techniques for, 395–396, 398–399
imaging as, 400, 411
medication administration as, 402–403
miscellaneous, 408–412
patient assessment as, 395–400
resources on, 389, 391
sample collection as, 405–408
species overview, 390
standard of care and, 389–390
triage as, 394–395

S

Salmonella vaccine, for avian species, 317

Salmonellosis, in reptiles, 262–263

Salt solutions, for fish environment, 226

Sample collection, in amphibians, 247, 250–252
  in avian species, 305–307
  in ferrets, 351–355
  in fish, 226–231
  in invertebrates, 211–213
  in nondomesticated species, 426–430
  in psittacines, 288–291
  in rabbits, 370–372
  in reptiles, 248–252
  in rodents, 405–408
  in wildlife, 441, 447

Sanitation assessment, for amphibians, 238–239
  for reptiles, 238–239

Scruffing, for examination, of ferrets, 349
  of rabbits, 367
  of rodents, 398–399

Sea snakes/kraits, common procedures in, 272
  safe handling techniques for, 274–281
  treatment techniques for, 281–284

Sedation, for examination, of fish, 225, 231
  of nondomesticated species, 420, 422, 427
  for miscellaneous procedures, in ferrets, 362–363

Septicemia, in neonatal wildlife, 450–451
  passive immunity and, 451

Sexing, of rodents, 393

Shedding, in reptiles, 261
  problems with. See *Dysecdysis.*

Shell trauma, repair procedures for, in invertebrates, 215–217

Shift boxes, for handling venomous reptiles, 280–281

Shock, in wildlife, as stress response, 440–441
  treatment of, in birds of prey, 332–333, 335
  in ferrets, 347–348
  in psittacines, 291–292
  in rabbits, 373

Sinuses, examination of, in birds of prey, 328

Skin examination, of amphibians, 240–242
  of ferrets, 349–350
  of hedgehogs, 430–431
  of invertebrates, 215–219
  of rabbits, 369
  of reptiles, 240–241, 257

of rodents, 397–398
of wildlife, 446
shedding problems and. See *Dysecdysis.*

Skin preparation, for surgical procedures, in avian species, 313
  in rodents, 410–411

Skin sampling/scraping, in fish, 229–230
  in invertebrates, 212–213
  in rabbits, 372
  in rodents, 406–407

Skin wounds. See *Wound entries.*

Snails, shell trauma in, repair procedures for, 216–217

Snake hooks, for handling venomous reptiles, 276–279

Snakes, common procedures in, blood collection as, 248
  dysecdysis and, 261–262
  intravenous catheter placement as, 255–256
  lung examination as, 252
  restraint and handling techniques for, 245, 276–279
  urogenital examination as, 242
  venomous. See *Venomous reptiles.*

Social behavior, of neonatal wildlife, 447–448

Soft tissue masses, examination of, in rodents, 397–398
  in wildlife, 447
  sample collection from, in ferrets, 355
  in rodents, 407

Soft tissue trauma. See *Wound entries.*

Sovereign red rubber feeding tube, for reptiles, 258–259

Spiders, examination handling techniques for, 206–208

Spinal trauma, in birds of prey, 342

Splay leg, in neonatal wildlife, 448

Spleen examination, in ferrets, 353, 364

Splenic aspiration, in ferrets, 353–354

Squeeze boxes, for handling venomous reptiles, 281

Stethoscope, for auscultation examination, of reptiles, 241
  of rodents, 397
  for endotracheal intubation, of rabbits, 380–381

Stress minimization, during examinations,
for amphibians, 242
for birds of prey, 323, 325, 327
for nondomesticated species, 420, 432
for rabbits, 367–368
for reptiles, 244
for rodents, 394–398
of wildlife, 441–443
during treatment, for birds of prey, 340
for rabbits, 374–375
for rodents, 400, 402

Stress response, in rodents, 395
in wildlife, minimization of, 441–443
neonatal, 448
physiology of, 439–441

Subcutaneous fluid administration, in avian species, 307
in birds of prey, 333–334
in nondomesticated species, 422–426
in psittacines, 292–293
in rabbits, 373–374
in reptiles, 257

Sugar gliders, common procedures in, anesthetics and analgesics for, 420–422
fluid therapy/injections as, 420, 422–424, 426
medication administration as, 424–427, 429
nutritional support as, 428
pain and distress recognition and, 419, 421
species-specific, 432–433

Supportive care procedures, for avian species, 307–310
for ferrets, 360–362
for fish, 226, 232–234
for psittacines, 295–299
for rabbits, 372–378
for rodents, 401–405

Surgical procedures, for aural abscesses, in turtles, 264–265
indications for, in avian species, 313
preparation for, in reptiles, 264
in rodents, 410–411
in venomous reptiles, 283–284
principles of, for avian species, 313–314
restraint for. See *Anesthesia;Restraint techniques.*

Sutures, placement and protection of, in rodents, 407–408

Sweat glands, of rodents, 393

Swivels, for birds of prey, 323–325

Sympathetic nervous system, stress response role of, in wildlife, 440–441

Syringe feedings, for rabbits, 375–376

T

Tail whipping, by reptiles, 243–244

Talon examination, of birds of prey, 329

Tarantulas, examination handling techniques for, 206–208
fluid deficit/therapy in, 210–211

Technical support staff, birds of prey handling by, 325–327

Teeth, anatomy of, of rodents, 390, 392–393
grinding of, in rodents, 393
trimming of, in rabbits, 384–385

Temperature, core. See *Hyperthermia;Hypothermia.*
environmental, for amphibians, 240, 261
for reptiles, 240, 258, 261
procedure for taking. See *Body temperature.*

Thermal support, for ferrets, 363
for neonatal wildlife, 449–450
for rabbits, 369
for reptiles, 258
for rodents, 410–411

Thermal zones. See *Preferred optimal temperature zone (POTZ).*

Thoracic cavity, assessment of, in ferrets, 364

Tongs, for handling venomous reptiles, 278–279

Topical anesthesia, in rabbits, 379

Total plasma protein (TPP), in birds of prey, 339–340

Towel restraint, for avian species, 303–304
for birds of prey, 326–327
for nondomesticated species, 416, 432
for psittacines, 287–288
for rabbits, 368, 371
for reptiles, 243–245

Toxin exposures, endotoxin, in neonatal wildlife, 450–451
environmental, in birds of prey, 342–343
of neurotoxins. See *Envenomation.*

Tracheal wash, in ferrets, 354–355
in psittacines, 290

Tranquilizers, for examination, of nondomesticated species, 420, 422

Transdermal route, for medications, in amphibians, 255

Transillumination, for amphibian examination, 243, 247

Transtracheal sample collection, in reptiles, 252

Trauma assessment, exoskeleton, of invertebrates, 215–217
  of birds of prey, 329, 342
    respiratory emergencies and, 341–342
  of fish, 229–230
  of wildlife, 442
    wound management and, 453–456

Triage, general, of avian species, 304–305
  of ferrets, 347–348
  of fish, 223–224
  of psittacines, 288
  of rabbits, 368–370
  of rodents, 394–395

Tricaine methanesulfonate (MS-222), for fish chemical restraint, 225

Tumor necrosis factor (TNF), septicemia and, in neonatal wildlife, 450

Turtles/tortoises, common procedures in, aural abscesses and, 263–266
    blood collection as, 249–250
    intravenous catheter placement as, 257
    restraint and handling techniques for, 246–247
    snapping, 437–460
      restraint and handling techniques for, 437–439
    urinary bladder and, 242

Tympanic cavity lavage, for aural abscess, in turtles, 264

U

Ultrasonography, diagnostic, in amphibians, 253–254
  in reptiles, 253–254
  for abdominal examination, in ferrets, 364
  for bladder examination, in rabbits, 371–372

Urates, in reptile urine, 252
  of birds of prey, 329

Uric acid level, in birds of prey, 338–339

Urinalysis. See *Urine collection/examination.*

Urinary bladder, catheterization of, in ferrets, 358–359
  examination of, in amphibians, 242
    in rabbits, 371–372
    in reptiles, 242

Urine collection/examination, in amphibians, 251–252
  in birds of prey, 329
  in ferrets, 352
  in rabbits, 371–372
  in reptiles, 251–252
  in rodents, 406

Urogenital examination, of amphibians, 242
  of reptiles, 242, 251

V

Vaccinations, for avian species, 317

Vagal-vagal response, in reptiles, 244

Vascular access. See *Catheter placement.*

Vasogenic shock, in birds of prey, 332

Venipuncture, in amphibians, 247
  in avian species, 305–307
  in birds of prey, 330–331
  in ferrets, 402
  in nondomesticated species, 426–430
  in psittacines, 288–289
  in rabbits, 370–371
  in reptiles, 248–250
  in rodents, 405–406
  in venomous reptiles, 281–282
  in wildlife, 447

Venomous reptiles, bagging/bagging systems for, 274–276
  common procedures in, **269–285**
    anesthesia as, 281
    bite outcomes and, 272–273
    emergency protocol for bites, 273
    examination planning for, 274
    hospitalization as, 281
    limitations of inexperienced veterinarians and, 269, 284
    necropsy as, 283
    paramyxovirus infection and, 282–283
    safe handling for, 274–281
    species overview, 269–272
    surgery as, 283–284
    treatment techniques as, 281–284
    venipuncture as, 281–282
  handling containers for, 276

restraint tubes for, 279–280
shift boxes for handling, 280–281
snake hooks for handling, 276–279
squeeze boxes for handling, 281
tongs for handling, 278–279

Viperidae reptiles, antivenoms for, 271
common procedures in, 270–272, 281–282
safe handling techniques for, 274–281
treatment techniques for, 281–284

Virus vaccines, for avian species, 317

Vitamin E, myopathy and, in wallabies, 433

W

Wallabies, common procedures in, anesthetics and analgesics for, 420–422
fluid therapy/injections as, 420, 422–424, 426
pain and distress recognition and, 420–421
species-specific, 433–434

Water quality testing, for fish, 223, 226
commercial tests for, 228
sample collection for, 226–228

Waterfowl, common procedures in, 437–460
bone healing and, 457–459
health examination as, 441–447
neonatal, 447–453
restraint and handling techniques for, 437–439
wound care as, 453–457

Weaning, of hand fed wildlife, 453

Websites, for rodent medicine, 390–391

Weight. See *Body weight.*

White blood cell count (WBC), in birds of prey, 340
in reptile urinalysis, 252

Wildlife, common procedures in, **437–460**
bone healing and, 457–459
fluid therapy as, 447
health examination as, 441–447
neonatal perspectives, 447–453
aspiration pneumonia and, 451–452
hand-rearing of orphans, 452
hypoglycemia and, 448–450
hypothermia and, 449
passive immunity and, 451
penile suckling and, 452
physiologic development and, 447–448
preputial suckling and, 452
septicemia and, 450–451
splay leg and, 448
restraint and handling techniques for, 437–439
sample collection as, 441, 447
stress response to, 439–441
wounds as, basic approach to, 457
initial stabilization for, 456–457
management of, 453–456

Wing feather trimming, for psittacines, 299–300

Wound care, for bites, by nondomesticated species, 416–417
postoperative, for chelonian aural abscesses, 265–266
trauma-related, for birds of prey, 342
for wildlife, 453–456
basic approach to, 457
initial stabilization for, 456–457

Wound cleansing, for wildlife trauma, 453–454, 457

Wound closure, for wildlife trauma, 453–454

Wound healing, classes of, 454
phases of, 454–456
suppression factors of, 456

Z

Zoonoses, potential, from nondomesticated species, 416–417